T0320893

Childbirth in South Asia

Endorsement

Childbirth in South Asia: Old Challenges, New Paradoxes is a sweeping overview of recent critical research on the transformations in the experience, management, and policymaking processes of maternal health in South Asia. This volume is the first of its kind to bring together interdisciplinary work on childbirth by anthropologists, sociologists, historians, and public health experts working across the region. Exploring reproductive care from the vantage point of mothers (or mothers-to-be) and families, a wide range of medical practitioners, and policymakers, the accessible chapters in this book elucidate enduring and novel challenges to providing humane high quality reproductive care in this rapidly changing and diverse part of the world in the early 21st century.

Cecilia C. Van Hollen, Professor of Anthropology, Yale-NUS College
Author of *Birth in the Age of AIDS: Women Reproduction and HIV/AIDS in India* and *Birth on the Threshold: Childbirth and Modernity in South India*

Childbirth in South Asia

Old Challenges and New Paradoxes

Edited by

CLÉMENCE JULLIEN AND ROGER JEFFERY

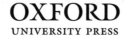

OXFORD
UNIVERSITY PRESS

OXFORD
UNIVERSITY PRESS

Great Clarendon Street, Oxford, OX2 6DP,
United Kingdom

Oxford University Press is a department of the University of Oxford.
It furthers the University's objective of excellence in research, scholarship,
and education by publishing worldwide. Oxford is a registered trade mark of
Oxford University Press in the UK and in certain other countries

© Oxford University Press 2021

The moral rights of the authors have been asserted

Impression: 1

All rights reserved. No part of this publication may be reproduced, stored in
a retrieval system, or transmitted, in any form or by any means, without the
prior permission in writing of Oxford University Press, or as expressly permitted
by law, by licence or under terms agreed with the appropriate reprographics
rights organization. Enquiries concerning reproduction outside the scope of the
above should be sent to the Rights Department, Oxford University Press, at the
address above

You must not circulate this work in any other form
and you must impose this same condition on any acquirer

Published in the United States of America by Oxford University Press
198 Madison Avenue, New York, NY 10016, United States of America

British Library Cataloguing in Publication Data
Data available

ISBN-13 (print edition): 978-0-19-013071-8

ISBN-10 (print edition): 0-19-013071-7

ISBN-13 (eBook): 978-0-19-099328-3

ISBN-10 (eBook): 0-19-099328-6

ISBN-13 (oso): 978-0-19-099329-0

ISBN-10 (oso): 0-19-099329-4

DOI: 10.1093/oso/9780190130718.001.0001

Typeset in Minion Pro 10/13
by Newgen KnowledgeWorks Pvt. Ltd., Chennai, India

Printed in India by
Rakmo Press Pvt. Ltd.

Links to third party websites are provided by Oxford in good faith and
for information only. Oxford disclaims any responsibility for the materials
contained in any third party website referenced in this work.

To all those south Asian women whose child-bearing experiences are represented, directly or indirectly, in this book. Without their willingness to share their views, our volume would not have been possible.

Contents

Preface

This project started as part of the 25th European Conference on South Asian Studies (ECSAS) that took place in Paris in July 2018. On this occasion we organized a panel on 'Childbirth in South Asia: Multiple Perspectives on Continuing Paradoxes' in order to discuss the changes taking place in health-care policies, as well as the contemporary conditions of childbirth and mid-wifery in South Asia. This meeting proved to be extremely fruitful. Not only were the approaches of medical anthropologists, historians, sociologists, and public health specialists complementary, but this panel also had the merit of bringing together senior and junior researchers from four different continents. This first stage of reflection has been crucial, and we are thus extremely grateful to the efforts the Centre d'Études de l'Inde et de l'Asie du Sud (CEIAS) put in to make the 25th ECSAS possible and successful. We would also like to express our gratitude to the panel participants—including Arunima Deka, Hasan Muhammad Baniamin, Haripriya Narasimhan, Bijoya Roy, Emma Varley, and Asmita Verma—who did not take part in this volume but greatly contributed to the conference panel and its discussions.

With a view to publishing an edited volume, we organized a two-day writing workshop called 'Transformation of Childbirth in South Asia: Ethical, Legal and Social Implications' at the Department of Social Anthropology and Cultural Studies at the University of Zürich (UZH), Switzerland, where Clémence Jullien was a post-doctoral researcher. Eleven scholars were invited to Zurich to attend the workshop. We sincerely thank the Swiss National Fund (SNF) as well as Professor Johannes Quack, University of Zurich, for facilitating this workshop through their financial support and continuous availability. This event allowed us to pursue the reflections initiated at the 25th ECSAS, to polish the argumentation of each author's text, and to enhance the coherence of the project.

Roger Jeffery would like to acknowledge the contributions of Patricia Jeffery in making this volume possible. From 1982 to 2010, we worked together on several projects that included research and publications on child bearing. This volume has benefited from that work in a general way, but does not draw directly from it, except where use is made of research material from already published joint works when citations have been made to the original source.

Roger Jeffery also acknowledges the support of the School of Social and Political Science, University of Edinburgh, Scotland, for its support on this project over the past two years.

In sum, as the background of the project clearly reveals, this edited volume is the result of international collaborations, joint efforts, and institutional support. We are thus extremely pleased to see this project completed and carried forward by Oxford University Press, India.

Not only do we believe this book offers new insights on a salient and timely topic, but we also hope it will be of use to researchers and policymakers interested in the ethical and social implications of health policies.

Clémence Jullien
and
Roger Jeffery

Abbreviations

AMTSL	active management of the third stage of labour (the period between delivery of the child and of the placenta)
AMWI	Association of Medical Women in India
ANC	antenatal care
ANM	auxiliary nurse midwife
ART	assisted reproductive technologies
ASHA	accredited social health activist (India)
AWC	ānganwādī (courtyard) Centre (India)
AWW	ānganwādī (courtyard) worker (India)
BHU	basic health units (Pakistan)
BPL	below poverty line (India)
CEHAT	Centre for Enquiry into Health and Allied Themes (Maharashtra, India)
CHC	community health centre
CHW	community health worker (India)
CMW	community midwife (Pakistan)
COPASAH	Community of Practitioners on Accountability and Social Protection in Health (India)
C-section	caesarean section or the use of surgery to deliver babies
CSSM	Child Survival and Safe Motherhood (India)
CY	Chiranjīvī Yojanā (Programme promoting institutional delivery) (Gujarat, India)
DF	Dufferin Fund
DFID	Department for International Development (UK)
DHO	district health officer (Pakistan)
DHQH	district headquarter hospital (Pakistan)
EmOC	emergency obstetric care
FLW	frontline worker
HIV/AIDS	human immuno-virus/acquired immune deficiency syndrome
HRC	Human Rights Council
ICDS	Integrated Child Development Services (India)
ILO	International Labour Organization
IMS	Indian Medical Service
INR	Indian National Rupee
IT	Information Technology
IV	intravenous

JSSK	Jananī Śiśu Surakṣā Kāryakram or Programme for Maternal and Infantile Protection (India)
JSY	Jananī SurakṣāYojanā or safe motherhood scheme (India)
LaQshya	Labour Room Quality Improvement Initiative (India)
LHV	lady health visitor (Pakistan now, earlier also in India and Bangladesh)
LHW	lady health worker (Pakistan)
LMO	lady medical officer (Pakistan)
LNHO	League of Nations Health Organization
MBBS	Bachelor of Medicine, Bachelor of Surgery
MCHC	Maternal Child Health Centre (Pakistan)
MCI	Medical Council of India
MD	Doctor of Medicine
MDGs	Millennium Development Goals
MMR	maternal mortality ratio
MoTeCH	Mobile Technology for Community Health
MS	medical superintendent (Pakistan); master of surgery
NABH	National Accreditation Board for Hospital and Healthcare Providers (India)
NFHS	National Family Health Survey (India)
NGO	non-governmental organization
NHM	National Health Mission (India)
NRHM	National Rural Health Mission (India)
NUHM	National Urban Health Mission (India)
ODI	Overseas Development Institute (London)
PHC	primary health centre (India) or primary healthcare (globally)
PM-JAY	Pradhan Mantri Jan Arogya Yojana (India)
PNDT Act	Pre-Natal Diagnostic Techniques Act (India)
PPH	post-partum haemorrhage (bleeding after giving birth)
RAS	Rural Ambulance Service (Pakistan)
RCH	Reproductive and Child Health (Indian health programme)
RF	Rockefeller Fund
RHC	rural health centre (Pakistan)
RMNCH+A	Reproductive Maternal Neonatal Child and Adolescent Health (India)
SBA	skilled birth attendant (includes MBBS doctor, registered nurse, nurse midwife, or community midwife)
SC	scheduled caste (ex-Untouchables) (India)
SDGs	Sustainable Development Goals
SDIP	Safe Delivery Incentive Programme (Nepal)
ST	scheduled tribe (India)
TBA	traditional (or trained) birth attendant

UN	United Nations
UNICEF	United Nations Children's Fund
USAID	United States Agency for International Development
WHO	World Health Organization
WMSI	Women's Medical Service in India

SECTION 1
HISTORICAL PERSPECTIVE

1

Changing Childbirth in
Twenty-First-Century South Asia

Clémence Jullien and Roger Jeffery

Across the world, the conditions of childbirth are changing—but not all in
the same direction. While women in Western countries have pressed for
more home deliveries, to mitigate the effects of male appropriation and the
over-medicalized experience of motherhood and childbirth, most developing countries are promoting institutionalized deliveries and are directly
or indirectly stigmatizing women who deliver at home. In addition, new information technologies are being pressed into service, such as identifying
high-risk mothers and offering them advice through social media. Such an
evolution is particularly visible in South Asia. Within the last decade, with
the influence of the Millennium Development Goals (MDGs; 2000–15), important new government schemes have been introduced, designed to address
the issues of safe motherhood and childbirth, often through offering women
cash payments or vouchers if they give birth in approved health facilities
(Jehan et al. 2012).

This book discusses how some of the old challenges—such as resource
constraints, poverty, high levels of exclusion of marginalized groups, and
high rates of maternal and infant mortality—have generated new paradoxes
linked to childbirth in India, Pakistan, Nepal, and Bangladesh. Providing
a broad panorama of the last 25 years, it brings together anthropologists,
historians, sociologists, and public health specialists working with both
quantitative (census analysis and national surveys) and qualitative data (ethnographic fieldwork and archival material).

This 'Introduction' sets out why childbirth is a salient and timely issue for
South Asia. New and unprecedented government schemes have emerged
from global initiatives, often introduced very rapidly and without taking
into account the local, regional, and national variations in contexts. We review key public health analyses relevant to childbirth as well as the main

Clémence Jullien and Roger Jeffery, *Changing Childbirth in Twenty-First-Century South Asia* In: *Childbirth in South Asia*. Edited by: Clémence Jullien and Roger Jeffery, Oxford University Press. © Oxford University Press 2021.
DOI: 10.1093/oso/9780190130718.003.0001

turning points of health policies over the last 25 years. We also review health inequities by gender, country, residence (urban, rural), and social position (class, caste, and religion), and show how these different bases interact in creating highly unequal health situations. The 'Introduction' will conclude by explaining the structure of the book, along with a brief summary of each chapter.

The Need for New Government Schemes

At the turn of the millennium, leading maternal health policymakers across the region began to argue that it was really time that something should happen with respect to maternal health policy in South Asia:

> Little has been achieved because of inadequate monitoring, poor ac-countability, and a failure to address underlying determinants of maternal health. Governments in [S]outh Asia have been reluctant to ad-dress these issues squarely. The reproductive health of women is closely intertwined with basic issues of social status, access to education, em-powerment, and fertility, and without tackling these issues other meas-ures are at best perfunctory. Issues such as gender imbalances in health and education as well as humane governance have been highlighted in several influential reports from [S]outh Asia, but the findings of these reports have not been translated into action through national or regional programmes.
>
> Bhutta 2000: 810

Some of this sense of urgency was driven by the perceived failure of the Safe Motherhood Initiative, a global policy promoted by the previous gen-eration of maternal health policymakers. The Safe Motherhood Initiative addressed health risks such as poor nutrition, illiteracy, lack of income and employment opportunities, inadequate health and family planning services, and women's low social status. Despite its strength through the breadth of issues it identified, one weakness was its close links with family planning. Another was the failure to emphasize strongly enough 'proximate' or im-mediate causes of maternal mortality, such as the 'three delays' in getting women into emergency obstetric care when necessary, and the need for schemes that would provide continuity of care between initial caregivers and specialized services. Although global agencies and private donors were supporters of these initiatives, maternal healthcare was rarely on the agenda of governments and other policymakers in South Asia, perhaps partly because the initiative lacked a 'clear, concise, feasible strategy' (Maine and Rosenfield 1999: 480).

Until around 1980, maternity health programmes across the region focused on improving obstetrics in medical education in large public hospitals and cities. For villages, rural health programmes delivered by nurses or nurse-midwives had little priority. Ongoing campaigns to improve the practices of traditional birth attendants had varying, but usually limited effects. These women were often nominally included by schemes, then trained, but then excluded, either formally or, for example, by failures to pay the promised honoraria. Towards the end of the 1970s, ideas of community health became popular among NGOs who delivered maternity care as well as, briefly, among governments who picked up on the 'comprehensive primary health care approach' elaborated by WHO and UNICEF in 1978. That window closed, in the face of the selective primary healthcare counter-revolution, sometimes characterized as neoliberal reform. The 1980s and 1990s saw a levelling-off in efforts to improve public health services, affecting maternal and child healthcare as well. Leading up to the conference that produced the MDGs in 2000, global pressures and local concerns highlighted the need for new government schemes.

Women's Birthing Experiences: A New Paradox

Our focus in this book is on how, in responding to resilient challenges, the innovations since 1990 have affected women's birthing experiences. Throughout what follows, we ask readers to keep in mind that birthing intersects with other social practices that are also in flux. For example, recent changes in the meaning of marriage have led to the institution becoming politicized in various ways, as young people attempt to have a greater say in who their elders decide they should marry. Similarly, contraception and abortion are contested topics across the subcontinent, as women and men struggle to find common ground in areas where spousal communication patterns change with education, urbanization, and rising aspirations.

Since 2000, there have been several paradoxes. On the one hand, indicators of maternal and neonatal mortality have shown substantial improvements—albeit at different rates between countries and by social categories within countries—on the other hand, more births take place in hospitals and clinics, but with few additional staff or resources. These births must often take place in settings that cannot cope adequately with the additional pressures of such rapid expansions.[1] Yet there is little evidence of how this has happened. There is little to explain why the decline in maternal and neonatal mortality has been below the expectations and objectives set. Most epidemiological surveys collect minimal information on the institutions—nothing, for example, on how long they have been in existence, how many staff they employ per delivery, the qualifications of the staff, and the maternity bed occupancy rates. Sociological and anthropological studies have continued to focus on traditional birth attendants or on the new reproductive technologies (surrogacy, for example, in Hodges and Rao 2016; Pande 2014) rather than exploring the (current) majority tendency (deliveries in government hospitals). At institutions where one or two deliveries took place per day, numbers have sometimes risen more than tenfold in less than 10 years.[2] New institutions—mostly private, sometimes not-for-profit, or occasionally governmental—have been established. Women may arrive for a delivery and leave soon after—or never arrive at all, but nonetheless claim a cash transfer, or this may be claimed by someone else, nominally on their behalf. Existing birth attendants have sometimes found new roles for themselves or else have been sidelined as new childbirth routines have taken over and biopower—with its associated increased surveillance of women and their bodies—has taken new forms. And during the same period, new social media have swept across South Asia, offering additional means of communication between women, birthing attendants, and medical institutions.

Despite the increased attention being paid to maternal and child health, and the steady rise in institutional deliveries in South Asia, rates of institutional delivery vary dramatically across regions and social groups. Little attention has been paid to the price of this change (for example, in terms of the support available for birthing women, and relationships between doctors, nurses, and marginalized women). Far from withering away, in some places traditional birth attendants have seen a resurgence, in part due to the demeaning conditions offered to poor, low-caste, rural women in formal health settings. Against this backdrop, the authors of this volume explore the social implications of the changes being introduced in the technologies and social arrangements of childbirth in South Asia.

The Context: Levels of Maternal and Neonatal Mortality

Evidence of the medical risks of childbirth is of mixed quality and precision, in the absence of robust recording of births and deaths. Across South Asia, more attention was paid to these issues after the agreements that set out the MDGs in 2000.

Target 4A of the MDGs was to reduce the under-five mortality rate by two-thirds, between 1990 and 2015, by focusing on the following indicators:

- 4.1 Under-five mortality rate
- 4.2 Infant mortality rate
- 4.3 The proportion of 1-year-old children immunized against measles

Unexpectedly, the neonatal mortality rate (the number of deaths of live-born children during the first 28 days of life per 1,000 live births in a given year) and the stillbirth rate (the number of stillbirths per 1,000 live births in a given year) were not targeted by the MDGs. In this chapter, we include these two indicators as they provide good evidence of child mortality that is linked to conditions of childbirth.

In addition, target 5A of the MDGs was to reduce the maternal mortality ratio by three-quarters, between 1990 and 2015, by focusing on the following indicators:

- 5.1 Maternal mortality ratio (MMR) (deaths of women due to complications from pregnancy or childbirth per 100,000 live births in a given year)
- 5.2 Proportion of births attended by skilled health personnel
- 5.3 Contraceptive prevalence rate
- 5.4 Adolescent birth rate
- 5.5 Antenatal care coverage (at least four visits)
- 5.6 Unmet need for family planning

For our purposes, indicators 5.1 and 5.2 are the most relevant, though others are also important indirectly.

Tables 1.1–1.4 provide summary overview figures for some of these key indicators. The 'achievements' in these tables represent the extent to which the country as a whole is estimated to have reached the MDG targets and provide no information about the extent of internal variation, for example,

Table 1.1 Neonatal mortality rates in largest South Asian countries, 1990–2015

Country	1990	2000	2015	MDG	Achievement (%)
Bangladesh	64	43	21	16	90
India	57	45	26	14	72
Nepal	58	40	22	14	82
Pakistan	64	60	47	16	35
Sri Lanka	13	10	5	3	80
South Asia	59	47	29	15	68

Source: Available at https://data.unicef.org/topic/child-survival/neonatal-mortality/; last accessed on 17 September 2018.

Table 1.2 Stillbirth rates in largest South Asian countries, 1990–2015

Country	1990	2000	2015	MDG	Achievement (%)
Bangladesh	37.8	42.3	25.4	9.5	44
India	29.5	33.3	23.0	7.4	29
Nepal	54.6	28.0	18.4	13.7	89
Pakistan	41.4	53.3	43.1	10.4	−5
Sri Lanka	9.6	7.5	4.9	2.4	65
South Asia	32.1	35	25	8.0	29

Source: Stanton et al. 2006 for the year 1990 and Blencowe et al. 2016 for the years for 2000 and 2015.
Note: The figures given for 1990 are for the nearest available year. Due to differences in methods of calculation and data collection, the 1990 figures are not strictly comparable with those for 2000 and 2015, and the estimates for decline over the whole period should only be used as rough estimates of rankings.

There was no MDG for stillbirths, but if the same targets had been set (a reduction by three-quarters from 1990 levels by 2015) then these are the figures that might have been applied.

Table 1.3 Maternal mortality ratios in largest South Asian countries, 1990–2015

Country	1990	2000	2015	MDG	Achievement (%)
Bangladesh	550	340	176	137	92
India	556	374	174	139	92
Nepal	901	548	258	225	95
Pakistan	431	306	178	108	78
Sri Lanka	75	57	30	19	80
South Asia	558	388	182	140	90

Source: Aziz et al. (2015: 65).

Table 1.4 Proportions of births not attended by skilled health personnel in largest South Asian countries, 1990–2015

Country	1990	2000	2015	MDG	Achievement (%)
Bangladesh	91	87	58	23	49
India	66	57	19	16	94
Nepal	93	89	42	23	73
Pakistan	81	77	48	20	54
Sri Lanka	6	4	1	1.5	111
South Asia	70	63	27	17	81

Source: Available at https://data.unicef.org/topic/maternal-health/delivery-care/; last accessed on 18 September 2018.
Notes:1. The dates of the estimates do not all align with the three chosen years, but usually include those mentioned or the nearest year available.

2. South Asia figures have been calculated by the authors using UN estimates.

by income, region, or ethnic origin. Estimates for all these rates are also subject to considerable uncertainty in South Asia.[3]

What these tables tell us is that all South Asian countries have made considerable progress since 1990 in reducing the burdens of deaths related to childbirth, whether of the child or the mother. But probing into detail reveals a more complex story. In brief, the current picture has been described as follows:

> While South Asia has reduced maternal mortality ratio across the region, mortality remains high in many countries including Afghanistan, Pakistan, and Nepal. Despite progress in delivering antenatal care and vaccinations, wide disparities exist across wealth groups and between rural and urban populations in many countries. Social determinants and health systems or policies are important contributors to observed improvement and differentials in the region. Ongoing challenges include conflict or insecurity, malnutrition, encouraging empowerment of girls and women, and supporting better and timely data collection.
>
> Akseer et al. 2017: 1

Due to its population size, dwarfing its neighbours, but also because its rapid economic growth has not been matched by equivalent progress in social development, in 2015 India still accounted for more than two-thirds of total maternal deaths in the region, or 17% of global maternal deaths. The country also shows wide disparity in MMRs across states and income groups. In Nepal and Bangladesh, by contrast, social development and its impact on the social determinants of health seem to have been very important. In Nepal, despite a 10-year civil war, MMR significantly dropped (Kerber et al. 2007; but see Chapter 11 in this volume, for some cautionary remarks). The decrease in MMR in Bangladesh can be attributed to an accelerated fertility decline: Bangladesh has been a pioneer in areas such as girls' education, employment of women, and micro-credit programmes. Despite introducing several maternal and child interventions, progress has been the slowest on many indicators in Pakistan. Female community health workers there have been effective in reaching women in rural and poor urban areas, yet Pakistan's MMR is the highest in South Asia (excluding Afghanistan). Slow fertility reduction, as well as deficits related to the health system, including lack of trained health staff and inadequate availability of emergency obstetric care, may have contributed to Pakistan's relatively slow progress, along with gender inequities in education and work (Alkema et al. 2016; El-Saharty 2015).

What these tables do *not* tell us are the changes in the constitution of maternity services, between public and private providers, or in who actually attends deliveries (Hodges and Rao 2016). Nor do they provide information on the impact of such changes on women's experience of deliveries or on the range of outcomes for different groups—for example, according to where people live, their social class, or other indicators of social difference such as religion or caste (on caste, see, for example, Bora et al. 2019). It is now normative in most of the region to give birth in a hospital or clinic if possible, even if pregnant women and their advisers cannot get access to the financial support promised by their governments (El-Saharty 2015). While all countries have seen a sharp increase in the number of private providers of maternity care, there are many differences across the region, leading, for example, to very different rates of caesarean section (C-section) (Boerma et al. 2018).

Beyond Healthcare

Furthermore, while governments often assume that higher rates of institutionalized deliveries will necessarily lead to reducing maternal and infant mortality, researchers provide a more nuanced view, in which non-health sector changes may be more significant. In other words, to understand these reductions, we must take account of interactions between globally-inspired reforms, local realities, entrenched public and private sector ways of working, and resource constraints (Hurst et al. 2015). Non-health policy decisions (such as decentralizing governments and privatizing some services) may impact on maternal health, even if unintentionally, as with the transfer of federal health ministry functions to the Pakistani provinces in 2011 (Lim et al. 2010; Sidney et al. 2016). The socio-economic factors that set a framework within which women can or cannot access quality maternal health services and impinge directly or indirectly on maternity outcomes include poverty, poor nutrition, low education levels, and gender inequities. Samer el-Saharty, senior health policy specialist, South Asia region for the World Bank, summarized these challenges facing countries in South Asia as follows (Randive et al. 2013):

- high early marriage and pregnancy rates in some countries;
- inequity in access to maternal health services;

- chronic malnutrition, a frequent underlying cause of maternal deaths, even among the wealthy;
- gender inequalities that persist in all domains of South Asian societies and have a daily impact on the lives and health of women.

Most of these challenges appear as issues to be addressed in the other MDGs, but the linkages to health are not explicitly acknowledged. Thus, the education sector might be keen to ensure that girls are attending school, but not necessarily be equally concerned with whether this leads to later marriages and a reduction in adolescent pregnancies. The impact of socio-economic factors also varies according to context. Significantly, some of the comparative results demonstrated in Tables 1.1–1.4 are counter-intuitive, in particular the relative successes of Bangladesh and Nepal.

Bangladesh has lower levels of institutional delivery than India and Nepal, yet MMR has declined more quickly. This has been attributed to 'reducing gender inequality in some crucially important respects'; 'women have also received special attention from Bangladesh's powerful non-governmental organisations'; 'the general acceptance of a multiplicity of instruments in the public and private sectors for rapid social advancement'; and 'the intelligent use of community-based approaches in the delivery of health services and medical care' (Mazhar and Shaikh 2012). Or as a *Lancet* review put it:

> Maternal health is affected by factors both directly linked and indirectly linked to health services such as improved transportation, access to mobile telephone technology (and thus communication channels for information and social assistance), as well as education and socioeconomic status. An almost doubling in the proportion of girls with at least some secondary education is believed to be empowering, raising their potential to respond effectively to maternal complications and navigate the health-care system.
>
> Alkema et al. 2016

Given that Nepal experienced a 10-year insurgency (1996–2006) and continuing political churning, and that its physical terrain makes access to health services very difficult over much of the country, Nepal's MDG achievements are remarkable, as can be seen in Tables 1.1–1.4. A review by the Overseas Development Institute (ODI) attributed this success to 'consistent policy focus and sustained financial commitment by the government and donors', but it also identified the remaining problems including continuing inequalities in access to care and to maternity indicators, poor accountability, and the need to maintain governmental and donor support (El-Saharty 2015). Similarly, a 2013 study underlines that 'despite the enormous efforts, Nepal is facing huge challenges for [sic] increasing the utilization rate of skilled birth attendance proportionally across the country' (Bhandari and Dangal 2013: 641; see also Engel et al. 2013). Across South Asia, fertility has been declining, reducing the number of higher parity births and adolescent births, due to increase in marriageable ages. Both trends could be expected to reduce MMR and child mortality rates on their own, without external intervention. Many of these explanations, while plausible, lack convincing supporting evidence and sometimes seem designed for propaganda purposes (see Chapter 11 in this volume). What then are these related policy reforms?

Overview of Policy Reforms

Drawing on McPake and Koblinsky (2009) and Lunze et al. (2015), we summarize the main innovations in maternity healthcare provisions across South Asia in Box 1.1:

Box 1.1: Maternal Health Policy Reforms in South Asia, 1990–2015

1. Demand-side enhancement
   a. Conditional cash transfers
   b. Subsidized or free delivery care, including maternal health voucher schemes
   c. Community-based awareness programmes
   d. Social media or mobile phone-based outreach programmes
2. Supply-side reforms
   a. Revamped schemes for birth attendants, female community health workers, and obstetric skills for doctors
   b. Building new or refurbishing maternity facilities
   c. Improved ambulance facilities for emergency obstetric care

Demand-Side Enhancement

Conditional Cash Transfers

The largest and best known of these is India's Janani Suraksha Yojana (JSY), a flagship scheme that provides financial entitlements as incentives for women to deliver in public (and some private) institutions and is being implemented nationwide. But there are significant variations between the so-called 'low-performing states', where money is given for every delivery, and the 'high-performing states' that provide money only for the first two deliveries. Furthermore, in most states the scheme does not cover all pregnant women, but only those with a below poverty line (BPL) certificate, and women from scheduled caste (SC) and scheduled tribe (ST) backgrounds. In addition, there may be age restrictions (only women above the age of 19, for example) and parity (only up to parity three) (Bhandari and Dangal 2013: 121). A recent analysis of challenges in the acceptance and use of institutional obstetric care facilities that need to be resolved by the JSY identifies continuing shortages in facilities, specialists, and staff; essential drugs; diagnostics; and necessary equipment. The authors point out that facilities receive very similar allocations despite widely varying caseloads and needs, and emergency transport is often unavailable (Gupta et al. 2018). At the beginning of the programme, because of the focus on 'poor-performing states', some studies showed that JSY made little impact on the poorest, for example, in Jharkhand (Thongkong et al. 2017), increasing rather than reducing the inequalities in access. A national study suggested that: 'Equity and uptake of institutional delivery and ANC improved in most states in late post-NRHM period 2011–12, the period when the targeted outreach of the most components of the NRHM was reached. Our study also found considerable inter-state variations in the impacts of the NRHM and the proportion of eligible women that received cash transfers' (Vellakkal et al. 2017: 87).

Not surprisingly, reductions in inequality in the use of maternal healthcare services were greatest where the programme was universalized, but in several low-performance states (such as Uttar Pradesh [UP]) significant inequalities nonetheless remain (Paul et al. 2019). Secondary analysis of the results of India's National Family Health Survey for 2015–16 (NFHS-4) similarly demonstrates that antenatal care (ANC) provision is far from universal: wealthier, urban, well-educated women who already have good relationships with the health services and some participation by the child's father are most likely to access the full available range of services (Ministry of Health and Family Welfare 2016). Again, inequities are greatest in states with the lowest overall rates of full ANC coverage, such as Bihar, UP, Madhya Pradesh (MP), and Assam, as compared with Andhra Pradesh (AP), Karnataka, Tamil Nadu, Telangana, and Kerala (Kumar et al. 2019).

In 2005, Nepal introduced the Safe Delivery Incentive Programme (SDIP), which included cash payments by the government of Nepal through hospitals or primary health centres to service users and service providers, to defray some of the patient's cost of transportation to health institutions. In 2007, this was reformulated as a Safer Mother Programme, and in 2009 changed again, to become the Aama-Suraksha-Karyakram (see further in the chapter). Baral (2012: 118) concluded that the effect of these cash payments was to increase, dramatically, the pressure on tertiary-care institutions: 'There is a gross discrepancy in non-targeted service delivery at the tertiary level health facility. Overflooding of maternity cases has hampered gynecological admission and surgical management delaying subspecialty care and junior physicians'. Service providers also receive cash to cover some of the costs associated with delivery, prescription drugs, and medical equipment (Pandey 2018). In Bangladesh, a demand-side financing scheme was trialled in 2007, providing vouchers (distributed by health workers) to women (mainly poor women) that entitle them to receive skilled care at home or at a facility, and also provide payments for transport and food (Schmidt et al. 2010). The trial did not, however, lead to a national programme.

Subsidized or Free Care, Including Maternal Health Vouchers

In India, individual states have piloted several schemes alongside or in place of JSY. Gujarat's Chiranjeevi Yojana (CY) involved only private practitioners and targeted poor women; the only cash transfer was for transport costs (see later in the chapter) (Engel et al. 2013). There has been an attrition of empanelled doctors, who did not find the rewards sufficient. A recent survey suggested that only about 50% of women were able to access the promised benefits (Doke et al. 2015). The system of recompensing doctors varies from state to state: in Gujarat, doctors were offered a flat rate per 100 deliveries, whereas in MP, there was an enhanced rate for C-sections, leading to an increase in C-sections in MP compared to a reduction in Gujarat (Bhat et al. 2009).

In Nepal, the Aama-Suraksha-Karyakram provided subsidized or free care for maternal and child health services (Vora et al. 2015). The preceding scheme was extended to not-for-profit institutions in early 2007 (Bogg et al. 2016; see also Rai 2016).

In Pakistan, a system of vouchers known as the Sehat (health) Voucher Scheme was launched in 2008–9 in two districts by Contech International and the Zahanat Foundation with the support of USAID (Jehan et al. 2012), but this does not seem to have led to any wider programme.

Community Awareness Programmes

In Nepal, 'behavioural and economic changes at the household level, driven by increased empowerment and education of women and greater awareness of how to mitigate pregnancy-related risks' have, it is claimed, helped reduce MMR (Ensor et al. 2009). A report on research in Nepal claimed that: 'In twelve of the Village Development Committees[,] a trained, locally based facilitator was employed to mobilize women's groups . . . Astonishingly, there was a reduction in neonatal mortality by 30% in intervention clusters, and an even larger and statistically significant effect on maternal mortality rates (78% reduction), although caution is required in interpretation given the relatively few maternal deaths' (Morrison et al. 2005: 2–3; see also Manandhar et al. 2004).

Similarly, a study of a project involving community-based activities carried out by an NGO in Jamalpur district, Bangladesh, succeeded in promoting women's access to and knowledge of maternal healthcare (Islam and Faruqye 2015). The generalizability of this finding has been questioned, however, in a review of the literature that found that: 'Exposure to women's groups was associated with a 23% non-significant reduction in maternal mortality and a 20% reduction in neonatal mortality, but with high statistical heterogeneity' (Prost et al. 2014: 1740).

Finally, India is particularly well represented in terms of community awareness programmes through grassroots health workers: the auxiliary nurse midwife (ANM), the anganwadi worker (AWW), and the accredited social health activist (ASHA) are expected to play a vital role in maternal and newborn healthcare in primary health sub-centres and rural areas.

Social Media–Based Initiatives

The field of maternal health has been a priority target for mHealth programmes (Noordam et al. 2011; Tamrat and Kachnowski 2012). The use of mobile phones to reduce delays in getting women to appropriate emergency obstetric care has been reported from Bangladesh (Prost et al. 2014) and in India (Hurst et al. 2015). The NGO ARMMAN (Advancing Reduction in Mortality and Morbidity of Mothers, Children and Neonates) went further by launching the Mobile Alliance for Maternal Action (Labrique et al. 2011) in Bangladesh (2012) and in India (2014): free oral messages are sent to pregnant women coming from underprivileged backgrounds, to give them advice and to remind them about the antenatal check-ups to be done. Similarly, ReMiND (reducing maternal and newborn deaths) was introduced in two blocks of rural UP, and seems to have been cost-effective as it represented only 6% of the annual budget for the Reproductive and Child Health (RCH) programme (Ilozumba et al. 2018). Yet, as Al Dahdah and Kumar underline in their studies in rural Bihar (this volume), focusing on the providers as well as the recipients involved in such programmes is required in order to grasp the complex and intertwined philanthropic and commercial interests at stake. Unintended effects such as gender reification are also worth noticing while exploring gendered technologies such as mobile phones.

Supply-Side Reforms

Revamped Schemes for Birth Attendants, Female Community Health Workers, and Obstetric Skills for Doctors

Most of these involved building the capacity of traditional birth attendants in the period up to 2005, with studies in Pakistan and Bangladesh suggesting considerable improvements in stillbirths and neonatal mortality (Mamata et al. 2015). In India, to help reach marginalized communities through female community health workers, the National Rural Health Mission (NRHM) introduced the ASHA category in 2006. The NRHM introduced the short-term training of MB BS doctors in emergency obstetric care in view of the grave shortages of medical and paramedical staff at health facilities. These shortages were seen as one of major reasons for delays in providing emergency care to pregnant and post-partum women and their babies, which contribute strongly to the high maternal and neo-natal mortality rates (Iyengar and Dholakia 2015).

Building New or Refurbishing Maternity Facilities

Apart from routine programmes of building (and occasionally maintaining) government facilities, new programmes have often included additional provisions. Some of these provisions involved public–private partnerships (PPPs) (Mian et al. 2018). Some field reports suggest that new buildings in rural areas have been sited far away from village residential areas, have taken several years to commission, and have rarely attracted skilled staff (Ministry of Health and Family Welfare 2008).

Ambulance and Transport Support

In India, the 'provision of transport in the form of various ambulance schemes', originally just for obstetric emergencies but now for all patients, was introduced under the NRHM (Mian et al. 2018). The Mamta Vahan scheme, an ambulance service for pregnant women, was introduced to reduce transportation barriers that prevent women from reaching health facilities. In Pakistan, the Primary and Secondary Healthcare Department launched a Rural Ambulance Service (RAS) in 2016 for pregnant women living in selected remote areas of Punjab.[4]

Overall, of course, these divisions into different kinds of policy interventions are somewhat artificial, since policies have often involved both demand- and supply-side activities. In the Sylhet district of Bangladesh, for example, financial incentives to cover expenses, a provision of emergency transport, and referral support to a tertiary-level hospital were combined with service-provider refresher training, 24/7 service coverage, additions of drugs and supplies, and incentives to the providers; doing all this together led to an increase in institutional deliveries from 25% in 2014 to 78% in 2016, compared with much lower increases with only some or only one of these interventions (Rahman et al. 2017).

Quality of Public and Private Sector Maternity Services

Across South Asia the balance between public and private facilities has shifted since the 1990s, with the growth in the private sector helping to fill the gap in provisions in urban areas. In India, private medical colleges, fuelled by rising urban middle-class incomes, have expanded urban maternity beds, more in south India than in the north (Bajpai et al. 2009: 82). The Indian government encourages PPPs through private investments in public health infrastructure, but the urban poor are increasingly reliant on non-formal private providers and 'traditional' healers. An RCH programme introduced integrated maternal and child health, family planning, and reproductive health services; quality concerns were voiced increasingly, but no action strategies were formulated. In 2000, a National Population Policy outlined a new RCH strategy and set specific maternal and infant mortality reduction goals; in the tenth (2002–7) and eleventh (2007–12) plan periods, strategies for quality assurance and appraisal were introduced. The NRHM expanded funding and decentralized programme implementation. Regular monitoring and feedback mechanisms were mandatory for funding streams, and other quality initiatives included Indian Public Health Standards for quality assurance in primary care and the National Accreditation Board for Hospital and Healthcare Providers (NABH) for quality certification of private providers (Ministry of Health and Family Welfare 2008; Lefebvre 2019).

The 'quality' of the health facilities that women are being encouraged to visit, whether for antenatal care, delivery services, or postnatal support and immunizations has generally been assessed on technical grounds, using checklists to assess physical clinic facilities and the knowledge of birthing staff. These assessments are often linked to schemes to train staff of various levels. Whether these schemes are effective is unclear. For example, emergency obstetric procedures may not be well understood, even among those who have been trained (Kamal et al. 2016). In Bihar, a programme of mentorship to address knowledge and skill deficiencies identified many barriers to improvement that they were not designed to address: 'including resource shortages, facility infrastructure, corruption, and cultural norms. These require government support, community awareness, and other systemic changes', while other barriers, such as 'hierarchy, violence against providers, and certain cultural taboos' needed adaptations to such programmes (Morgan et al. 2018: 12).

When 'satisfaction' and 'perceptions of health care providers' are considered, they have been assessed through focus group discussions, and short interviews with women or their companions as they leave a facility. Some recent examples include studies in several districts of Bangladesh that concluded that shortages of staff and logistical support, lack of laboratories, failures to follow patient protocols because of the pressure of patient numbers, and poor management contributed to poor quality of healthcare at all maternity facilities (Islam et al. 2015; Srivastava et al. 2014). In India, studies have mentioned poor hygiene standards (Bajpai et al. 2009), chaotic conditions that are not woman-friendly (Chaturvedi et al. 2015), and have drawn attention to:

> poor access, infrastructure constraints, high costs, ineffective treatment and insensitive behaviour as major reasons for low utilization of public facilities . . . Maternal care particularly suffered because of lack of trained human resources, poor communication, and poor referral and blood bank linkages . . . major deficiencies in physical and human resources with respect to handling the increased numbers of institutional deliveries.
>
> Chaturvedi et al. 2014

Women's experiences of 'quality' in the new birthing regimes are not standard, but are refracted through prisms of caste, class, and religion, depending on context. In India, for example, Dalit and Adivasi women, along with poor Muslims, are particularly likely to experience poorer quality of care and treatment (Jeffery et al. 2007), which rights-based approaches have specifically struggled to ameliorate.

Change and Ambivalence in the Medicalization of Childbirth

While various procedures aimed at improving the quality of maternal services have flourished, obstetrical technologies have been increasingly and often unjustifiably routinized, sometimes affecting the health of mothers and infants. For many years, there has been controversy on the effectiveness of induced labour, the relevance of routinized episiotomies (a surgical cut made at the opening of the vagina during childbirth, to aid a difficult delivery and prevent rupture of tissues), and more particularly the rationale behind the rise in C-sections. As *The Lancet* underlined, worldwide the number of babies born through C-sections almost doubled between 2000 and 2015, going from 12% to 21% of all births (Boerma at al. 2018).[5] The most rapid increase happened in South Asia (6.1% per year), especially in private hospitals in urban settings. India appears as a relevant example: in 1998–9, only 7.1% of all births in India were C-sections. This increased to 9% in 2005–6 and then shot up to 18.1% in 2015–16. Furthermore, most of the C-sections are occurring among affluent women who are at lower risk and supposedly need less intervention (Guilmoto and Dumont 2019). In other words, there is 'a dichotomy of not enough intervention in some populations with the consequences of high morbidity and mortality, and needless intervention in other populations where there is no real need for them. Either way, both groups suffer' (Pai 2000: 2760). Short-term and long-term risks of C-section—such as bleeding, placenta complications, ectopic pregnancies, as well as future stillbirths—are indeed well documented.

Beside issues of overuse, some medical technologies, such as amniocentesis and ultrasound, have been adversely diverted from their primary function by facilitating gender discrimination. Both amniocentesis and ultrasound were created to assess the condition of the foetus. Yet, shortly after their introduction in South Asia in the 1970s, prenatal diagnoses were largely used for sex detection and sex-selective abortion. The magnitude of the problem varies according to the abortion laws of each country: cases of sex-selective abortion are well known in India where abortion laws are relatively liberal (see the Medical Termination of Pregnancy Act, 1971), whereas they are less reported in Pakistan and Bangladesh where stricter laws only allow abortion if the life of the woman is endangered (Abrejo et al. 2009). The misuse of sex detection has led to antenatal gender discrimination and familial conflicts. It also appears as a serious public health issue in South Asian countries: sex-selective abortion constitutes an important proportion of induced abortions, which are the major cause of maternal mortality (Abrejo et al. 2009). In 1994, India passed the Pre-Natal Diagnostic Techniques (PNDT) Act. Despite this law that bans the use of prenatal technologies for sex selection, and despite awareness campaigns led by the government and NGOs, the Census shows that the child sex-ratio (0–6 years) imbalance has continued to deteriorate and that practices of female-selective abortion have spread throughout India. From 962 girls per 1,000 boys in 1981, the child sex-ratio dropped to 945 girls per 1,000 boys in 1991, 927 girls per 1,000 boys in 2001, and 919 girls per 1,000 boys in 2011. By comparison, in Bangladesh, according to the 2011 Census, the 0–5 sex–ratio was 972 girls per 1,000 boys (Bangladesh Bureau of Statistics 2015).

Like prenatal diagnosis, the emergence of assisted reproductive technologies (ART) has had mixed effects. During the last two decades, growing transnational demand for ART combined with a legal vacuum has resulted in rapidly growing numbers of Indian clinics specializing in surrogacy. The Indian surrogacy industry enabled infertile and homosexual couples to start families. With a flourishing commercial surrogacy industry offering good infrastructures and affordable prices (three times cheaper than in the USA, for example), it also attracted a substantial transnational clientele. Surrogacy is reported to bring between $400 million and $1 billion per year to the Indian economy (Rudrappa 2017). Yet, according to many researchers, this industry is controversial as it feeds upon the patriarchal stigmatization of childlessness (Banerjee 2012), the constrained choices of women from disadvantaged backgrounds (Pande 2014), and the commodification of women's bodies and energy (Vora 2009). After intense debates between politicians, feminists, and bioethicists, India introduced a surrogacy law in 2016: nowadays only altruistic surrogacy for infertile heterosexual Indian couples is allowed. But it seems that doctors practising in private clinics have already found ways to circumvent the law. By asking surrogate mothers to move across international borders (like Nepal) or by recruiting surrogate mothers from Kenya, not only is surrogacy maintained in India but the women are in more vulnerable situations (Rudrappa 2017).

These different examples show that the medicalization of maternal healthcare has significantly intensified over the last four decades in South Asia. This medicalization operates at various levels, such as childbirth practices (C-sections, episiotomies, inductions), pregnancy follow-up (ultrasounds), and infertility remedies (surrogacy). These examples further point to frictions between medical discoveries, the logics of economic rationality, and concerns for patients' health or well-being. Accounting for the medicalization of childbirth involves exploring the interests (financial, practical) of the medical profession, as well as understanding the regulatory and legislative power of the state.

Growing Concerns over Obstetric Violence

Apart from the shortcomings inherent in the medicalization of childbirth (such as non-medically justified interventions or iatrogenic effects of obstetric practices), there is growing evidence of patient abuse (see, for example, Jeffery et al. 2007) and increasing concern that the principle of informed consent is being flouted in obstetrical wards. The term 'obstetric violence' has been coined precisely to encompass all the forms of dehumanized care that women face in hospitals and clinics during pregnancy and childbirth. It gained popularity in Latin America in 2007 as Venezuela (followed later by Argentina and some states in Mexico) formally included obstetric violence within broader laws on gender inequalities. In South Asia, such landmark events have not yet occurred, but, since 2015, an increasing number of academic studies address the issues of obstetric violence with a particular focus on India (Shrivastava and Sivakami 2019) and Sri Lanka (Perera et al. 2018). In a study conducted in Ahmedabad, Gujarat, 40% of the women reported physical abuse, up to 55% faced verbal abuse, and 57% mentioned non-consented clinical care (Patel et al. 2018). A study based on focus group discussions in Colombo district revealed the widespread prevalence of verbal, emotional, and sometimes sexual violence perpetrated by caregivers in Sri Lankan state health institutions (Perera et al. 2018). As the authors rightly underline, this obstetric violence often silences and targets mainly Muslim and Tamil-speaking women, and undermines the trust that users should be able to place in the caregivers and the health system. These interdisciplinary or quantitative studies echo some well-known ethnographical studies that described and analysed in detail different practices of abuse in delivery rooms of Indian government hospitals, without referring to the recent concept of obstetric violence (Jeffery and Jeffery 2010; Jeffery et al. 1989, 2007; Pinto 2008; Van Hollen 2003).

It has been fairly argued that obstetric violence has particular features that require an analysis of their own: 'it is a feminist issue, a case of gender violence; labouring women are generally healthy and not pathological; and labour, and birth can be framed as sexual events, with obstetric violence being frequently experienced and interpreted as rape' (Sadler et al. 2016: 50). Yet the term 'obstetric violence' also has two main drawbacks. First, it prompts readers to hold the health workers responsible, potentially generating more hostility towards them and further reinforcing the dichotomy between caregivers and caretakers. Professionals and institutions tend to favour the term 'humanizing childbirth' (Sadler et al. 2016).[6] Second, while the concept 'obstetric violence' refers explicitly to the pervasiveness of gender-domination mechanisms, it also minimizes the intersectional dimension of the violence at stake. In South Asia (Jeffery and Jeffery 2008; Jullien 2019a; Perera et al. 2018), as elsewhere (Fassin 2001; Jaffré and Olivier de Sardan 2003), studies show that gender as well as criteria of age, language, religion, social position, and cultural background need to be jointly considered to understand the structural violence in obstetrical wards. Roger Jeffery's discussion (2018) of the relevance of Farmer's concept of 'structural violence' and Bourdieu's notion of 'symbolic violence' provides a way to approach the ethical issues of obstetrics, and to account for the 'ability of people to misrepresent their subjugation'. We suggest that further discussions are required to better understand the specificities of the terms 'structural violence' and 'obstetric violence', as well as their impact on pregnant and labouring women. Nonetheless, our point here is that hostile treatment of women in labour remains a substantial issue that needs to be addressed as countries in South Asia turn to the implementation of the norms of good governance of health services that is mandated by the Sustainable Development Goals (SDGs).

Although initiatives for humanizing childbirth remain limited in South Asia, the growth of NGOs and programmes promoting natural birth or positive birth since 2010 should be highlighted. In India, for example, not only NGOs (such as the White Ribbon Alliance, Society for Midwives India, and Birth India) but also less-formalized support groups based in the major cities of the country work to ensure that women are aware of their rights and experience humane childbirths.[7] Some NGOs, such as the Centre for Enquiry into Health and Allied Themes (CEHAT), are planning to launch courses for medical students in order to alert them to these concerns (Nayak and Nath 2018).

Some birth centres are now run by independent professional midwives and doulas, offering personalized and more spiritual approaches to labour in southern India.[8] So far, the government has not made substantial efforts to assure humanized childbirth. Yet new initiatives such as the LaQshya guidelines (Ministry of Health and Family Welfare 2017), aiming at promoting safe and respectful childbirth practices, as well as the Guidelines on Midwifery Services of 2018 initiated by the Ministry of Health and Family Welfare, suggest the possibility of properly educating and training nurse-practitioner midwives (National Health Mission 2018).

Rights-Based Approaches

The rhetoric of those supporting reforms in maternity provisions has increasingly referred to 'rights-based' approaches and 'empowering women to make the right choice'. Bangladesh's 2001 National Policy for Maternal Health has been described as rights-based (Islam et al. 2005) and the Government of India described the JSY in the same way. As has often been pointed out, however, rights-based approaches sit uneasily with conditional cash transfers. Some argue that incentives such as those in the JSY are used in a coercive way instead of empowering women (Srivastava et al. 2014: 36). Alternatively, JSY may have generated a sense of entitlement to the cash transfer, rather than to available, accessible, acceptable, and good-quality health services (Unnithan 2015). A study of 22 maternal deaths in MP concluded that 'normative elements of a human rights approach to maternal health (i.e. availability, accessibility, acceptability, and quality of maternal health services) were not upheld' (Jat et al. 2015). What Mishra and Roalkvam call an 'institutionalisation of motherhood' involves a contract in which the state provides services, but women must embrace 'acceptable motherhood' in return (Mishra and Roalkvam 2014: 126). They argue that in rural, tribal Odisha, 'JSY and its cash incentives are seen as linked to the act of delivering in the institution *per se*, and not to the quality of care received' (Mishra and Roalkvam 2014: 133) and that by paying women to give birth in institutions, their entitlement to quality maternity care is obscured (Mishra and Roalkvam 2014: 134).

In addition to perception problems, there are also issues of implementation. A study carried out in five Indian states showed that 81% of the women were aware of the scheme, but only 76% of JSY beneficiaries received any money after delivery (Mishra and Roalkvam 2014: 127). A study in West Bengal found that delays in providing the cash incentive resulted in women making multiple visits to claim their JSY entitlement, and funds are often diverted to other uses (United Nations Population Fund 2009: 8). In the absence of community-level monitoring of the scheme, these procedural complexities for beneficiaries reduce its impact. In Varanasi, JSY reimbursement helped fewer than 1 in 10 households to escape the catastrophic costs often associated with maternity payments (Tripathy et al. 2017: 409).[9] A nationwide comparison of costs associated with maternity in 2004 and 2014, however, suggests that catastrophic health spending declined over this period, especially for poorer mothers, but out-of-pocket expenditures rose, and the benefits were restricted to the costs associated with deliveries, rather than antenatal or postnatal care (Mohanty and Kastor 2017). In Bangladesh, use of maternal and child health (MCH) services remains biased along social class and urban–rural lines (Mukhopadhyay et al. 2018: 29). In Pakistan, 'the selection criteria and adverse attitude of healthcare workers, along with inadequacy of programmatic resources to sustain outreach activities' contribute to the exclusion of lower-caste poor women and nomads from community spaces (including clinics) (Mukherjee and Singh 2018). All these studies suggest that equity issues have barely begun to be addressed across the region.

While health policies in South Asia have mainly addressed maternal health issues by focusing on institutionalization (and medicalization) of childbirth deliveries, since the 1980s a growing number of international institutions and NGOs have been advocating rights-based approaches in maternal healthcare. Such approaches aim at accelerating the fight against maternal and infant mortality and morbidity by broadening the perspective and addressing directly the economic, social, cultural, and political forces linked to maternal healthcare. In rights-based approaches, investment in maternal care is not fruitful if other factors are not tackled simultaneously: special attention should be paid to providing a fully functional healthcare system, ensuring access to healthcare (tackling access, cost, and negative perceptions of care), and enhancing women's status (through improved education, women's decision-making, raising the age of marriage, and fostering positive evaluations of women).

For example, it is well known that women need sufficient physical (and emotional) maturity to cope with pregnancy and deliver safely. Yet South Asian governments generally do not check the effective implementation of the legal minimum age of marriage, even though most countries have officially set one. Regarding India, the Human Rights Council (HRC) explained that: 'While acknowledging measures taken to outlaw child marriages (Child Marriage Restraint Act) [which sets the minimum age of marriage at 18 for girls and 21 for boys] . . . the Committee remains gravely concerned that legislative measures are not sufficient and that measures designed to change the attitudes which allow such practices [child marriages] should be taken' (WHO 2001: 36).

In fact, by taking human rights into development discourses and by underlining the indivisibility of health and rights (Correa et al. 1994), rights-based approaches seek to empower rights-holders as well as strengthen the capacity of duty-bearers, by pressuring state authorities (WHO 2001). Advocates in domestic courts have successfully referred to constitutional and human rights laws to show that the Indian state was not fulfilling its legal obligations to prevent maternal mortality and morbidity. In a case in 2010 (*Laxmi Mandal* v. *Deen Dayal Hari Nager Hospital & Ors*), where two impoverished women died during childbirth, the High Court recognized the state's failure to implement various programmes to reduce maternal and infant mortality (HRC 2011: 15). Compensation for human rights violations was also required.

By encouraging governments to consider societal factors and include comprehensive reproductive health services in their policies, rights-based approaches have also encouraged the realization of reproductive health rights. Since 1990, 'reproductive rights' have been presented as a new international standard. In the milestone Cairo Programme of Action, agreed in 1994, 179 countries signed up to reproductive rights, defined as 'the recognition of the basic rights for all couples and individuals to decide freely and responsibly the number, spacing and timing of their children and to have the information and means to do so' (United Nations 1994: 13). Since then, the focus has shifted from policies targeting population control and mortality ratios to programmes that prioritize individual consent, choices, and rights, without governmental control or coercion. In Bangladesh, for example, the status of maternal mortality (and morbidity) was addressed at the national policy level as human rights in 1990. Since then, 'the role of husbands, family and community are recognized as being essential to improve maternal health and, as a result, strategies to improve community engagement were developed' (HRC 2011: 15). Similarly, in Nepal, efforts are being made to ensure respect for a woman's decision to seek care promptly when she feels in need of assistance. According to a 1998 study of maternal mortality in Nepal, husbands were the main decision-makers in whether to go to the hospital for maternity care, and maternal family members made the decision in only 11.5% of the cases (WHO 2001: 41).

There is certainly no consensus on the notion of reproductive rights, and there is often a gap between countries' international commitments and their local implementation (Gautier and Grenier-Torres 2014). Nonetheless, states are now sensitized to the question of fundamental reproductive rights, and they are invited (sometimes pressured) to ensure that these rights are guaranteed in their countries. In this regard, Indian policies on family planning show an interesting evolution (Rao 2004). As a signatory to the Cairo Programme of Action, India officially supports the right to voluntary and informed choice in matters related to contraception. This concern is stipulated in the National Population Policy of 2000, marking a significant turning-point after India's well-known repressive policies of sterilization during the period of Emergency in the 1970s. Yet, a target-free approach varies considerably across regions, with some states unwilling to abandon targets and incentives (Kosgi et al. 2011). The current 'two-child norm policy' implemented locally by some Indian states goes explicitly against the national resolutions. Furthermore, in public hospitals, entrenched attitudes among doctors and nurses have been difficult to change, as some continue to hold the poor or Muslim communities responsible for demographic and development issues. Their practices are then determined by nationalistic considerations rather than by any concerns for the individual freedom of their patients (Jeffery et al. 2007; Jullien 2019b).

Structure of the Book

This book includes chapters that are designed to illuminate different aspects of the changes in childbirth since the early 2000s. One of the strengths of this book is our inclusion of material drawing out the perspectives of caregivers, and not just those of women giving birth (or unable to do so). Samiksha Sehrawat's chapter gives a historical overview of maternal health policies in South Asia, returning to their genesis and providing a 100-year perspective. She highlights the continuities between colonial discourses and initiatives and post-colonial policies aimed at improving maternal healthcare. This historical perspective partly continues in Section 2 of this book, 'Continuing Relevance of "Traditional Birth Attendants"', dedicated to the ongoing relevance (but more often, dismissal) of traditional birth attendants. Based on ethnographic fieldwork in Balochistan, Pakistan, Fouzieyha

Towghi examines how the medicalization of childbirth in hospitals (which often involves unnecessary and risky practices) has enhanced the perceived benefits of Balochi medicines and midwifery. Similarly, Pascale Hancart-Petitet uses her research in Tamil Nadu, India, to show how the role and knowledge of traditional midwives have been legitimized, delegitimized, or merely acknowledged in successive health policies. Contrary to what one might assume, given the contemporary pressure to use only skilled birth attendants and hospital deliveries, these two authors show that traditional midwives resist state pressures and continue to assist childbirths in India as well as in Pakistan, by strategically reconfiguring their practices and by affirming their ethical stance.

Categories of birth attendants are further discussed in Section 3, 'Contested Categories'. Through an ethnographic case study in slums in New Delhi, India, Helen Vallianatos compares how trained and traditional birth attendants consider childbirth and how their respective perspective and practices affect women's birth experiences. Based on interviews of migrant women living in slums in Maharashtra, also in India, Deepra Dandekar shows that childbirth practices are 'in transit' between urban medical facilities and rural home birthing, a transit that reflects other aspects of women's socio-economic positions and everyday lives. Not only do these chapters underline the logics of power relations and social networks embedded in childbirth, they also assess more broadly whether (and how) the institutionalization of birth promoted by state policies is spreading among slum-dwellers in India.

Section 4, 'Contemporary Birth Attendants', addresses the training, role, and status of staff involved in institutionalized obstetrics. Based on ethnographic research on women doctors' avoidance of village clinics in Jaipur district, Rajasthan, India, Jocelyn Killmer explores the reasons why rural spaces are marked as dangerous sites for urban middle-class women. Drawing on ethnographic fieldwork in private clinics in Rajasthan and UP, India, Isabelle L. Lange, Sunita Bhadauria, Sunita Singh and, Loveday Penn-Kekana examine the vulnerability and precarious status of unlicensed medical staff working in these clinics. By focusing on a leading government medical college in Mumbai, India, Neha Madhiwala examines the contribution of obstetrical postgraduate students coming from rural areas in terms of knowledge production. When South Asia—and India in particular—is strongly supporting hospital delivery to reduce maternal and infant mortality and meet its MDG and SDG targets, these ethnographies on the (dys)functioning of rural and urban hospitals are particularly valuable to understand the constraints of current health policies.

Section 5, 'Institutionalization of Childbirth', looks more specifically at the (un)intended consequences of the institutionalization of childbirth, as well as on the ambivalent effects of new technologies. Drawing on her ethnographic fieldwork in Rajasthan, Clémence Jullien shows how campaigns condemning preference for male child and the institutionalization of childbirth have reinforced medical and moral surveillance within obstetrical wards, while affecting how preferences for male children are discussed and experienced. Jeevan Sharma and Radha Adhikari show that in Nepal, foreign donors have established many schemes and programmes. They all claim to have contributed to Nepal's apparent success in reducing maternal mortality, rarely acknowledging the role of non-health sector changes. Very different—much higher—recent maternal mortality estimates place a question mark against how far these reductions are real.

Section 6, 'New Technologies', considers two different forms of technological innovations. Using interviews with childless women who sought fertility treatments in Bangladesh, Mirza Taslima Sultana reminds us that infertility and non-birthing are essential frames to understand birthing practices. She emphasizes the continuities and transformations in biomedical power, paying particular attention to patients' agency and how they negotiate doctor–patient relationships. In their study of mHealth programmes on safe motherhood in Bihar, India, Marine Al Dahdah and Alok Kumar examine the impact mobile phone technologies have on the status and practices of the community health workers in charge of such programmes.

Through different angles these authors show how medical procedures change women's perception of their reproductive health and how they alter the role of the medical staff within communities, often in unintended and ambiguous ways.

This volume provides new and revealing perspectives on childbirth in twenty-first-century South Asia—perspectives that need to be taken seriously in planning future changes. South Asian countries are now grappling with a new set of goals—the SDGs, with targets set for 2030. These include several targets that impact on maternal and reproductive health, and therefore have implications for the contexts and outcomes of childbirth. Target 3.1 is, by 2030, to 'reduce the global maternal mortality ratio to less than 70 per 100 000 live births' (UN Sustainable Development Summit 2015). Target 3.2 is, by 2030, 'to end preventable deaths of newborns, with all countries aiming to reduce neonatal mortality to at least as low as 12 per 1000 live births' (UN Sustainable Development Summit 2015). Target 3.7 is, by 2030, to 'ensure universal access to sexual and reproductive health-care services, including for family planning, information and education, and the integration of reproductive health into national strategies and programmes' (UN Sustainable Development Summit 2015). Target 3.8 is to 'achieve universal health coverage, including financial risk protection, access to quality essential health-care services and access to safe, effective, quality and affordable essential medicines and vaccines for all' (UN Sustainable Development Summit 2015). These are to be achieved within a framework dedicated to the 'eradication of poverty', 'gender equality and the empowerment of all women and girls', and 'peaceful, just and inclusive societies which are free from fear and violence' (UN Sustainable Development Summit 2015). Once again, quantitative targets are employed. While there is certainly a case to be made that such targets focus the mind and provide yardsticks against which governments can be held accountable, they also lay themselves open to the possibility of unintended consequences. Despite the hopes that all countries will achieve good governance, there is an increased need to be aware of the downside of programmes that ignore *processes* of change (Hamal et al. 2018). New patterns of inequities are emerging, and continuing gaps in transparency and accountability in public and private provisions are being reinforced. We hope that the chapters in this volume will contribute to the debates that are essential if all women in South Asia are to experience safe and humane conditions of childbirth.

Notes

1. Over South Asia as a whole, the total number of births was stable between 1990 and 2000, slightly declining from 2000 to 2015 because fertility rates have declined more rapidly than the total population has risen. Official and UN estimates suggest that the number of births taking place in institutional settings has risen from c. 11 million in 1990 to c. 14 million in 2000 and to c. 25 million in 2015 (authors' calculations).

2. For example, in Bijnor (Uttar Pradesh) the District Female Hospital in 2006–7 saw an average of 35 women give birth per month; in 2015 (between April and September), average monthly deliveries were 326 (GBD Child Mortality Collaborators 2016: Appendix tables). See also World Health Organization (2015: 4–11), for comparable information from elsewhere in UP and in MP.

3. The figures in these tables are the median estimates: compared to the estimates given in Tables 1.1–1.3, the real figures could easily be 10% above or below (approximately equal to the lower and upper bounds of 90% uncertainty intervals).

4. Available at: https://en.dailypakistan.com.pk/23-Nov-2016/punjab-to-introduce-rural-ambulance-service-for-pregnant-women-in-remote-areas, last accessed 9 March 2021.
5. As a reminder, medical experts estimate that only 10–15% of births require surgical intervention (Betrán et al. 2016).
6. An international conference held in Fortalezal, Brazil, in 2000 was entitled 'First Conference for the Humanization of Birth', https://www.orgasmicbirth.com/humanization-conference-brazil/, last accessed 9 March 2021.
7. We would like to thank sincerely Sreya Majumdar (Department of Liberal Arts, Indian Institute of Technology, Hyderabad), whose unpublished paper 'The Positive Birth: Emergence of Professional Midwifery in India' (Majumdar 2020), is the source for this section on positive birth.
8. Case studies of two doulas (women providing social and emotional support for women in pregnancy, childbirth, and the post-partum period) trained beyond South Asia, are discussed in a paper on Hyderabad presented at the Paris Conference by Haripriya Narasimhan (2018). More details are available from her on request.
9. Illness-related costs, for patients, that are ≥20% of the pre-illness annual household income are defined as 'catastrophic'.

References

Abrejo, Farina Gul, Babar Tasneem Shaikh, and Narjis Rizvi. 2009. ' "And They Kill Me, Only Because I Am a Girl": A Review of Sex-Selective Abortions in South Asia'. *The European Journal of Contraception & Reproductive Health Care* 14 (1): 10–16.

Akseer, Nadia, Mahdis Kamali, Shams E. Arifeen, Ashar Malik, Zaid Bhatti, Naveen Thacker, Mahesh Maksey, Harendra D'Silva, Inacio C.M. da Silva, and Zulfiqar A. Bhutta. 2017. 'Progress in Maternal and Child Health: How Has South Asia Fared?' *British Medical Journal* 357: j1608.

Alkema, Leontine, Doris Chou, Daniel Hogan, Sanqian Zhang, Ann-Beth Moller, Alison Gemmill, Doris Ma Fat, Ties Boerma, Marleen Temmerman, Colin Mathers, and Lale Say. 2016. 'Global, Regional, and National Levels and Trends in Maternal Mortality between 1990 and 2015, with Scenario-Based Projections to 2030: A Systematic Analysis by the UN Maternal Mortality Estimation Inter-agency Group'. *The Lancet* 387 (10017): 462–74.

Aziz, Ayesha, Fazal Ali Khan, and Geof Wood. 2015. 'Who Is Excluded and How? An Analysis of Community Spaces for Maternal and Child Health in Pakistan'. *Health Research Policy and Systems* 13 (1): S56.

Bajpai, Nirupam, Jeffrey D. Sachs, and Ravindra H. Dholakia. 2009. 'Improving Access, Service Delivery and Efficiency of the Public Health System in Rural India'. In *CGSD Working Paper 37*. New York: Center on Globalization and Sustainable Development.

Banerjee, Sneha. 2012. 'Emergence of the "Surrogacy Industry"'. *Economic and Political Weekly* 47 (11): 27–9.

Bangladesh Bureau of Statistics. 2015. *Population Monograph of Bangladesh: Age–Sex Composition of Bangladesh Population*. Dhaka: Ministry of Planning.

Baral, Gehanath. 2012. 'An Assessment of the Safe Delivery Incentive Program at a Tertiary Level Hospital in Nepal'. *Journal of Nepal Health Research Council* 10 (20): 118–24.

Betrán, A.P., Torloni, M.R., Zhang, J.J., Gülmezoglu, A.M., WHO Working Group on Caesarean Section, Aleem, H.A., Althabe, F., Bergholt, T., de Bernis, L., Carroli, G. and Deneux-Tharaux, C., 2016. WHO statement on caesarean section rates. *BJOG: An International Journal of Obstetrics & Gynaecology* 123 (5): 667–670.

Bhandari, T. Ram, and Ganesh Dangal. 2013. 'Safe Delivery Care: Policy, Practice and Gaps in Nepal'. *Journal of the Nepal Medical Association* 52 (192): 637–44.

Bhat, Ramesh, Dileep V. Mavalankar, Prabal V. Singh, and Neelu Singh. 2009. 'Maternal Healthcare Financing: Gujarat's Chiranjeevi Scheme and Its Beneficiaries'. *Journal of Health, Population, and Nutrition* 27 (2): 249–58.

Bhutta, Zulfiqar Ahmed. 2000. 'Why Has So Little Changed in Maternal and Child Health in South Asia?' *British Medical Journal* 321 (7264): 809.

Boerma, Ties, Carine Ronsmans, Dessalegn Y. Melesse, Aluisio J.D. Barros, Fernando C. Barros, Liang Juan, Ann-Beth Moller, Lale Say, Ahmad Reza Hosseinpoor, and Mu Yi. 2018. 'Global Epidemiology of Use of and Disparities in Caesarean Sections'. *The Lancet* 392 (10155): 1341–8.

Blencowe, Hannah, Simon Cousens, Fiorella Bianchi Jassir, Lale Say, Doris Chou, Colin Mathers, Dan Hogan, Suhail Shiekh, Zeshan U. Qureshi, and Danzhen You. 2016. 'National, Regional, and Worldwide Estimates of Stillbirth Rates in 2015, with Trends from 2000: A Systematic Analysis'. *The Lancet Global Health* 4 (2): e98–e108.

Bogg, Lennart, Vishal Diwan, Kranti S. Vora, and Ayesha DeCosta. 2016. 'Impact of Alternative Maternal Demand-Side Financial Support Programs in India on the Caesarean Section Rates: Indications of Supplier-Induced Demand'. *Maternal and Child Health Journal* 20 (1): 11–15.

Bora, Jayanta Kumar, Rajesh Roshan, and Wolfgang Lutz. 2019. 'The Persistent Influence of Caste on Under-Five Mortality: Factors That Explain the Caste-Based Gap in High Focus Indian States'. *PloS One* 14 (8): e0211086.

Chaturvedi, Sarika, Ayesha De Costa, and Joanna Raven. 2015. 'Does the Janani Suraksha Yojana Cash Transfer Programme to Promote Facility Births in India Ensure Skilled Birth Attendance? A Qualitative Study of Intrapartum Care in Madhya Pradesh'. *Global Health Action* 8 (1): 27427.

Chaturvedi, Sarika, Sourabh Upadhyay, and Ayesha De Costa. 2014. 'Competence of Birth Attendants at Providing Emergency Obstetric Care under India's JSY Conditional Cash Transfer Program for Institutional Delivery: An Assessment Using Case Vignettes in Madhya Pradesh Province'. *BMC Pregnancy and Childbirth* 14 (1): 174.

Correa, Sonia, Rebecca Lynn Reichmann, Gigi Francisco, and Rebecca Reichmann. 1994. *Population and Reproductive Rights: Feminist Perspectives from the South*. New Delhi: Kali for Women in Association with DAWN.

Doke, Prakash P., U.H. Gawande, Shailesh R. Deshpande, and Mukta Gadgil. 2015. 'Evaluation of Janani Suraksha Yojana (JSY) in Maharashtra, India: Important Lessons for Implementation'. *International Journal of Tropical Disease & Health* 5 (2): 141–55.

El-Saharty, Sameh. 2015. 'South Asia's Quest for Reduced Maternal Mortality: What the Data Show'. *Investing in Health: News and Views in Healthy Development*, 17 September. Accessed 9 March 2021. http://blogs.worldbank.org/health/south-asia-s-quest-reduced-maternal-mortality-what-data-show

Engel, Jakob, Jonathan Glennie, Shiva Raj Adhikari, Sanju Wagle Bhattarai, Devi Prasad Prasai, and Fiona Samuels. 2013. 'Nepal's Story: Understanding Improvements in Maternal Health'. In *Research Reports and Studies*. London: Overseas Development Institute.

Ensor, Tim, Susan Clapham, and Devi Prasad Prasai. 2009. 'What Drives Health Policy Formulation: Insights from the Nepal Maternity Incentive Scheme?' *Health Policy* 90 (2–3): 247–53.

Fassin, Didier. 2001. 'Le culturalisme pratique de la santé publique: Critique d'un sens commun'. In *Critique de la santé publique: Une approche anthropologique*, edited by Jean-Pierre Dozon and Didier Fassin, 181–208. Paris: Balland.

GBD Child Mortality Collaborators. 2016. 'Global, Regional, National, and Selected Subnational Levels of Stillbirths, Neonatal, Infant, and Under-5 Mortality, 1980–2015: A Systematic Analysis for the Global Burden of Disease Study 2015'. *The Lancet* 388 (10053): 1725–74.

Gautier, Arlette, and Chrystelle Grenier-Torres. 2014. 'Controverses autour des droits reproductifs et sexuels'. *Autrepart* 2 (70): 3–21.

Guilmoto, Christophe Z., and Alexandre Dumont. 2019. 'Trends, Regional Variations, and Socioeconomic Disparities in Cesarean Births in India, 2010–2016'. *JAMA Network Open* 2 (3): e190526.

Gupta, Adyya, Jasmine Fledderjohann, Hanimi Reddy, V.R. Raman, David Stuckler, and Sukumar Vellakkal. 2018. 'Barriers and Prospects of India's Conditional Cash Transfer Program to Promote Institutional Delivery Care: A Qualitative Analysis of the Supply-Side Perspectives'. *BMC Health Services Research* 18 (1): 40.

Hamal, Mukesh, Marjolein Dieleman, Vincent De Brouwere, and Tjard de Cock Buning. 2018. 'How Do Accountability Problems Lead to Maternal Health Inequities? A Review of Qualitative Literature from Indian Public Sector'. *Public Health Reviews* 39 (9). doi: 10.1186/s40985-018-0081-z.

Hodges, Sarah, and Mohan Rao, eds. 2016. *Public Health and Private Wealth: Stem Cells, Surrogates, and Other Strategic Bodies*. Delhi: Oxford University Press.

Human Rights Council (HRC). 2011. *Practices in Adopting a Human Rights-Based Approach to Eliminate Preventable Maternal Mortality and Human Rights, Report of the Human Rights Committee (A/HRC/18/27)*. Geneva: Office of the United Nations High Commissioner for Human Rights.

Hurst, Taylor E., Katherine Semrau, Atul Gawande, and Lisa R. Hirschhorn. 2015. 'Demand-Side Interventions for Maternal Care: Evidence of More Use, Not Better Outcomes'. *BMC Pregnancy and Childbirth* 15(1): 297.

Ilozumba, Onaedo, Marjolein Dieleman, Nadine Kraamwinkel, Sara Van Belle, Murari Chaudoury, and Jacqueline E.W. Broerse. 2018. '"I am Not Telling. The

Mobile Is Telling": Factors Influencing the Outcomes of a Community Health Worker mHealth Intervention in India'. *PloS One* 13 (3): e0194927.

Islam, Farzana, Aminur Rahman, Abdul Halim, Charli Eriksson, Fazlur Rahman, and Koustuv Dalal. 2015. 'Perceptions of Health Care Providers and Patients on Quality of Care in Maternal and Neonatal Health in Fourteen Bangladesh Government Healthcare Facilities: A Mixed-Method Study'. *BMC Health Services Research* 15 (1): 237.

Islam, M.T., M.M. Hossain, M.A. Islam, and Y.A. Haque. 2005. 'Improvement of Coverage and Utilization of EmOC Services in Southwestern Bangladesh'. *International Journal of Gynecology & Obstetrics* 91 (3): 298–305.

Islam, Rezaul and Cathleen Jo Faruqye. 2015. 'Safe Motherhood Promotion in Bangladesh: Evidence from a NGO's Local Level Health Monitoring and Advocacy Project'. *Journal of Family Medicine & Community Health* 2 (2): 1–7.

Iyengar, Shreekant, and Ravindra H. Dholakia. 2015. Specialist Services in the Indian Rural Public Health System for maternal and child healthcare—a study of four states. Working Paper 2015-07-04. Ahmedabad: Indian Institute of Management. Accessed 4 March 2021. http://vslir.iima.ac.in:8080/jspui/bitstream/11718/16594/1/WP2015-07-04.pdf

Jaffré, Yannick, and Jean-Pierre Olivier de Sardan, eds. 2003. *Une médecine inhospitalière: Les difficiles relations entre soignants et soignés dans cinq capitales d'Afrique de l'Ouest*. Paris: Karthala Editions.

Jat, Tej Ram, Prakash R. Deo, Isabel Goicolea, Anna-Karin Hurtig, and Miguel San Sebastian. 2015. 'Socio-cultural and Service Delivery Dimensions of Maternal Mortality in Rural Central India: A Qualitative Exploration Using a Human Rights Lens'. *Global Health Action* 8 (1): doi: 10.3402/gha.v8.24976

Jeffery, Patricia, and Roger Jeffery. 2008. '"Money Itself Discriminates": Obstetric Emergencies in the Time of Liberalisation'. *Contributions to Indian Sociology* 42 (1): 59–91.

Jeffery, Patricia, and Roger Jeffery. 2010. 'Costly Absences, Coercive Presences: Health Care in Rural North India'. In *Diversity and Change in Modern India: Economic, Social and Political Approaches*, edited by Anthony F. Heath and Roger Jeffery, 47–71. Oxford: Oxford University Press.

Jeffery, Patricia, Roger Jeffery, and Andrew Lyon. 1989. *Labour Pains and Labour Power: Women and Childbearing in India*. London: Zed Books.

Jeffery, Roger. 2018. 'War against Disease Without Violence to Clinical Trial Participants?' In *Violence and Non-violence across Time: History, Religion and Culture*, edited by Sudhir Chandra, 222–46. New Delhi: Routledge India.

Jeffery, Roger, Patricia Jeffery, and Mohan Rao. 2007. 'Safe Motherhood Initiatives: Contributions from Small-Scale Studies'. *Indian Journal of Gender Studies* 14 (2): 285–94.

Jehan, Kate, Kristi Sidney, Helen Smith, and Ayesha de Costa. 2012. 'Improving Access to Maternity Services: An Overview of Cash Transfer and Voucher Schemes in South Asia'. *Reproductive Health Matters* 20 (39): 142–54.

Jullien, Clémence. 2019a. *Du bidonville à l'hôpital: Nouveaux enjeux de la maternité au Rajasthan*. Paris: Éditions de la Maison des sciences de l'homme, collection le (bien) commun.

Jullien, Clémence. 2019b. ' "Bien-être familial": Une notion illusoire? L'envers de la rhétorique en milieu hospitalier indien'. *In L'hôpital en Asie du Sud. Politiques de santé, pratiques de soins*, edited by Jullien, Clémence, Lefebvre, Bertrand, and Fabien Provost, 36: 57–79. Purushartha.

Kamal, Nahid, Sian Curtis, Mohammad S. Hasan, and Kanta Jamil. 2016. 'Trends in Equity in Use of Maternal Health Services in Urban and Rural Bangladesh'. *International Journal for Equity in Health* 15 (1): 27.

Kerber, Kate J., Joseph E. de Graft-Johnson, Zulfiqar A. Bhutta, Pius Okong, Ann Starrs, and Joy E. Lawn. 2007. 'Continuum of Care for Maternal, Newborn, and Child Health: From Slogan to Service Delivery'. *The Lancet* 370 (9595): 1358–69.

Kosgi, Srinivas, Satheesh Rao, Shrinivasa Bhat Undaru, and Nagesh B. Pai. 2011. 'Women Reproductive Rights in India: Prospective Future'. *Online Journal of Health and Allied Sciences* 10 (1): 1–5.

Kumar, Gunjan, Tarun Shankar Choudhary, Akanksha Srivastava, Ravi Prakash Upadhyay, Sunita Taneja, Rajiv Bahl, Jose Martines, Maharaj Kishan Bhan, Nita Bhandari, and Sarmila Mazumder. 2019. 'Utilisation, Equity and Determinants of Full Antenatal Care in India: Analysis from the National Family Health Survey 4'. *BMC Pregnancy Childbirth* 19 (1): 327.

Labrique, A.B., R. Paul, S. Sikder, L.S. Wu, N. Jahan, and K.P. West Jr. 2011. 'Mobile Phones as Disruptive Agents in the Pathway to Mortality During Emergency Obstetric Crises in Rural Bangladesh'. *60th Annual Meeting of the American Society of Tropical Medicine and Hygiene*, Philadelphia, PA.

Lefebvre, Bertrand. 2019. 'L'accréditation hospitalière et la qualité des soins en Inde. Entre logiques commerciales et objectifs de santé publique'. In *L'hôpital en Asie du Sud. Politiques de santé, pratiques de soins*, edited by Jullien, Clémence, Lefebvre, Bertrand, and Fabien Provost, 36: 31–56. Purushartha.

Lim, Stephen S., Lalit Dandona, Joseph A. Hoisington, Spencer L. James, Margaret C. Hogan, and Emmanuela Gakidou. 2010. 'India's Janani Suraksha Yojana, a Conditional Cash Transfer Programme to Increase Births in Health Facilities: An Impact Evaluation'. *The Lancet* 375 (9730): 2009–23.

Lunze, Karsten, Ariel Higgins-Steele, Aline Simen-Kapeu, Linda Vesel, Julia Kim, and Kim Dickson. 2015. 'Innovative Approaches for Improving Maternal and Newborn Health: A Landscape Analysis'. *BMC Pregnancy and Childbirth* 15 (337): 1–19.

Maine, Deborah, and Allan Rosenfield. 1999. 'The Safe Motherhood Initiative: Why Has It Stalled?' *American Journal of Public Health* 89 (4): 480–2.

Majumdar, Sreya. 2020. 'The Positive Birth: Emergence of Professional Midwifery in India' (presentation, unpublished), *Reproduction, Demography and Cultural Anxieties in India and China in the 21st Century*. IIT: Delhi.

Mamata, Deenadayal, Subrat K. Ray, Kumar Pratap, Parikh Firuza, Ashish Ramesh Birla, and Banker Manish. 2015. 'Impact of Different Controlled Ovarian Stimulation Protocols on the Physical and Psychological Burdens in Women Undergoing In Vitro Fertilization/Intra Cytoplasmic Sperm Injection'. *Journal of Human Reproductive Sciences* 8 (2): 86–92.

Manandhar, Dharma S., David Osrin, Bhim Prasad Shrestha, Natasha Mesko, Joanna Morrison, Kirti Man Tumbahangphe, Suresh Tamang, Sushma Thapa, Dej Shrestha, and Bidur Thapa. 2004. 'Effect of a Participatory Intervention with Women's Groups on Birth Outcomes in Nepal: Cluster-Randomised Controlled Trial'. *The Lancet* 364 (9438): 970–9.

Mazhar, Arslan, and Babar Tasneem Shaikh. 2012. 'Reforms in Pakistan: Decisive Times for Improving Maternal and Child Health'. *Healthcare Policy* 8 (1): 24–32.

McPake, Barbara, and Marge Koblinsky. 2009. 'Improving Maternal Survival in South Asia: What Can We Learn from Case Studies?' *Journal of Health, Population, and Nutrition* 27 (2): 93.

Mian, Naeemuddin, Muhammad Adeel Alvi, Mariam Zahid Malik, Sarosh Iqbal, Rubeena Zakar, Muhammad Zakria Zakar, Shehzad Hussain Awan, Faryal Shahid, Muhammad Ashraf Chaudhry, and Florian Fischer. 2018. 'Approaches towards Improving the Quality of Maternal and Newborn Health Services in South Asia: Challenges and Opportunities for Healthcare Systems'. *Globalization and Health* 14 (1): 17.

Ministry of Health and Family Welfare. 2008. *Directory of Innovations Implemented in the Health Sector*. New Delhi: Ministry of Health and Family Welfare and Department for International Development (DfID).

Ministry of Health and Family Welfare. 2016. *India Fact Sheet: National Family Health Survey (NFHS-4)*. Mumbai: International Institute for Population Science.

Ministry of Health and Family Welfare. 2017. 'LaQshya: Labour Room Quality Improvement Initiative Guidelines'. Ministry of Health and Family Welfare. Accessed 23 March 2020. http://nhsrcindia.org/updates/laqshya-%E0%A4%B2%E0%A4%95%E0%A5%8D%E0%A4%B7%E0%A5%8D%E0%A4%AF-labour-room-quality-improvement-initiative-guideline

Mishra, Arunima, and Sidsel Roalkvam. 2014. 'The Reproductive Body and the State: Engaging with National Rural Health Mission in Tribal Odisha'. In *Women, Gender and Everyday Social Transformation in India*, edited by Anne Waldrop and Kenneth Bo Nielsen, 123–38. London: Anthem Press.

Mohanty, Sanjay K., and Anshul Kastor. 2017. 'Out-of-Pocket Expenditure and Catastrophic Health Spending on Maternal Care in Public and Private Health Centres in India: A Comparative Study of Pre and Post National Health Mission Period'. *Health Economics Review* 7 (1): 31.

Morgan, Melissa C., Jessica Dyer, Aranzazu Abril, Amelia Christmas, Tanmay Mahapatra, Aritra Das, and Dilys M. Walker. 2018. 'Barriers and Facilitators to the Provision of Optimal Obstetric and Neonatal Emergency Care and to the Implementation of Simulation-Enhanced Mentorship in Primary Care Facilities in Bihar, India: A Qualitative Study'. *BMC Pregnancy and Childbirth* 18 (1): 420.

Morrison, Joanna, Suresh Tamang, Natasha Mesko, David Osrin, Bhim Shrestha, Madan Manandhar, Dharma Manandhar, Hilary Standing, and Anthony Costello. 2005. 'Women's Health Groups to Improve Perinatal Care in Rural Nepal'. *BMC Pregnancy and Childbirth* 5 (6): 1–12.

Mukherjee, Saradiya, and Aditya Singh. 2018. 'Has the Janani Suraksha Yojana (a Conditional Maternity Benefit Transfer Scheme) Succeeded in Reducing the

Economic Burden of Maternity in Rural India? Evidence from the Varanasi District of Uttar Pradesh'. *Journal of Public Health Research* 7 (1): 1–8.

Mukhopadhyay, Dipta K., Sujishnu Mukhopadhyay, Sarmila Mallik, Susmita Nayak, Asit Kumar Biswas, and Akhil B. Biswas. 2018. 'Exploring the Bottlenecks: An Assessment of the Implementation Process of Janani Suraksha Yojana in the State of West Bengal, India'. *International Journal of Medicine and Public Health* 8 (1): 29–33.

Narasimhan, Haripriya. 2018. 'The Midwife and the Dula: Changing Professional Birthing Practices in Contemporary Indian Obstetrics and Gynaecology' (presentation, unpublished), *Panel Gender, Health and Childbirth in South Asia: Colonial Perspectives and Continuing Paradoxes*, ECSAS, Paris.

National Health Mission. 2018. *Guidelines on Midwifery Services in India*. New Delhi: Ministry of Health and Family Welfare.

Nayak, Akhaya Kumar, and Shivani Nath. 2018. 'There Is an Urgent Need to Humanise Childbirth in India'. *Economic and Political Weekly* 53 (2). Accessed 23 February 2020. https://www.epw.in/engage/article/urgent-need-to-humanise-childbirth-in-india

Noordam, A. Camielle, Barbara M. Kuepper, Jelle Stekelenburg, and Anneli Milen. 2011. 'Improvement of Maternal Health Services through the Use of Mobile Phones'. *Tropical Medicine & International Health* 16 (5): 622–6.

Pai, Madhukar. 2000. 'Unnecessary Medical Interventions: Caesarean Sections as a Case Study'. *Economic and Political Weekly* 35 (31): 2755–61.

Pande, Amrita. 2014. *Wombs in Labor: Transnational Commercial Surrogacy in India*. New York: Columbia University Press.

Pandey, Shanta. 2018. 'Women's Knowledge about the Conditional Cash Incentive Program and Its Association with Institutional Delivery in Nepal'. *PloS One* 13 (6): e0199230.

Patel, Shailee Girish, Rajkumar Pareshbhai Patel, Niral Rajnibhai Patel, and Khush Patel. 2018. 'Awareness of the Patterns of Delivery in Urban Slums of Ahmedabad City'. *International Journal of Community Medicine and Public Health* 5 (9): 3860.

Paul, Sohini, Sourabh Paul, and K.S. James. 2019. 'Universalisation Versus Targeting in Maternal and Child Health Care Provisioning: Evidence from India'. *SSM— Population Health* 9: 100502.

Perera, Dinusha, Ragnhild Lund, Katarina Swahnberg, Berit Schei, and Jennifer J. Infanti. 2018. '"When Helpers Hurt": Women's and Midwives' Stories of Obstetric Violence in State Health Institutions, Colombo District, Sri Lanka'. *BMC Pregnancy and Childbirth* 18 (1): 211.

Pinto, Sarah. 2008. *Where There Is No Midwife: Birth and Loss in Rural India*. New York & Oxford: Berghahn Books.

Prinja, Shankar, Pankaj Bahuguna, Aditi Gupta, Ruby Nimesh, Madhu Gupta, and Jarnail Singh Thakur. 2018. 'Cost Effectiveness of mHealth Intervention by Community Health Workers for Reducing Maternal and Newborn Mortality in Rural Uttar Pradesh, India'. *Cost Effectiveness and Resource Allocation* 16(1): 25.

Prost, Audrey, Tim Colbourn, Nadine Seward, Kishwar Azad, Arri Coomarasamy, Andrew Copas, Tanja A.J. Houweling, Edward Fottrell, Abdul Kuddus, Sonia Lewycka, Christine MacArthur, Dharma Manandhar, Joanna Morrison, Charles Mwansambo, Nirmala Nair, Bejoy Nambiar, David Osrin, Christina Pagel, Tambosi Phiri, Anni-Maria Pulkki-Brännström, Mikey Rosato, Jolene

Skordis-Worrall, Naomi Saville, and Neena Shah More. 2014. 'Women's Groups Practising Participatory Learning and Action to Improve Maternal and Newborn Health in Low-Resource Settings: A Systematic Review and Meta-Analysis'. *Lancet* 383 (9931): 1806.

Pulok, Mohammad Habibullah, Md Nasim-Us Sabah, Jalal Uddin, and Ulrika Enemark. 2016. 'Progress in the Utilization of Antenatal and Delivery Care Services in Bangladesh: Where Does the Equity Gap Lie?' *BMC Pregnancy and Childbirth* 16 (1): 200.

Rahman, Sayedur, Aziz Ahmed Choudhury, Rasheda Khanam, Syed Mamun Ibne Moin, Salahuddin Ahmed, Nazma Begum, Nurun Naher Shoma, Mohammed Abdul Quaiyum, Abdullah H. Baqui, and Projahnmo Study Group in Bangladesh. 2017. 'Effect of a Package of Integrated Demand- and Supply-Side Interventions on Facility Delivery Rates in Rural Bangladesh: Implications for Large-Scale Programs'. *PLoS One* 12 (10): e0186182.

Rai, Pramila. 2016. 'Aama Programme of Nepal'. *Dimensions of Public Health*, 9 October. Accessed 9 March 2021. http://publichealthinnepal.blogspot.com/search?q=aama+programme

Randive, Bharat, Vishal Diwan, and Ayesha De Costa. 2013. 'India's Conditional Cash Transfer Programme (the JSY) to Promote Institutional Birth: Is There an Association between Institutional Birth Proportion and Maternal Mortality?' *PLoS One* 8 (6): e67452.

Rao, Mohan, ed. 2004. *The Unheard Scream: Reproductive Health and Women's Lives in India*. New Delhi: Zubaan.

Rudrappa, Sharmila. 2017. 'India Outlawed Commercial Surrogacy: Clinics Are Finding Loopholes'. *The Conversation* 23.

Sadler, Michelle, Mário J.D.S. Santos, Dolores Ruiz-Berdún, Gonzalo Leiva Rojas, Elena Skoko, Patricia Gillen, and Jette A. Clausen. 2016. 'Moving beyond Disrespect and Abuse: Addressing the Structural Dimensions of Obstetric Violence'. *Reproductive Health Matters* 24 (47): 47–55.

Schmidt, Jean-Olivier, Tim Ensor, Atia Hossain, and Salam Khan. 2010. 'Vouchers as Demand Side Financing Instruments for Health Care: A Review of the Bangladesh Maternal Voucher Scheme'. *Health Policy* 96 (2): 98–107.

Shrivastava, Surbhi, and Muthusamy Sivakami. 2019. 'Evidence of "Obstetric Violence" in India: An Integrative Review'. *Journal of Biosocial Science* 52 (4): 610–28.

Sidney, Kristi, Rachel Tolhurst, Kate Jehan, Vishal Diwan, and Ayesha De Costa. 2016. '"The Money Is Important but All Women Anyway Go to Hospital for Childbirth Nowadays": A Qualitative Exploration of Why Women Participate in a Conditional Cash Transfer Program to Promote Institutional Deliveries in Madhya Pradesh, India'. *BMC Pregnancy and Childbirth* 16 (1): 47.

Srivastava, Aradhana, Sanghita Bhattacharyya, Christine Clar, and Bilal I. Avan. 2014. 'Evolution of Quality in Maternal Health in India: Lessons and Priorities'. *International Journal of Medicine and Public Health* 4 (1): 33–9.

Stanton, Cynthia, Joy E. Lawn, Hafiz Rahman, Katarzyna Wilczynska-Ketende, and Kenneth Hill. 2006. 'Stillbirth Rates: Delivering Estimates in 190 Countries'. *The Lancet* 367 (9521): 1487–94.

Tamrat, Tigest, and Stan Kachnowski. 2012. 'Special Delivery: An Analysis of mHealth in Maternal and Newborn Health Programs and Their Outcomes around the World'. *Maternal and Child Health Journal* 16 (5): 1092–101.

Thongkong, Nattawut, Ellen van de Poel, Swati Sarbani Roy, Shibanand Rath, and Tanja A.J. Houweling. 2017. 'How Equitable Is the Uptake of Conditional Cash Transfers for Maternity Care in India? Evidence from the Janani Suraksha Yojana Scheme in Odisha and Jharkhand'. *International Journal for Equity in Health* 16 (1): 48.

Tripathy, Jaya Prasad, Hemant D. Shewade, Sanskruti Mishra, A.M.V. Kumar, and A.D. Harries. 2017. 'Cost of Hospitalization for Childbirth in India: How Equitable It Is in the Post-NRHM Era?' *BMC Research Notes* 10: 409. doi: 10.1186/s13104-017-2729-z.

United Nations. 1994. 'International Conference on Population and Development Programme of Action'. International Conference on Population and Development, Cairo.

United Nations Population Fund. 2009. *Concurrent Assessment of Janani Suraksha Yojana (JSY) in Selected States: Bihar, Madhya Pradesh, Orissa, Rajasthan, Uttar Pradesh*. New Delhi: United Nations Population Fund.

UN Sustainable Development Summit. 2015. 'Transforming Our World: The 2030 Agenda for Sustainable Development'. Division for Sustainable Development Goals: New York, NY, USA. Accessed 10 November 2020. https://sustainabledevelopment. un.org/post2015/transformingourworld

Unnithan, Maya. 2015. 'What Constitutes Evidence in Human Rights-Based Approaches to Health? Learning from Lived Experiences of Maternal and Sexual Reproductive Health'. *Health and Human Rights* 17 (2): 45–56.

Van Hollen, Cecilia. 2003. *Birth on the Threshold: Childbirth and Modernity in South India*. Berkeley & Los Angeles: University of California Press.

Vellakkal, S., A. Gupta, Z. Khan, D. Stuckler, A. Reeves, S. Ebrahim, A. Bowling, and P. Doyle. 2017. 'Has India's National Rural Health Mission Reduced Inequities in Maternal Health Services? A Pre-post Repeated Cross-Sectional Study'. *Health Policy and Planning* 32: 79–90.

Vora, Kalindi. 2009. 'Indian Transnational Surrogacy and the Disaggregation of Mothering Work'. *Anthropology News* 50 (2): 9–12.

Vora, Kranti Suresh, Sandul Yasobant, Amit Patel, Ashish Upadhyay, and Dileep V. Mavalankar. 2015. 'Has Chiranjeevi Yojana Changed the Geographic Availability of Free Comprehensive Emergency Obstetric Care Services in Gujarat, India?' *Global Health Action* 8 (1). doi: 10.3402/gha.v8.28977.

World Health Organization (WHO). 2001. *Advancing Safe Motherhood Through Human Rights*. Geneva: Department of Reproductive Health and Research.

World Health Organization (WHO). 2015. *Trends in Maternal Mortality: 1990–2015. Estimates from WHO, UNICEF, UNFPA, World Bank Group and the United Nations Population Division: Executive Summary*. Geneva: World Health Organization.

2

Colonial Legacies and Maternal Health in South Asia

Samiksha Sehrawat

The persistence of certain aspects of the 'problem of childbirth' over a long period of time requires a historical analysis that includes in its ambit the colonial era. Sociological assessments of contemporary measures to lower maternal mortality tend to assume that these are substantially different from those in the distant colonial past.[1] This chapter challenges this assumption by analysing the historical origins of biomedical and development discourses on childbirth. Concern regarding maternal and infant health in colonial South Asia emerged in the 1920s, pushed by British women doctors active in three major organizations linked to colonial Indian women's healthcare— the Dufferin Fund (DF), the Women's Medical Service in India (WMSI), and the Association of Medical Women in India (AMWI). Their interventions marked the culmination of two important discourses—gendered ideological justifications of the Empire that cast the British as saviours of oppressed Indian womanhood; and British women doctors' professional project,[2] which in colonial South Asia was cast as representing the medical needs of Indian women. This chapter, therefore, analyses the important role played by British women doctors in shaping what Cecilia Van Hollen has called the 'problem' of childbirth (Van Hollen 2003). Due to a growing eugenicist framing of nationalism from the 1920s, discourses of childbirth also came to be vitally linked with the relationship between health and governance from the interwar period in South Asia (Hodges 2008). Devolution of power in colonial South Asia gave elected Indian ministers greater influence over healthcare. During the interwar period, elected Indian ministers and nationalist politicians revisited aspects of colonial medical policy and anticipated later initiatives by the developmental state to solve problems of public health and medical care (Sehrawat 2022).

The medicalization of childbirth in South Asia was embedded in discursive networks with local and global contexts. The medicalization of

Samiksha Sehrawat, *Colonial Legacies and Maternal Health in South Asia* In: *Childbirth in South Asia.*
Edited by: Clémence Jullien and Roger Jeffery, Oxford University Press. © Oxford University Press 2021.
DOI: 10.1093/oso/9780190130718.003.0002

childbirth in the 1920s and 1930s took place amidst rising concern regarding conditions of childbirth in eugenicist and maternalist ideologies internationally. The emergence of several international health organizations—including the League of Nations Health Organization (LNHO), the Rockefeller Fund (RF), and the International Labour Organization (ILO) —not only created the conditions necessary for the framing of health issues globally, but was also marked by linking the conditions of maternity with poverty and regulation of labour. Internationally, US imperialism was becoming more assertive, leading to the forging of an Anglo–American imperial cooperation that has survived into the contemporary period. Since US imperial ideologies gave more weight in this period to questions of public health, it can be argued that British ideologies of rule that had criticized colonial societies for the poor treatment of women were recast in the 1920s and 1930s in terms of using maternal and infant health as measures of development.

Two other longer processes also left important colonial legacies that determine the conditions in which contemporary maternal health measures are deployed—the embedding of scientism as a sign of modernity for South Asian elites (including medical professionals) and the importance given to credentialism by the South Asian medical profession. These were privileged over an ethical concern for patients or a commitment to more equitable distribution of medical resources. Further, international epistemic communities of medical professionals shaped the agendas of international health organizations.[3] International networks of medical professionals privileged credentialist and technocratic approaches, which have continued to pervade discourses on health and development since the interwar period, within both international health organizations and post-colonial states in South Asia. As a result of this professional influence, major international organizations promoting healthcare have remained historically tied to scientist conceptions. These conceptions have proved difficult to dislodge, despite countervailing historical initiatives and critiques by sociologists and anthropologists. Another important factor was that discourses of modernity were linked with gendered discourses on social reform and revivalist politics of nationalism and communalist mobilization. Increasingly imbricated in eugenicist concerns, these hegemonic discourses on modernity have continued to shape South Asian discourses on childbirth.

The prevalence of culturalist attitudes to patients is, thus, a colonial legacy that haunts the practice of contemporary South Asian biomedical professionals. It permeates the development discourse on childbirth of many international organizations and post-colonial states' initiatives. Medical professional projects shaped by imperial exigencies have perpetuated culturalism in developmental discourses, contributing to the poor serving of marginalized groups. It is also important to interrogate the continued impact of colonial expertise emerging from networks of medical professionals forged in the late imperial era on national and international health policies after decolonization. This is important since colonial experts were influential in shaping developmental discourses even after the decline of formal empires (Hodge 2007: 117–25; Kothari 2005).

The neoliberal restructuring of health sectors in South Asia has led to the resurgence of several funding initiatives that had proved singularly ineffective in improving healthcare during the colonial era. Policy changes in post-colonial South Asian health sectors following guidelines from international bodies, such as the World Bank and the International Monetary Fund, have led to the contraction of the state sector and expansion of the private sector since the 1990s (Baru 2001). This emphasis on the private sector as a way of ensuring accountability and empowering patients with consumer choice is especially problematic as it echoes discourses about the limits of the colonial state. See Chapter 8 for more on the current limits of state regulation of the private sector. Since colonial policies of leaving the health sector to voluntary and private provision were responsible for the anaemic health infrastructure inherited by post-colonial South Asian states (Sehrawat 2013a), it is important to acknowledge the similarities between the two discourses. Imperial ideologies of fiscal conservativism, modernization, scientism, and culturalism have survived in post-colonial state policy and in international health discourses, despite strong challenges to them from proponents of universal healthcare internationally from the 1940s to the 1970s (Basilico et al. 2013; Chakrabarti 2009; Gorsky and Sirrs 2018; Jeffery 1988a: 112–14; Sirrs 2020).

British Women Doctors and the Colonial Medicalization of Childbirth

From 1918, several programmes to improve maternal and infant health commenced under the auspices of the Women's Medical Service and the DF. These initiatives were spearheaded by British women doctors keen to push forward their claims as colonial medical experts responsible for Indian women's health. British women doctors were important interlocutors who provided the earliest biomedical research on childbirth and who shaped initial international and national understandings of the Indian 'problem' of childbirth (Srivastava 2018; Trivedi 2019). They were instrumental in constructing the framework of Indian public health initiatives on maternal and infant health. Their initiatives replicated British schemes arising from maternalist and eugenicist concerns regarding childbirth in colonial India. The medical profession had emerged as one of the key players in the medicalization of childbirth and motherhood in interwar Britain, with an important role given to health visitors—to mould working-class mothers' domestic behaviour and teach them mothercraft (Davin 1978; Dyhouse 1978; Lewis 1980). It is important to explore the colonial professional project of British women doctors and its links with the nineteenth-century struggles of women to enter the medical profession in Britain, as both were significant in medicalizing childbirth in India.

British women's professional project emerged in the nineteenth century in response to attempts by the male establishment of the British medical profession to exclude women from medical education and qualifications, as a strategy of occupational closure. Witz (1992) describes the British female professional project as initially using usurpatory tactics, countervailing credentialist and equal rights tactics, and, when these failed, legalistic tactics that ultimately won them entrance into the profession. Employment opportunities in the Empire, especially in colonial India, proved crucial for the success of this project. The quasi-governmental DF provided a valuable source of funding for students at the newly founded London School of Medicine for Women (Burton 1996) and opened up India as a source of employment for many British women doctors struggling for employment after graduation (Elston 1986). It was founded at the direction of Queen Victoria in 1885 as an imperial charity managed by vicereines (Arnold 1993: 262–6; Harrison 1994: 92–6; Lal 1994). The DF's privileging of an orientalist construction of the zenana patient as unable to seek medical help from male professionals (Sehrawat 2013a: 102–10) provided invaluable support to the arguments used by British women doctors that women's medical work was an expression of middle-class Victorian feminine values, such as benevolence, moral goodness, and self-sacrifice (Bashford 1998: 85–107).

The experience of this struggle was to inform the professional project pursued by British women doctors in India and their advocacy of improved healthcare for Indian women, including conditions of childbirth. British women doctors who were employed in India became dissatisfied with their pay and work conditions by the turn of the twentieth century and established a professional organization—the Association of Medical Women in India

(AMWI)—in 1907. Acting as an imperial lobbying group in colonial India and Britain, the AMWI demanded state intervention to improve Indian women's health. This resulted in the formation of a cadre of women doctors in the Women's Medical Service in India (WMSI), run by the DF on state subsidies (Sehrawat 2013a: 172–86; Sehrawat 2013b). British women doctors active in the AMWI formed the core of the employees of the WMSI and were quick to consolidate their hold on the DF and other quasi-governmental medical charities associated with childbirth (Sehrawat 2013a: 182–4). Margaret Balfour held positions at the apex of the four major organizations associated with Indian women's health between 1919 and her retirement in 1924—as joint-secretary to the DF (1916–24), as the chief medical officer of the WMSI (1920–4), as president of AMWI (1918–25), and from 1919, as the chief architect of the Lady Chelmsford All-India League for Maternity and Child Welfare.[4] Indian institutional responses to maternal mortality from 1918 were crafted by British women doctors, such as Margaret Balfour, and mirrored contemporary British concerns regarding maternal and infant mortality. These British discourses had scrutinized working-class women's childcare and sought to 'correct' working women's activities both outside and inside the home by imposing middle-class norms of correct mother-hood (Davin 1978; Dyhouse 1978; Lewis 1980). Colonial Indian interwar initiatives included public campaigns to disseminate mothercraft; 'scientific' medical research on infant and maternal mortality by British women doctors employed in the WMSI; training of South Asian female sub-assistant surgeons (who belonged to a lower cadre); as well as advocating the training and use of health visitors and maternity supervisors by provincial governments.[5] The Chelmsford League distributed small grants to regional centres under-taking child welfare work, but its primary success was in promoting child welfare propaganda.[6] Like the 'Child Welfare Movement' in Britain, such initiatives conceived maternal and child welfare in terms of a series of discrete personal health problems, to be solved by providing health visitors, infant welfare centres, and better maternity services; encouraging breastfeeding; and improving domestic hygiene (Srivastava 2018: 223–8). Although the ma-ternalist framing of childbirth (Plant and van der Klein 2012) was abandoned over time, these early activities proved historically significant in several ways. British women doctors cast themselves as colonial experts and were im-portant participants within an international epistemic community on ma-ternal and infant health that emerged in the 1920s. As participants in this epistemic community, British women doctors provided research and infor-mation for international health bodies. The colonial biases that had shaped the professional project of these British women doctors were thus embedded in both nationalist discourses on childbirth and in international medical discourse on the links between medical and developmental health.

By developing and proclaiming their specialist knowledge of maternal health, British women doctors in India were emulating strategies employed by British and US women doctors to improve their professional status. Both in Britain and the USA, women doctors had been pushed by a lack of employment opportunities into low-status areas of 'female' specialities and social medical services. The specialization of women doctors in women's health generally, and maternal health especially, was an extension of the separatist strategies that women had pursued to gain access to medical education (Drachman 1986: 71; Elston 1986: 248–59). Continued pursuit of opportunities for the advancement of careers and public worth by women doctors in Edinburgh had led them to place themselves in the vanguard of the infant and maternal welfare movement in the city (Thomson 1998: 214–21). Thus, Balfour and her colleagues were part of an international network of women doctors and were aware of the growing efforts in Britain by the state to monitor, control, and repress working-class mothers to improve neonatal health. Participation in the international discourse on maternal and infant health expanded career openings for these British female professional elites in the colonies, while augmenting their social status and power.

British women doctors active in the AMWI were important contributors to a wider international epistemic community of medical professionals specializing in maternal health. The AMWI and its members were actively engaged with activities of the Association of Registered Medical Women (founded in London in 1879) and the Medical Women's International Association, which sought to promote the professional interests of medical women and the cooperation of medical women in matters connected with international health. Maternal and infant welfare was an important cause championed by these organizations. The imperial and inter-colonial connections of infant welfare work in the interwar years were also significant. In 1932, on behalf of the British Medical Association, Balfour advised on the medical aspects of the report of the Indian Round Table Conference, which had been convened to deliberate on devolution of power to Indian politicians.[7] The Chelmsford League provided expert advice to other colonies, including the Malay States and East Africa (Balfour and Young 1929: 148). British women doctors were active in colonial Indian initiatives to improve maternal and neonatal health and provided expert advice on infant and maternal 'welfare' in colonies such as Ethiopia in the 1940s (Weis 2015: 42–3).

The AMWI had contributed to tropes depicting British women doctors as representing the medical needs of 'dumb' Indian women oppressed by Indian patriarchal traditions since the early twentieth century (Sehrawat 2013a). In the interwar period, it recast such imperial discourses in the context of the medicalization of childbirth in colonial India. In doing so, it provided the early monolithic, universalizing, and essentializing constructions of women—the survival of which in Western feminist and ethnocentric scholarship on development has been critiqued by Mohanty (1988). Burton (1994) provides evidence of similar appropriations of the figure of the colonized woman by early Victorian feminists. Ahluwalia (2008) points out that in late colonial India, Western feminists like Stopes and Sanger also claimed to speak for universal sisterhood while ignoring the particular problems of impoverished women under colonial rule. Forbes (1994a) shows that dais—also known as traditional birth attendants (TBAs) or native midwives—were blamed for the problem of childbirth even as it was being medicalized in a move that increasingly came to ignore the role of poverty in creating poor maternal health. The politicization of South Asian childbirth practices was further exacerbated by the international controversy created by Katherine Mayo's book *Mother India* (1927), written with the aim of discrediting nationalist demands for self-rule (Sinha 2006). The book criticized Indian society and culture and focused on the eugenicist impact of child marriage on girls. It was imbricated in international shifts in the framing of public health and maternity and created a controversy which led to a more prominent role for Indian women's organizations in nationalist politics (Sinha 2006). This controversy also led to elite Indian women's involvement in the medicalization of childbirth (Forbes 1994a).

Van Hollen (2003: 36) has argued that 'colonial sympathizers and [Indian] nationalists alike depicted the conditions of childbirth as deplorable and used these images to legitimize their own political and economic goals in the name of protecting the "vulnerable" members of society, i.e., women and children'. Both colonial and nationalist discourses converged in locating the professionalization of obstetrics as an antidote to this 'problem'. Van Hollen's location of contemporary difficulties to improving maternal health in South Asia within a longer historical continuum (Van Hollen 2003: 36–7) is welcome, and her analysis of nationalist marginalization of women and colonial justifications for imperial rule in terms of the uplift of Indian women follows consensus among gender historians. However, her analysis does not include the professional project of British women doctors in colonial South Asia. When, like Engels (1996), she goes on to argue that the pollution

associated with childbirth in India also helps to explain the contrasts between how childbirth was viewed in Europe and South Asia, she is on weaker
ground.[8] Pollution concerns are not universal but rather specific to some
ethnic groups, and it would be more pertinent to consider how Indian male
doctors' strategies to combat professional closure arguably deviate from the
model of professional control over midwifery in Europe that Van Hollen
relies on to explain why they tended to disassociate themselves from childbirth. A renewed attention to the importance of British women doctors' professional project in colonial India can provide a more robust explanation of
how culturalist assumptions were embedded in development discourses on
childbirth at the historical moment when it came to be medicalized. Thus, the
questioning of the reliability or otherwise of auxiliaries, including TBAs, and
the thorny questions of their regulation marks continuities with colonial orientalist discourses on dais (Forbes 1994a; Lang 2005).[9] See Chapters 3, 4, and
5 for more detail on current policy towards indigenous midwifery. British
women doctors also initiated the discursive flattening of the considerable regional variation in the practice of indigenous midwives, which is echoed in
some contemporary development discourses criticizing TBAs, despite evidence provided by sociologists and anthropologists regarding the considerable variation in TBAs' skill and practice. See Chapters 3 and 5 for more on
current patterns of training of TBAs. As examined later in the chapter, such
discourses on medicalization of childbirth also had an important impact on
South Asian middle-class attitudes towards childbirth, which have persisted
in the post-colonial period.

Training South Asian women to work as medical staff who would replace
the dai was a persistent problem through the colonial period, whether elite
female medical professionals or subordinate female medical staff such as
hospital assistants and nurses (Forbes 1994b).[10] Dais or TBAs were blamed
for high levels of maternal mortality, even though adequate resources to train
and support subordinate female medical staff to replace TBAs did not materialize. As British women doctors consolidated their professional status
through claims to equality with male British doctors, they also turned to
demarcatory strategies of occupational closure against South Asian male
doctors and South Asian female medical subordinates, using exclusion on
the grounds of ethnicity as well as a lack of credentials (Sehrawat 2013b).
This use of credentialism and medical training of South Asian medical auxiliaries by British women doctors promoted adherence to colonial medical
discourses regarding childbirth. Some of the challenges that prevented more
women from seeking medical training and employment, especially in remote

rural areas in north India, have also persisted from the colonial period. Both British and Indian female medical practitioners were vulnerable to sexual harassment when they were seen as having stepped out of the 'symbolic shelter' (Papanek 1982) provided by practices of veiling and female segregation in South Asia in pursuit of professional medical work (Forbes 2000: 29, 41–2).[11] This meant that a medical career remained a challenge for women, especially in North India, where purdah practices were more widely prevalent. The regional variations in treatment and status of female medical professionals in South Asia may have been shaped, at least partially, by the survival of such social norms, which vary considerably by ethnicity, caste, religion, and class.

The relative importance of maternal health within a broader healthcare strategy also continues to be marked by legitimizing ideologies that claim to uplift South Asian women while failing to allocate resources to their healthcare, as in colonial times. Colonial gendered ideologies of rule that marked South Asian societies as backward due to their poor treatment of women underwent a transformation over the twentieth century by yoking colonial rule to the improvement of health provision for South Asian women (Sehrawat 2013a). The next section considers how such assumptions have been embedded in international health and development discourses at the moment of their genesis.

The Emergence of International Health Organizations and a Development Discourse on Childbirth

The interwar period witnessed several changes that transformed the international context of health policies. These included the emergence of several international health organizations, the rise of maternalism, and the increasing importance given to development and public health in new justifications for Western imperialism with the rising international power of the USA. Thus, post-1950s development discourses on health built upon a 'new civilizing mission in India' in the interwar period, with the League of Nations and the RF acting as its 'agents' (Sinha 2006: 40). These institutional and political developments took place within a context of the international rise of maternalist and eugenicist ideas, which influenced nationalist and other political discourses in South Asia. Seth Koven and Sonya Michel (1990: 1079) defined maternalism as 'ideologies that exalted women's capacity to mother and extended to society as a whole the values they attached to that role: care, nurturance and morality'. Whether or not such maternalist ideas were instrumental in introducing welfare regimes in Europe and the USA, their framing of initiatives to improve maternal and neonatal health was to prove significant for India.

The 'problem of childbirth' gained political attention and resources in India during the interwar period, just as the LNHO, ILO, and RF establishing international networks of communication among medical experts. The formation of international health organizations during the interwar period addressed multiple pressures to regulate medical matters between states, across whole regions, and on a global basis. This was done by imposing quarantine, collecting international public health statistics, setting international health standards and health indices and proved crucial to interwar efforts to provide aid to the diseased and famished (Weindling 2015: 194). The LNHO's initiatives in the 1920s to document mortality trends internationally included statistics on maternal and infant mortality. Initial attempts, in the 1920s, by the ILO to protect women and children and secure paid maternity leave were important in framing legislation in interwar colonial India. They gave rise to political debates about the extent of employers' and the state's responsibility for maternal health (Sen 1999; Srivastava 2018), even though as Weindling (1995: 138–9) points out these initiatives were 'largely inappropriate for non-European and non-industrial states'. Dagmar Engels shows that the ILO's guidelines in the Maternity Convention of 1919 had an important impact on colonial legislation on the organized economic sector (Engels 1996: 142; also Sen 1999: 142–7), even though employers resisted the guidelines on maternity benefit and leave in the mills and mines throughout the 1920s (Engels 1996; Srivastava 2018).

The RF became involved in improving the public health administrations in various European colonies, including British India, in a bid to bring to them the more 'scientific and efficient' tenor of US intervention in its colonies.[12] The emergent discipline of 'tropical medicine' was viewed as proof of the benefit of Western imperialism (Arnold 1988). Sinha argues that the rise of international health organizations in the interwar period was accompanied by the transformation of the economic basis of colonial rule, leading up to a time in the post–Second World War period 'when the survival of the British Empire would become pegged less ambiguously to a "special relationship" with the United States' (Sinha 2006: 40). The US imperial rhetoric cast itself as the global disseminator of Western civilization on scientific lines by foregrounding public health policy as a tangible boon to colonized societies. The RF was particularly attuned to the value of public health initiatives as a means of expanding the commercial and industrial penetration of tropical regions by the USA, both at home and abroad. It sought to internationalize US models of public health—its activities in East Asia and South America have been linked to regions of strategic importance to the USA and interpreted as an informal extension of US imperialism (Brown 1976; Parmar 2012). Mayo's critique of conditions of maternity in colonial India arose from such imperial ambitions of the RF and produced a strong backlash from Indian nationalists and elite South Asian feminists (Sinha 2006). The resulting nationalist discourses significantly extended the hegemonic reach of discourses on the medicalization of childbirth in South Asian society.

During this interwar period, the LNHO and ILO together created a new international public health consensus that was dominated by an elite of expert advisers, basing their interventions in social policy on physiological and biochemical research within a positivistic scientific framework (Weindling 1995: 144–6). The LNHO's approach of training public health experts to deliver essential medical solutions for social problems of chronic ill-health arising from poor diet and poverty (Weindling 1995: 137) was embedded in its elaborate institutional structures and proved remarkably durable. The dominance of this technocratic approach was inscribed in global health discourses—including those about maternal and neonatal health—that emerged through new international health and welfare organizations in the interwar period. Paul Weindling describes the LNHO's approach as 'social medicine in a technic and elitist mode', shaped by medical researchers and 'driven by the scientific preoccupation of the laboratory' (Weindling 1995: 143). Its influence was formative and deep, operating at a time when developmental discourses were just beginning to take the orientation that has persisted in post-1950s development thought and infrastructure, locally and internationally. Dubin points out that the LNHO shaped national administrative, research, and educational agencies by drawing them into an international biomedical/public health infrastructure. The LNHO 'developed new intellectual resources essential for systematic public health work' (Dubin 1995: 73). Weindling argues that the ILO's approach was also based on a 'scientific universalism', which privileged scientific experts and empirically-based approaches limited to 'what could be proven in the laboratory' (Weindling 1995: 139). Similar technocratic approaches inflected proposals by British women doctors who fashioned themselves as expert advisers to the colonial state. Research by British women medical professionals, such as Margaret Balfour and Dagmar Curjel, into maternity conditions in mills in Bombay and Calcutta (now Kolkata) arose from an awareness of medical discourses leading to the 1918 Maternity and Child Welfare Act in

Britain, and was spurred on by the colonial state's interest in ILO maternity guidelines to conduct research (Arnold 2001: 35–44; Srivastava 2018: 153–79).[13] While technocratic approaches came to dominate international health initiatives during the interwar period, scientism became an organizing value for the colonial state in South Asia as well as for modernizing elites driving post-colonial states' development initiatives. The next section examines the enduring influence of these ideas on governing elites and the medical profession in South Asia.

Modernization and Development through Scientism, Culturalism, and the South Asian Professional Project

Given strident nationalist critiques of colonial rule in South Asia and a decolonization driven by popular anti-colonialism, it is surprising that colonial discourses on health and childbirth have persisted. An explanation may be found by reflecting on the enduring appeal of scientism for South Asian elites and the deepening of the disciplinary regime spawned by the 'hegemonic project of colonial rule' after decolonization. Like scientism, what Didier Fassin (2001) has called practical 'culturalism' has proved to be more significant in decisions about medical care by governing elites and medical professionals than ethical concerns or commitment to normative standards of biomedical practice and equitable distribution of resources. While Fassin has examined the importance of culturalism in justifying the marginalization of migrant communities in public health and health provision in multicultural settings in the West, and his work has proved influential in analysing contemporary development discourses, it is argued here that the origins of culturalism can be traced back to colonial health policies, which gave rise to such discourses internationally. Culturalism as a strategy emerged in colonial contexts where the introduction of biomedicine and public health was dominated by the policing of the population, and marked by a refusal to provide for the welfare of the population. In such settings, the state inaugurated a discourse that disavowed any responsibility for providing for the healthcare of the population due to commitment to a fiscally conservative political economy (Sehrawat 2013a). The impact of these discourses on South Asian medical professionals has proved significant due to the form that the South Asian medical profession took in response to exclusionary strategies of occupational closure practised by British doctors employed in colonial India.[14] In colonial settings, where biomedicine was promoted as part of an imperial civilizing mission, biomedical professionals produced discourses that denigrated indigenous medical practitioners in pursuance of strategies of occupational closure against them—creating a wider discourse regarding the malpractice of indigenous practitioners and the ignorance of colonized populations regarding Western science, medicine, and hygiene (Hume 1977).[15] This meant that Indian biomedical professionals became increasingly complicit in the creation of such culturalist discourses, along with British doctors employed in the colonial Indian Medical Service (IMS).[16] Such discourses were especially potent in the context of childbirth, as they were given higher visibility by British women doctors' professional project. They were also incorporated in the discourse produced by Indian biomedical professionals as a nationalist critique of the underinvestment of the colonial state and healthcare for its Indian subjects. The credentialist strategies of Indian biomedical professionals to counter exclusion from the higher echelons of the profession also provided a strong incentive to mimic culturalist discourses of British professionals, which were increasingly being circulated within the international epistemic community to which Indian doctors sought affiliation (Jeffery 1979; Monnais and Wright 2016).

Partha Chatterjee (1994: 81) analyses the hegemonic project of colonialism in terms of the 'legitimization of "rationality" as the central thematic of a new social order'. This required the institutionalization of rational-bureaucratic norms in South Asian societies, including those related to science and medicine. Chatterjee (1994: 83) argues that 'education'—in its wider sense of disseminating of rational-bureaucratic norms beyond the small group of alien rulers to increasingly large sections of the colonized people— became the 'chief instrument' of the hegemonic project of the colonial state. The 'small section of the colonized elite' who could 'set about the task of enlightening their fellow countrymen', sought to transform South Asian society by discarding tradition and adopting universal forms of a rational and scientifically ordered social life. This colonized elite included Indian doctors, who were expected to disseminate biomedical understandings of disease, health, and childbirth. Indian doctors and other Western-educated elites, thus, emerged as what Chatterjee has termed a 'crucial mediating agency', turning the external force of the colonial critique of indigenous tradition into an internal critique' (Chatterjee 1994: 83). South Asian elites thus came to participate—to varying degrees—in the 'great experiment . . . [of] the education of a backward people in the ways of modern social life' (Chatterjee 1994: 83). This project survived colonialism to continue in post-colonial

South Asia, and its imprint is evident in the social framing of neonatal health by South Asian elites.

The impact of scientism on post-colonial healthcare discourses in South Asia is manifested in the reduction of public health and medical care problems to terms of scientific methods, practices, and attitudes; obfuscating the extent to which these are social and political problems. It also becomes apparent in the pursuit of the highest forms of medical technologies as a matter of national pride, allowing South Asian elites to project parity with developed countries within an international context (Phillips 1990).[17] Science in India was not only institutionalized as a colonial practice under British colonial rule but came to provide 'cultural authority as the legitimating sign of progress and rationality' for Indian nationalism (Prakash 1999: 7). Nationalist scientism envisioned a broad social regeneration of India based on scientific principles.[18] Thus, Indian medical professionals have advocated setting up regional centres of medical excellence which seek to maintain the highest world standards as an expression of national self-reliance and reduced dependence on foreign technology (Frankenberg 1981). This scientism has influenced public expectations and has resulted in the privileging of the needs of elites in metropolitan urban centres over the needs of the rural and peri-urban population. Thus, scientism in nationalist ideology has been in tension with the post-colonial Indian state's commitment to democratizing access to healthcare for the majority of the Indian population unable to access medical facilities concentrated in metropolises. Indeed, nationalist leaders' acceptance of scientism as a core value has contributed to a technocratic conception of medical care which contradicts and undermines the post-colonial state's ideological commitment to providing universal healthcare. As mentioned earlier, scientism also has a long history of permeating international development discourse on health. Weindling argues that both the LNHO and the industrial health section of the ILO had shifted to a narrowly technical approach that rejected broader concerns with welfare and, as early as the mid-1920s, had ceased to acknowledge the importance of social inequalities in shaping public health outcomes (Weindling 1995: 141).

The use of culturalism by biomedical providers and state functionaries continues to shape the practice of biomedicine in the Global South and for immigrants in post-imperial Western countries. Culturalism involves explaining the behaviour of individuals or communities in terms of their cultural beliefs in ways that essentialize these beliefs and treat them as ahistorically static. By making 'culture the ultimate interpretation of human behaviour' (Fassin 2001: 302), culturalism limits the analytical focus to target communities, excluding the context and content of interventions from analysis. Those who are at the receiving end of health interventions are blamed for difficulties in delivering health outcomes, since these are believed to arise from behaviours that result from cultural norms. Such attitudes can be seen as legacies of colonial discourses that denied the right of colonized people to understand their bodies and illness in ways that diverged from biomedical understandings. Colonial doctors and medical institutions were engaged in stimulating a public circulation of reason in order to undermine and disqualify indigenous knowledge of health and illness (Harrison 1994: 88, 90; Sehrawat 2013a: xx–xxiii). As a condition of participation in the medical profession, Indian medical professionals had to contribute to the colonial project of creating a rational public by demonstrating their fluency in 'scientific' medical knowledge and pointing out the unreason of indigenous medical knowledge. Both the IMS and the dispensary system were meant to discredit 'irrational', 'unscientific', and 'superstitious' indigenous medicine and often explained poor health and non-compliance among South Asian patients as a result of these attitudes. It is not surprising, therefore, that various chapters in this volume show that poor reproductive health is often explained away by medical professionals in terms of the ignorance and superstition of rural patients. Indeed, as Akhil Gupta has pointed out, such attitudes reproduce colonial dichotomies in the present. Of these, the dichotomy between modernity and tradition has proved especially enduring—associating modernity with progress, development, the hyperreal West, science and technology, high standards of living, rationality, and order; and tradition with stasis, stagnation, underdevelopment, conventional tools, rudimentary technologies, poverty, superstition, and disorder (Gupta 1998: 9). In simplistically dismissing patients' concerns as arising from traditional and irrational understandings of the body, contemporary Indian medical professionals are reproducing a colonial discourse that has been institutionalized in medical education in India and broadly accepted by Indian elites. Colonial medical educational ethos and the credentialist strategies of ethnic exclusion have survived in South Asian professional culture and social control processes. As a result, South Asian medical professionals tend to privilege high technical competence while dismissing typical Indian patients as traditional and unscientific. See Chapters 7 and 9 for further detail on current medical education in India. In doctor–patient relationships, sickness is perceived as an untoward accident which will yield to individually applied treatment and medical care. Within public discourse, depictions of illness as an isolated, individual, deviant phenomenon that can be medically treated persist, despite the existence of public health, development, and other expert discourses regarding the social roots of illness and the importance of collectivist interventions to prevent and manage these. Given that it has been acknowledged that medical socialization can encourage professionals to treat the socially powerless or medically unrewarding patients in ways that are at odds with the ideals enshrined in professional codes of ethics, it is worth revisiting sociological literature on the South Asian medical profession and education. See Chapter 10 for further discussion of attitudes towards marginalized patients in contemporary Rajasthan.

South Asian medical professionals tend to self-identify as belonging to the axis of modernity and relegate patients not from elite 'Westernized' social backgrounds to the axis of tradition. This effect is partly produced by the South Asian professional project that emerged during the colonial period. Under colonialism, South Asian medical practitioners were involved in struggles for market control, negotiation of social mobility, and assertion of a political–professional status that had important implications for the development of both the medical profession and healthcare in South Asia. The involvement of colonial South Asia's physicians in a professional project of their own required the challenging of the colonial state and its discriminatory institutions; accommodation of nationalist ideologies regarding indigenous medicine (Ayurveda, Unani, Siddhi, and homeopathy in particular); and acceptance of a circumscribed role within the developmental state. These moves deeply transformed the medical profession and continue to inform the social role of biomedical practitioners in South Asia.[19] The South Asian medical professions' privileging of high technical competence while dismissing typical Indian patients as traditional and unscientific is a result of the colonial medical educational ethos and credentialist strategies of ethnic exclusion employed by IMS officers. The marginalization of ethical concerns in this project is also significant. Roger Jeffery (1978: 102–6) has argued that one indication of 'deprofessionalization' of the post-colonial Indian medical profession is how complaints about malpractice are dealt with, in which professional bodies play a minor role. Indeed, professional bodies, such as the Medical Council of India (MCI), which are required to act as vehicles for self-regulation and the enforcement of an ethical code of conduct for doctors, were created in colonial South Asia not for these purposes but primarily to ensure British recognition of Indian medical qualifications (Jeffery 1979).

Also important is the deep impact of colonial medical education in establishing contemporary medical education standards that are designed to ensure international recognition of Indian medical degrees rather than to address the medical needs of the Indian population (Jeffery 1979). Thus, Indian medical education produces practitioners who are curative-oriented, dependent on expensive technology, and focused on the diseases of the affluent elite rather than towards providing healthcare that privileges a preventive or community approach and the needs of a rural population. British medical professionals used educational qualifications and accreditation to monitor and restrict access to the medical profession in colonial India (Jeffery 1979). To counter the racialization of the medical profession in colonial India, Indian biomedical practitioners engaged in their own professional project, which on the one hand sought the support of anti-colonial nationalism, and on the other, employed what Anne Witz calls 'countervailing credentialist tactics' of a 'usurpationary response' by seeking sufficient biomedical and technical skills, knowledge, entry credentials, or technical competence (Witz 1992: 70–1, 84–8). Such countervailing credentialist tactics have defined the South Asian medical profession—they were used initially to seek entry to the peaks of the medical profession's occupational hierarchy in colonial India (Sehrawat 2022) and later for seeking parity internationally in the post-colonial era. It is not surprising then that in an effort to pursue this professional project, South Asian medical professionals perceive themselves as without ideology, trained in the concept of the neutral quality of scientific knowledge, and yet hedged around with a society that is unscientific and irrational and which resists their worldview. The importance of amassing credentials by rising through a university career and privileging of medical and scientific knowledge as the key to advancement leads them to blame the irrational nature of patients —especially those not belonging to their own strata—to explain their patients' failure to accept a biomedical model of disease. Observations by Lange (Chapter 10) of the deployment of culturalism by Indian biomedical professionals towards socially and economically marginalized patients mark continuities in the continued prevalence of scientist and culturalist attitudes. It is also significant that these are produced to explain patient choice, in ways that tie in with neo-liberal marketization of the relationship between patients and practitioners. This marketization produces a systemic absence of ethical concerns for the patient—a reflection of the historic marginalization of subaltern patients when the private sector is expected to fill in gaps left by the state's disavowal of welfare spending on health due to fiscal conservatism. The backwardness of rural South Asian societies is frequently used by South Asian medical professionals to explain their inability in rural regions to implement technocratic solutions they have been trained in. See Chapters 8 and 10 for further examples of this point.

Thus, South Asian medical professionals can be seen as belonging to a class, which Rajni Kothari explains 'has been used to abstract[ing] itself away from the people, has always had access to privileges which it has considered its *rights,* and has usually identified itself with the flow of history, not its refuse' (Kothari 2000: 203). The next section revisits such questions of power through analysis of the politicization and medicalization of childbirth in gendered discourses of reform and development.

Middle-Class Gendered Discourses of Reform and Childbirth in South Asia

As Sarah Hodges points out, reproduction was targeted as 'a strategic site for reform' despite regional and temporal variations on discourses on childbirth (2006). The *social* history of reproduction has interpreted how it was 'constituted and reconstituted in political and social reform agendas' and was 'intimately bound up with the representational politics of caste, nation, community and family' (Hodges 2006: 11–16). Such constructions have endured in post-colonial political and social discourse. They have centred on Malthusian concerns, marriage reform, communalist demography, and national efficiency—informed by a preoccupation with eugenics in the interwar period, both internationally and in South Asia. Hodges points out that from the 1920s to the 1950s, eugenic thinking permeated social and political debate. In South Asia, eugenics did not provide 'an explicit model for understanding heritability', leaning instead towards Malthusian anxieties about overpopulation and poverty. It has provided 'a powerful and enduring template for connecting reproductive behaviour to the task of revitalizing the nation as a whole' (Hodges 2010: 228).

The social reframing of childbirth by regional politicians and elite middle-class groups was shaped by their engagement with a South Asian gendered politics of nationalism that was interpreting modernity. Anshu Malhotra (2003) has argued that the newly emerging upper-caste middle classes in Punjab reconfigured biomedical notions of pathogenicity from the early twentieth century to relate to South Asian concepts of caste. Such discourses sought to discipline women's bodies to the reproductive and eugenicist requirements of the nascent nation, a newly emergent middle-class, and communal discourses that sought muscular strength for religious communities. The introduction of biomedical midwifery practices in colonial Punjab overlapped with Punjabi Hindu and Sikh middle-class projects of asserting control over women's reproductive health in the nineteenth and twentieth centuries. The Punjabi middle-class's efforts to fashion itself as modern led to the appropriation of the colonial discourse regarding dais and their unhygienic practices during childbirth and its refashioning in line with communal and casteist discourses. This middle-class modernizing discourse sought to appropriate new ideas of pathogenicity and hygiene by reconceptualizing the pollution associated with childbirth and the parturient woman as centred in the unclean dai and her unhygienic practices. These discourses were used to sequester the homes of middle-class Punjabis from lower-caste and Muslim dais. By attacking the traditional ways of the dai, middle-class reformers displaced her from *jajmani* relationships that lasted over a lifetime. Dais were reduced to a low-caste servant of the emerging middle classes, while the profession of obstetrics was simultaneously opened up to upper-caste women. Although this discourse opened up spaces for Indian women to become medical professionals that supervised childbirth, the discourses of middle-class 'scientific' modernity that enabled this also alienated women from their bodies and restricted their access to a women's popular culture that had cut across class lines. Ahluwalia (2008) argues that all five constituencies producing discourses on female reproductive health in late colonial India—the colonial state, the medical profession, Indian nationalists advocating a 'eugenic patriotism', elite Indian women activists, and British and US feminists—emphasized surveillance and restraint, critiquing subaltern fertility while asserting upper-caste, upper-class, and colonial interests.[20] Similar concerns showing the overlapping of caste and communal politics were evident in the United Provinces. Communal discourses in the United Provinces responded to the coupling of demographic size of communities with political representation by raising fears of 'Muslim offspring of "Hindu wombs"' (Gupta 2006).

The class inflection in the British discourse on maternal and infant welfare—brought to interwar South Asia by British women doctors active in an international epistemic community and maternalist discourse—was adopted enthusiastically by middle-class women (for Bengal, see Engels 1996: 146–50, and Samita Sen 1999: 148–50; for Bombay presidency, see Srivastava 2018: 175–82). Bengali social reform organizations working to further the nationalist village reconstruction programme espoused by Gandhi and Tagore adopted a maternalist approach to improving conditions of childbirth, targeting lower-middle-class women. These initiatives provided maternity clinics as well as classes on hygiene for TBAs, midwifery training programmes, and activities to disseminate mothercraft in the 1920s and

1930s. Thus, Indian middle-class interventions also pressed their own class values and practices onto working-class and rural dais and mothers, without any attention to the appropriateness of their initiatives (Engels 1996: 147–50; also Srivastava 2018: 153–229). Indeed, Dagmar Engels has argued that in colonial Bengal, Indian reformists' efforts to improve conditions of childbirth were *more* successful than those by colonial institutions such as the DF because they did not suffer from the racial bias of the latter. The question of childbirth became closely tied to the nationalist ideals of gender roles and motherhood. An important consequence of colonial, nationalist, and reformist interventions was that the privileging of childbearing and infant care in their discourses accentuated tensions between women's productive and reproductive labour. These tensions have survived into the post-colonial era and are especially problematic when they inform state schemes targeting subaltern groups. The development discourse on childbirth is driven by colonial and post-colonial elites and medical professionals who deploy it to serve broader political and ideological purposes, deepening further the historical exclusion of socially and economically marginalized groups.

Conclusion

I will conclude by acknowledging that the persistence of earlier denouements of issues surrounding maternal healthcare may be only one factor among many shaping the contemporary problem of childbirth. But if it *is* a factor, it ought to be taken into account and its relative weight examined. Historians of South Asia, especially medical historians, have tended to privilege historical analysis of the means of enunciation, production, and legitimization of discourse—colonial *and* nationalist—as well as the power dynamics underlying these discourses. This preoccupation has prevented critical examination of the continuities in state medical interventions in public health from the colonial to the post-colonial period. Since the 1920s, medical and developmental experts and the state—both colonial and post-colonial—have accepted that improving maternal health is vital. Yet, such claims have also been marked by failures to heed expert advice, even though this advice has changed considerably (for the colonial period, see Arnold 2001). Neoliberal reforms of health have drawn on discourses about the limits of the state's role that are remarkably congruent with colonial discourses on the fiscally conservative minimalist state (Sehrawat 2013a). Since they have been championed by a multiplicity of actors, even mounting proof of the ineffectiveness of policies produced by these discourses has been insufficient to lead to the abandoning of ideological frameworks that drive them.

It is important to examine the historical roots of the impact of social and economic marginalization on the health of the population and the healthcare available to it. This is especially significant given that neoliberal reforms have reintroduced colonial limits on post-colonial states' initiatives to provide universal healthcare. Historical studies of public–private partnerships in the Bombay presidency to improve conditions of childbirth suggest that they failed signally (Srivastava 2018: 204–6, 212–15). Yet, public–private partnerships have been reintroduced since the 1990s, despite overwhelming evidence that they would have a detrimental impact on the healthcare of marginalized groups (Qadeer et al. 2001). Neoliberal policies are discursively and structurally very similar to the colonial state's emphasis on the private and voluntary sector as a justification for a minimalist and fiscally conservative conception of the state (Sehrawat 2013a). The state's withdrawal from healthcare investment began much before the structural adjustment programme of the 1990s, with the latter making even more pronounced what had been the policy of favouring the medical profession and its ambitions for increased income through the private sector (Baru 2001: 211–34; Qadeer 2005: 88–92). Indeed, it might be possible to argue that there was only a brief hiatus when universal healthcare was declared to be the aim of state policy in India (Banerji 2001: 44–6; Jeffery 1988b: 112–18, 143–66; Qadeer 2005: 88). Thus, public debates in South Asia about the allocation of resources to healthcare have privileged efficiency over equity. Equity, requiring a collectivist approach and initiatives for an egalitarian distribution of healthcare resources among different strata of the population, has also been seen as competing with the contrasting value of individual autonomy by the medical profession in South Asia. The value of autonomy—representing the ability for self-determination and independence in healthcare—has been interpreted in post-colonial India as consonant with nationalist ideals of self-determination and independence from reliance on Western centres of technical expertise, leading to investment in high-technology medicine. Under neoliberal constraints, the emphasis on individual autonomy has been interpreted in terms of increasing patient choice by expanding the number and role of private providers (Baru 1998). Thus, the systemic marginalization of concern with the welfare of the patient—in professional neglect of ethical commitments to patients *and* in the state's refusal to allocate resources to provide healthcare for subaltern groups—has colonial roots. It is salutary to remember that the continued manifestation of culturalist attitudes towards subaltern South Asian groups, and the privileging of fiscal conservatism over the healthcare and welfare of the population, are aspects of a medical system produced to serve the needs of a colonial elite. The use of the state medical infrastructure and the medical profession to cement power for this colonial elite historically tied biomedicine in South Asia to a medical system that neglected the mass of the South Asian population. Ideological commitments to champion the needs of this population—in the discourses of post-colonial states borne out of anti-colonial nationalism; organizations committed to development, and South Asian medical professionals—will continue to fail to escape the neglect embedded in South Asia's medical system unless colonial legacies are confronted and renounced by the post-colonial elites who stand to benefit from them.

Contemporary initiatives to address neonatal health share considerable similarity with initiatives taken a hundred years ago when the improvement of maternal health emerged as a central concern for the colonial Indian state, British women doctors, and South Asian elites. This chapter has taken on the important task of showing how the structures of post-colonial initiatives have been moulded by the colonial histories of medical institutions and infrastructure and how nationalist critiques failed sufficiently to democratize access to public health and healthcare.[21]

Notes

1. Some important exceptions are: Hume (1977), Jeffery (1979, 1988b), and Qadeer (2005).
2. I have borrowed here from Anne Witz's (1992) definition of professional projects as projects of occupational closure, as well as her fourfold distinction of strategies of occupational closure—exclusionary, inclusionary, demarcationary, and dual closure.
3. I borrow the concept from Neill 2012.
4. 'Medical Aid for Indian Women', *The Times,* December 1945, p. 7.
5. 'The Maternity and Infant welfare Exhibition', *Journal of the Association of Medical Women in India,* 8(1), March 1920, p. 13.
6. 'Medical Aid for Indian Women', *The Times,* December 1945, p. 7.
7. 'Margaret Balfour: Obituary', *British Medical Journal,* 15 December 1945, p. 867.
8. Dagmar Engels (1996) is also vulnerable to the same criticism.
9. Several chapters in this volume unpack the contested and ambiguous meanings of this term in the current context.

10. Also see repeated discussions in *Punjab Hospital Reports* from the 1890s to the 1930s about the challenges of persuading women to take up medical education and professional work.

11. As Chapter 7 shows, these challenges continue to effect female medical professionals in India.

12. The aggressively modernizing discourse of early-twentieth-century US imperialism had foregrounded public health in its governance of the Philippines as a US colony. The US lead in tropical medicine was established by treating the Philippines as an imperial laboratory to establish a 'sanitary regime'.

13. A fuller treatment of these initiatives within strategies of professional advancement is yet to be undertaken, though Curjel and Balfour's research and its impact on colonial debates regarding maternal health has been discussed in Engels (1996: 132–4) and Sen (1999: 150–1).

14. I have assumed here for the sake of analytic convenience that there is one monolithic South Asian profession. However, it is important to disaggregate this profession regionally and along gender, ethnic, and class lines to examine whether such a disaggregation produces a range of professional projects in a region as culturally and socially diverse as South Asia. Historically, efforts by practitioners of biomedicine that led to its vernacularization might also have challenged the emergence of a profession in the western sense.

15. Indigenous practitioners were part of the nationalist movement, and Congress provincial governments in the 1920s and 1930s were able to provide them with financial and symbolic support, but they remained marginalised and ineffective (Jeffery 1979, 1988a: 168).

16. Indian biomedical practitioners may have been less committed to this discourse as the nationalist movement championed indigenous medicine (Jeffery 1988b, Kumar 1997; for nationalist politics around Ayurveda see Berger 2013 and Sivaramakrishnan 2006). Some South Asian biomedical practitioners are known to have engaged in the process of translating/vernacularizing it to make it commensurable to local and indigenous understandings of health and disease. Mukharji (2009) has showed that the practice of Bengali *daktars* (practitioners of 'Western' medicine) interpreted 'western' medicine through localized therapeutics and played an important role in its dissemination. Since the practice of daktari medicine by these colonial medical subordinates led to the vernacularization of Western medicine, it may be argued that such practitioners—often designated as quacks in colonial official discourse—did not equate science and modernity with Westernization. Given the importance of professional projects in embedding credentialism as an important usurpationary strategy adopted by South Asian doctors, it is important to remember that Mukharji shies away from defining daktars in terms of a specific profession, conceiving the category as a fluid identity. Irrespective of such qualifications, it can be argued that the South Asian professional project—shaped by colonial exigencies—exercises a structural

influence resulting in the adoption of scientist and culturalist attitudes, especially towards marginalized social groups.

17. For a more nuanced appraisal of the extent to which high-technology curative facilities dominated over preventive approaches in the post-colonial Indian state's expenditure for the 1950s to 1980s, see Jeffery (1988b, 143–66).

18. Jawahar Lal Nehru believed that 'expertise' and 'scientific temperament' were essential for building the postcolonial Indian nation (Zachariah 2004: 152–3, 192).

19. Hume shows that demarcationary strategies of occupational closure were pursued by IMS officers towards practitioners of indigenous medicine and racialized and credentialist strategies to relegate Indian medical professionals to the subordinate medical services (Hume 1977).

20. These historical concerns continue to be manifested in the contemporary surveillance of patients examined in Chapter 10.

21. I would like to thank all the participants for their lively and enlightening discussion at the 'Transformation of Childbirth in South Asia: Ethical, Legal, and Social Implications' workshop at the Department of Social Anthropology and Cultural Studies (ISEK), Zurich, Switzerland. I would like to express my gratitude to Roger Jeffery, Clémence Jullien, Manu Sehgal, Fouzhieya Towghi, and Emma Varley who have been especially crucial in helping me formulate my ideas in this chapter. I am also grateful for the support I have received from the Leverhulme Trust and the Newcastle University Humanities and Social Sciences Faculty Research Fund.

References

Ahluwalia, Sanjam. 2008. *Reproductive Restraints: Birth Control in India, 1877–1947.* Urbana and Chicago: University of Illinois Press.

Arnold, David. 1988. 'Introduction: Disease, Medicine and Empire'. In *Imperial Medicine and Indigenous Societies*, edited by David Arnold, 1–26. Manchester: Manchester University Press.

Arnold, David. 1993. *Colonizing the Body.* Berkeley and Los Angeles: University of California Press.

Arnold, David. 2001. 'Official Attitudes to Population, Birth Control and Reproductive Health in India, 1921–1946'. *Reproductive Health in India: History, Politics, Controversies*, edited by Sarah Hodges, 22–50. Hyderabad: Orient Longman.

Balfour, Margaret Ida, and Ruth Young. 1929. *The Medical Work of Women in India.* London: Humphrey for Oxford University Press.

Banerji, Debabar. 2001. 'Landmarks in the Development of Health Services in India'. In *Public Health and the Poverty of Reforms*, edited by Imrana Qadeer, Kasturi Sen, and K.R. Nayar, 39–50. New Delhi and Thousand Oaks: Sage.

Baru, Rama V. 1998. *Private Health Care in India: Social Characteristics and Trends.* New Delhi: Sage.

Baru, Rama V. 2001. 'Health Sector Reforms and Structural Adjustment: A State-Level Analysis'. In *Public Health and the Poverty of Reforms: The South Asia Predicament*, edited by Imrana Qadeer, Kasturi Sen, and K.R. Nayar, 211–34. New Delhi and Thousand Oaks: Sage.

Bashford, Alison. 1998. *Purity and Pollution: Gender, Embodiment, and Victorian Medicine*. Basingstoke: Macmillan.

Basilico, Matthew, Jonathan Weigel, Anjali Motgi, Jacob Bor, and Salmaan Keshavjee. 2013. 'Health for All? Competing Theories and Geopolitics'. In *Reimagining Global Health: An Introduction*, edited by Paul Farmer, Julia Kim, Arthur Kleinman, and Matthew Basilico, 74–110. Berkeley, London: University of California Press.

Berger, Rachel. 2013. *Ayurveda Made Modern: Political Histories of Indigenous Medicine in North India, 1900–55*. Basingstoke: Palgrave Macmillan.

Brown, E. Richard. 1976. 'Public Health in Imperialism: Early Rockefeller Programs at Home and Abroad'. *American Journal of Public Health* 66 (9): 897–903.

Burton, Antoinette M. 1994. *Burdens of History: British Feminists, Indian Women, and Imperial Culture, 1865–1915*. Chapel Hill & London: University of North Carolina Press.

Burton, Antoinette M. 1996. 'Contesting the Zenana: The Mission to Make "Lady Doctors for India," 1874–1885'. *Journal of British Studies* 35 (3): 368–97.

Chakrabarti, Pratik. 2009. ' "Signs of the Times": Medicine and Nationhood in British India'. *Osiris* 24 (1): 188–211.

Chatterjee, Partha. 1994. 'Was There a Hegemonic Project of the Colonial State?' In *Contesting Colonial Hegemony: State and Society in Africa and India*, edited by Dagmar Engels and Shula Marks, 79–84. London: I.B. Tauris.

Davin, Anna. 1978. 'Imperialism and Motherhood'. *History Workshop* 5: 9–65.

Drachman, Virginia G. 1986. 'The Limits of Progress: The Professional Lives of Women Doctors, 1881–1926'. *Bulletin of the History of Medicine* 60 (1): 58–72.

Dubin, Martin David. 1995. 'The League of Nations Health Organisation'. In *International Health Organisations and Movements, 1918–1939*, edited by Paul Weindling, 56–80. Cambridge: Cambridge University Press.

Dyhouse, Carol. 1978. 'Working-Class Mothers and Infant Mortality in England, 1895–1914'. *Journal of Social History* 12 (2): 248–67.

Elston, Mary Ann C. 1986. 'Women Doctors in the British Health Services: A Sociological Study of Their Careers and Opportunities'. PhD, Sociology, University of Leeds.

Engels, Dagmar. 1996. *Beyond Purdah? Women in Bengal 1890–1939*. Delhi: Oxford University Press.

Fassin, Didier. 2001. 'Culturalism as Ideology'. In *Cultural Perspectives on Reproductive Health*, edited by Carla Makhlouf Obermeyer, 300–18. Oxford & New York: Oxford University Press.

Forbes, Geraldine. 1994a. 'Managing Midwifery in India'. In *Contesting Colonial Hegemony: State and Society in Africa and India*, edited by Dagmar Engels and Shula Marks, 152–72. London: British Academic Press.

Forbes, Geraldine. 1994b. 'Medical Careers and Health Care for Indian Women: Patterns of Control'. *Women's History Review* 3 (4): 515–30.

Forbes, Geraldine. 2000. 'Introduction'. In *The Memoirs of Dr. Haimabati Sen: From Child Widow to Lady Doctor*, edited by Geraldine Forbes and Tapan Raychaudhuri, 9–45. New Delhi: Roli Books.

Frankenberg, Ronald. 1981. 'Allopathic Medicine, Profession, and Capitalist Ideology in India'. *Social Science & Medicine. Part A: Medical Psychology & Medical Sociology* 15 (2): 115–25.

Gorsky, Martin, and Christopher Sirrs. 2018. 'The Rise and Fall of "Universal Health Coverage" as a Goal of International Health Politics, 1925–1952'. *American Journal of Public Health* 108 (3): 334–42.

Gupta, Akhil. 1998. *Postcolonial Developments: Agriculture in the Making of Modern India*. Durham: Duke University Press.

Gupta, Charu. 2006. 'Hindu Wombs, Muslim Progeny: The Numbers Game and Shifting Debates on Widow Remarriage in Uttar Pradesh 1890s–1930s'. In *Reproductive Health in India: History, Politics, Controversies*, edited by Sarah Hodges, 167–98. Hyderabad: Orient Longman.

Harrison, Mark. 1994. *Public Health in British India: Anglo-Indian Preventive Medicine 1859–1914*. Cambridge: Cambridge University Press.

Hodge, Joseph Morgan. 2007. *Triumph of the Expert: Agrarian Doctrines of Development and the Legacies of British Colonialism*. Athens, OH: Ohio University Press.

Hodges, Sarah. 2006. 'Towards a History of Reproduction in Modern India'. In *Reproductive Health in India: History, Politics, Controversies*, edited by Sarah Hodges, 1–21. Hyderabad: Orient Longman.

Hodges, Sarah. 2008. *Contraception, Colonialism and Commerce: Birth Control in South India, 1920–1940*. London: Routledge.

Hodges, Sarah. 2010. 'South Asia's Eugenic Past'. In *The Oxford Handbook of the History of Eugenics*, edited by Alison Bashford and Philippa Levine, 228–42. Oxford and New York: Oxford University Press.

Hume, John C. 1977. 'Medicine in the Punjab, 1849–1911: Ethnicity and Professionalization in the Control of an Occupation'. PhD thesis in History, Duke University.

Jeffery, Roger. 1978. 'Allopathic Medicine in India A Case of Deprofessionalisation?'. *Economic and Political Weekly* 13 (3): 101–13.

Jeffery, Roger. 1979. 'Recognizing India's Doctors: The Institutionalization of Medical Dependency, 1918–39'. *Modern Asian Studies* 13 (2): 301–26.

Jeffery, Roger. 1988a. 'Doctors and Congress: The Role of Medical Men and Medical Politics in Indian Nationalism'. In *The Political Economy of Indian Independence and the Indian National Congress, 1885–1985*, edited by Mike Shepperdson and Colin Simmons, 160–73. London: Gower.

Jeffery, Roger. 1988b. *The Politics of Health in India*. Berkeley: University of California Press.

Kothari, Rajni. 2000. 'The Decline of the Moderate State'. In *Politics and the State in India*, edited by Zoya Hasan, 177–205. New Delhi: Sage.

Kothari, Uma. 2005. 'From Colonial Administration to Development Studies: A Post-colonial Critique of the History of Development Studies'. In *A Radical History* of Development Studies: Individuals, Institutions and Ideologies, edited by Uma Kothari, 47–66. London: Zed Books.

Koven, Seth, and Sonya Michel. 1990. 'Womanly Duties: Maternalist Politics and the Origins of Welfare States in France, Germany, Great Britain, and the United States, 1880–1920'. American Historical Review 95 (4): 1076–108.

Kumar, Deepak. 1997. 'Unequal Contenders, Uneven Ground: Medical Encounters in British India, 1820–1920'. In Western Medicine as Contested Knowledge, edited by Andrew Cunningham and Bridie Andrews, 172–211. Manchester: Manchester University Press.

Lal, Maneesha. 1994. 'The Politics of Gender and Medicine in Colonial India: The Countess of Dufferin's Fund, 1885–1888'. Bulletin of the History of Medicine 68 (1): 29–66.

Lang, Seán. 2005. 'Drop the Demon Dai: Maternal Mortality and the State in Colonial Madras, 1840–1875'. Social History of Medicine 18 (3): 357–78.

Lewis, Jane. 1980. The Politics of Motherhood: Child and Maternal Welfare in England, 1900–1939. London: Harvester Wheatsheaf.

Malhotra, Anshu. 2003. 'Of Dais and Midwives: "Middle-Class" Interventions in the Management of Women's Reproductive Health—A Study from Colonial Punjab'. Indian Journal of Gender Studies 10 (2): 229–59.

Mohanty, Chandra. 1988. 'Under Western Eyes: Feminist Scholarship and Colonial Discourses'. Feminist Review 30 (1): 61–88.

Monnais, Laurence, and David Wright. 2016. Doctors beyond Borders: The Transnational Migration of Physicians in the Twentieth Century. Toronto: University of Toronto Press.

Mukharji, Projit Bihari. 2009. Nationalizing the Body: The Medical Market, Print and Daktari Medicine. London and New York: Anthem Press.

Neill, Deborah. 2012. Networks in Tropical Medicine: Internationalism, Colonialism, and the Rise of a Medical Specialty, 1890–1930. Stanford: Stanford University Press.

Papanek, Hanna. 1982. 'Purdah: Separate Worlds and Symbolic Shelter'. In Separate Worlds: Studies of Purdah in South Asia, edited by Hanna Papanek and Gail Minault, 3–53. Delhi: Chanakya.

Parmar, Inderjeet. 2012. Foundations of the American Century: The Ford, Carnegie, and Rockefeller Foundations in the Rise of American Power. New York: Columbia University Press.

Phillips, David R. 1990. Health and Health Care in the Third World. Burnt Mill, Essex: Longman.

Plant, Rebecca Jo, and Marian van der Klein. 2012. 'Introduction: A New Generation of Scholars on Maternalism'. In Maternalism Reconsidered: Motherhood, Welfare and Social Policy in the Twentieth Century, edited by Marian van der Kleinet, 1–21. New York: Berghahn.

Prakash, Gyan. 1999. Another Reason: Science and the Imagination of Modern India. Delhi: Oxford University Press.

Qadeer, Imrana. 2005. 'Continuities and Discontinuities in Public Health: The Indian Experience'. In Maladies, Preventives and Curatives: Debates in Public Health in India, edited by Amiya Kumar Bagchi and Krishna Soman, 79–96. New Delhi: Tulika Books.

Qadeer, Imrana, Kasturi Sen, and K.R. Nayar. 2001. *Public Health and the Poverty of Reforms: The South Asian Predicament*. New Delhi & Thousand Oaks: Sage.

Sehrawat, Samiksha. 2013a. *Colonial Medical Care in North India: Gender, State, and Society, c.1830–1920*. New Delhi: Oxford University Press.

Sehrawat, Samiksha. 2013b. 'Feminising Empire: The Association of Medical Women in India and the Campaign to Found a Women's Medical Service'. *Social Scientist* 41 (5/6): 65–81.

Sehrawat, Samiksha. 2022. *Biomedicine for the Colony: Institutions, Patients and Professionals in India, 1850-1930*. Manchester: Manchester University Press.

Sen, Samita. 1999. *Women and Labour in Late Colonial India: The Bengal Jute Industry*. Cambridge: Cambridge University Press.

Sinha, Mrinalini. 2006. *Specters of Mother India: The Global Restructuring of an Empire*. New Delhi: Zubaan.

Sirrs, Christopher. 2020. 'Promoting Health Protection Worldwide: The International Labour Organisation and Health Systems Financing, 1952–2012'. *International History Review* 40 (2): 1–20.

Sivaramakrishnan, Kavita. 2006. *Old Potions, New Bottles: Recasting Indigenous Medicine in Colonial Punjab, 1850–1945*. Hyderabad: Orient Longman.

Srivastava, Priyanka. 2018. *The Well-Being of the Labor Force in Colonial Bombay: Discourses and Practices*. Basingstoke, Hampshire: Palgrave Macmillan.

Thomson, Elaine. 1998. 'Women in Medicine in Late Nineteenth- and Early Twentieth-Century Edinburgh: A Case Study'. PhD, Science Studies Unit, University of Edinburgh.

Trivedi, Lisa. 2019. 'Maternal Care and Global Public Health: Bombay and Manchester, 1900–1950'. *Social History of Medicine* (online). doi: 10.1093/shm/hkz080.

Van Hollen, Cecilia. 2003. *Birth on the Threshold: Childbirth and Modernity in South India*. Berkeley and Los Angeles: University of California Press.

Weindling, Paul. 1995. 'Social Medicine at the League of Nations Health Organization and the International Labour Office Compared'. In *International Health Organisations and Movements, 1918–39*, edited by Paul Weindling, 134–53. Cambridge: Cambridge University Press.

Weindling, Paul. 2015. 'International Health between Public and Private in the Twentieth Century'. In *Healthcare in Private and Public from the Early Modern Period to 2000*, edited by Paul Weindling, 194–214. London: Routledge.

Weis, Julianne Rose. 2015. 'Women and Childbirth in Haile Selassie's Ethiopia'. DPhil, History of Science and Medicine, University of Oxford.

Witz, Anne. 1992. *Professions and Patriarchy*. London: Routledge.

Zachariah, Benjamin. 2004. *Nehru*. London: Routledge.

SECTION 2

CONTINUING RELEVANCE OF 'TRADITIONAL BIRTH ATTENDANTS'

3

Forms and Ethics of Baloch Midwifery

Contesting the Violations of Biomedicalized Childbirth in Pakistan

Fouzieyha Towghi

I tell them that Allāh will take care of the birth and bring the child safely into the world. Allāh is the bringer.

A dhīnabog

Drawing from ethnographic research in Balochistan, Pakistan, in this chapter, I show how *dhīnabogs* (Baloch midwives) and their *dhīnabogiri/* midwifery aid women and their kin to remedy and resist injuries of biomedicalized obstetrics. Dhīnabogs' mediations of the increasing iatrogenic effects of biomedical interventions reflect a form and ethics of their care, despite near two centuries of disparaging policy construction of South Asian indigenous midwives (Lal 1994; Towghi 2004, 2018). In Panjgur district of Balochistan, I met dhīnabogs, *kawwās* (expert midwives), *and bolluks* (grandmothers) who had escaped the reifying effect of "categories, acronyms, and discursive effacements" given the general absence of reference to them as a *dai* (South Asian midwife) or TBA (traditional birth attendant) in Panjgur (Pigg 1995).

Despite the long-standing presence of allopathy,[1] dhīnabogs remain vital in the antenatal, childbirth, and post-partum care of Panjguri women. As I accompanied them during their rounds to women's homes, walked with them through towns, fields, and valleys, and climbed mountains searching for wild herbs and plants, I learned about their distinctive importance in women's lives. They were reputed for their exceptional techniques of antenatal massage, used to shift and reposition the foetus both before and during delivery to ensure safe childbirth. They prescribed and administered *Balochi dhawā* (medicine), such as herbal formulas aiding women to avert immediate and long-term postnatal reproductive problems.

Fouzieyha Towghi, *Forms and Ethics of Baloch Midwifery:* In: *Childbirth in South Asia.* Edited by: Clémence Jullien and Roger Jeffery, Oxford University Press. © Oxford University Press 2021. DOI: 10.1093/oso/9780190130718.003.0003

One dhīnabog told me that no child or mother had ever died in her hands, nor in the hands of her great-aunt, someone who in her view was a 'true kawwās' who taught her the art of dhīnabogiri. Here, Bibi-Zarina was not exactly boasting about her aunt's specialized herbal knowledge and competence, characteristics reflecting the embodied ethical imperatives of dhīnabogiri; rather she was explicating the unpredictable outcome of all childbirth in which *khudhrath* (God's nature or the force of God) is viewed to have a central though empirically inexplicable place.[2] This was a recurrent philosophical outlook that many dhīnabogs echoed, as they relegated their own dignified, assiduous care of women as a calling, a vocation guided by Allāh, as well as a work of necessity. Bibi-Zarina continues, 'God's nature brings the child to the world. If s/he might bring death, then there is death. If there is no death, then the child lives'. This consciousness about the potentiality of death in and around childbirth did not form dhīnabogs into passive observers of childbirth-related emergencies that they linked to the inappropriate labour induction with the *sūch-chin* [uterotonic injection] (Towghi 2014, 2018). In such emergencies, women's kin would often turn to dhīnabogs for care, before risking the long journey to reach a tertiary hospital in Quetta or Karachi, due to the absence of a functional emergency obstetric care in the district headquarter hospital (DHQH).

Anthropological studies of reproduction and maternity, and histories of colonial medicine, have examined the embodied consequences of health policies and practices experienced by reproductive women and their midwives, known as dais in South Asia (Jeffery et al. 1984, 1989; Pinto 2008; Ram and Jolly 1998). Anthropologists have noted how spaces of modern reproduction manifest as zones of obstetric violence and terror for childbearing women (Castro and Savage 2018); a trend echoed in the narratives of women and dhīnabogs I interviewed, and confirmed in studies outlining the global escalation of unnecessary interventions during pregnancy, birth, and the early weeks of life-'risking iatrogenic harm to women and newborns' (Renfrew et al. 2014: 1129). Anthropologists have also cautioned against romanticizing the TBA at the expense of the labouring woman (Jeffery et al. 1984, 1989; Rozario 1998). Dhīnabogs, however, criticized the misuses of injections by lady medical officers (LMOs) and lady health visitors (LHVs) in their private clinics along with mismanaged births by inexperienced 'dais' who, they suggested, were not dhīnabogs, in so far as they qualified the role and its attendant expertise and practices. Their experiences are radically different from the government's view, which assumes the absence of institutional births and skilled birth attendants (SBAs) as a chief cause of maternal deaths, concomitantly disparaging homebirths and TBAs (Government of Pakistan 2005, 2012). The SBA defines a doctor, nurse, LHV, or Western midwife.

Panjguri Baloch women were clear about wanting to give birth at home, but not against seeking biomedicine in case of complications; and for antenatal care to receive the tetanus toxoid vaccine. Antenatal visits become an occasion for LMOs to pressure pregnant women to give birth in their clinic, with verbal and physical tactics of control, including the premature induction of labour (Towghi 2018: 679–82). Women might also visit an LMO or LHV for delivery in the absence of a dhīnabog. With about 9.6 million people in 31 districts, Balochistan province comprises 44% of Pakistan's territory and 5% of the national population (National Institute of Population Studies [NIPS] 2013). Until the 2010s, nearly all births in Panjgur, as elsewhere in Balochistan, occurred at home. Institutional deliveries are now rising but have reached only 26% of rural and 55% of urban births in Balochistan (NIPS 2019: 25).

Maternal mortality remains high in Pakistan, particularly in rural areas. In Balochistan, which is predominately rural, key factors associated with mortality were lack of transport, long distance to a hospital, and the absence of emergency obstetric care (EmOC) in district hospitals (2008). Panjgur and several other districts were not surveyed due to political unrest (NIPS 2008) and excluded in the latest national demographic and health survey (NIPS 2019). However, a district baseline survey of 734 households in 2003 identified 34 deaths in Panjgur in the previous 5-year period.[3] The deaths were not attributed to homebirths. The survey found that among the 722 women interviewed about their last pregnancy, 70% had dais or dhīnabogs attend the 'normal and complicated' childbirths, all live births. Other women with complications had visited public and private facilities, including in referrals to Quetta or Karachi where 14 women had forceps delivery and 8 needed a caesarean section. The circumstances of maternal deaths I learned about were all entangled with visits to biomedical facilities and uterotonics injections. Many of these women had first visited the DHQH for antenatal care, assessed to have a healthy pregnancy, and encouraged to give birth in a facility assisted by an LMO (Towghi 2018).

Because post-partum haemorrhage (PPH) is considered a direct medical cause of approximately 25% of maternal mortalities worldwide, policies to reduce maternal mortality have advocated routine AMTSL (active management of the third stage of labour, the period between delivery of the child and the placenta) with synthetic uterotonics (oxytocin, ergometrine, or misoprostol). Practitioners are asked to administer a uterotonic in all childbirth cases, irrespective of an apparent risk of PPH (Society of Obstetricians and Gynaecologists of Canada 2004; International Federation of Gynecology Obstetrics 2012). A respected gynaecologist in Quetta explained this to be a necessary PPH prevention policy.

In Panjgur, the AMTSL policy serves to compound the risks women experience in a pre-existing context of structural constraints entailed in obtaining timely obstetric care. Malnutrition, poor quality of biomedical care, and lack of emergency obstetric services combine to shape the iatrogenic consequences of the excessive uterotonic injections resulting in morbidities or death because women cannot reach a functioning hospital on time. If they do reach a hospital following a 12-hour or longer journey, they may experience further iatrogenesis, such as 'unnecessary hysterectomies' due to a diagnosis of abnormal vaginal bleeding, uterine tear, or a *kharāb* (bad) uterus (see Towghi 2012: 232).

In what follows, I first locate the dhīnabogs in the broader context of the female health worker force responsible for reproductive healthcare in Pakistan, delineating the factors underlying the continued preference by women for TBAs. Next, I discuss the historical and contemporary governmental policies designed to discipline the 'culture of homebirths' (Towghi 2014: 123–7). I highlight how these policies remain blind to the harmful effects of modern obstetrics in their quest to disappear a generic constructed TBA/dai. This is followed by an analysis of why some Panjguri childbearing women and their kin are soliciting the uterotonics during childbirth. I delineate dhīnabogs' responses to this trend that is linked to their ethics of care and sense of self as Baloch. The concluding section details the significance of the embodied affective work of dhīnabogs—embedded in their forms and ethics of care—towards women confronting iatrogenic effects of uterotonics.

My analysis is informed by 2 years (2004–6) of ethnographic research in Pakistan, archival research at the WHO and the United Nations in Geneva, and the British and Wellcome Trust libraries in London in 2006, subsequent ongoing communications with some of my interlocutors (2010–15), and the review of governmental and non-governmental national reports and policy documents. A significant proportion of research was in Panjgur; field research in Pakistan also took me to Khuzdar, Quetta, Karachi, Hub, Dera Bugti, Gwadar, Turbat, Peshawar, and Islamabad. Research in Panjgur involved participant observation in hospital wards and in the context of midwives' work in home and hospital settings, and individual and group interviews and conversations with 86 midwives; approximately 200 women; 4 *hakīms* (physician of Unani medicine); a range of allopathic practitioners including women and men medical doctors, LHVs, LHWs, and compounders; local artists; historians; politicians; government officials; social justice activists; *pensārs* (herb gatherers/sellers; pharmacists/herbalists) shop owners.

Located in Southwest Balochistan, bordering Iran, Panjgur has one DHQH, a rural health centre (RHC), 13 dispensaries, 15 basic health units (BHU), and four Maternal Child Health Centres (MCHC). A secondary level facility, the DHQH provides acute, ambulatory, inpatient care and is supported by tertiary care hospitals in Quetta. Having clusters of villages, Panjgur is connected with other parts of Pakistan by air and road, with limited air travel several times a week to three destinations only. Quetta (the provincial city) is reachable only by road—much of it (90%) unpaved in 2005 and to date. Some residents use their motorcycle or bicycle for inter-village travel. Public buses travel daily to and from Karachi, Quetta, and other cities. The roads are difficult to travel on during rains, crossing small streams and flood channels without any bridge, halting traffic for long periods until water levels are low enough to travel safely. A bus journey from Panjgur to Karachi can take up to 20 hours, and sometimes up to 24. The less affordable journey on a pickup truck is about 12 hours.

'Lady Doctors Say, "Don't Go to the Dais"'

They [the women] don't call us [for homebirths].

A lady health visitor

In rural and urban Balochistan, dais coexist with LMOs and LHVs, and most childbirths continue to be assisted by dais/TBAs (NIPS 2019). In Balochistan, about 75% of all births occur at home (NIPS 2019). Despite the requirement to assign women health workers in every government facility, approximately 33% have no women health staff, a persistent ratio since first noted by the Pakistan Federal Bureau of Statistics in 1996 (Bhutta 2004; Ghaffar et al. 2013; WHO 2007). While approximately a third of all physicians registered are women, they are concentrated in the cities—and only a small percentage of women are trained in obstetrics and gynaecology, and even fewer are trained to perform caesarean sections. When LMOs and LHVs are available, they assist with delivery only and exclusively in a clinical setting. The Pakistan Nursing Council registers three categories of midwives; dais and TBAs are not registered. The nurse-midwife is a registered nurse and a registered midwife with 3 years of training in general nursing and a year in post-basic allopathic training in 'modern' midwifery. They are a small number working in urban maternity institutions. The non-nurse-midwife receives a year of training in midwifery. The LHV receives 2 years of training, in midwifery and basic public health. They are the majority of women biomedical practitioners followed by LMOs.

Introduced in colonial India, the term *lady* (plr: *ladyān*) remains the official prefix in Pakistan's medical nomenclature, referring to LMOs, LHVs, and LHWs. The LHVs are non-physician paramedics introduced in Pakistan in 1951 to supplement the LMOs (MBBS—Bachelor of Medicine and Surgery graduates) (Hezekiah 1993). While permitted to attend 'normal' births in institutional or home settings, in Panjgur as in the rest of Pakistan, LHVs rarely if ever were called to attend homebirths. Unlike medical doctors, LHVs are prohibited from having a private practice, yet many ignore this regulation (WHO 2007). In terms of numbers, though concentrated in the cities, LHVs are the next important women's reproductive health providers to LMOs. Thus, the absence of women health workers in rural areas is not entirely due to insufficient government personnel. For example, over the years since Pakistan's independence in 1947, 10,000 'midwives' have been trained in Western obstetrics, yet no one can effectively track or locate them to ascertain if they are working (Shah et al. 2016; WHO 2007).

Reflecting Pakistan's broader context, in Balochistan, a majority of the LMO and LHV posts are vacant, despite ongoing matriculation of women medical workers (Arshad et al. 2017; WHO 2007). This is a trend that I observed in the 1990s and subsequently in Balochistan (Towghi et al. 2000). In 2005, a number of Punjabi LHVs assigned to work in Panjgur were preparing to transfer to districts located near their hometowns. Much to the displeasure of the district health officer (DHO), two of the LHVs received their transfer notice to BHUs in the Punjab. To prevent the gaps in services to women and children, the DHO attempted to block this transfer. Such politics surrounding transfers of men and women medical personnel is common in Pakistan (Shah et al. 2016; WHO 2007).

Generally, LHVs do not belong to the community they are assigned to serve, impeding the provision of proper care. Trust between them as outsiders and the community is difficult to develop, evident in Panjgur by the fact that the LHVs were rarely solicited for homebirths. I discussed this point with a group of LHVs. Several LHVs in their late twenties and thirties told me with a degree of humour that over their approximately 4 years of assignment in Panjgur, they assisted no more than one or two births—if any at all. 'They don't call us', one LHV states, giggling, having no apparent feelings of resentment, given they received a regular monthly salary from the government. Moreover, they were prohibited from accepting cash payment if assisting women in homes or clinics during working hours.

To overcome women's evident enduring reliance on dais, government-sponsored training programmes have attempted to employ 'trained' dais to work in government facilities, where a TBA might receive a scheduled monthly salary. The percentage of dais in such positions remains minimal, however (Tanner et al. 2013; Towghi 2004; WHO 2007). Often their work is reduced to running errands, maintaining order in the waiting halls of clinics and hospitals, and sweeping and tidying up the clinic, even if they may sometimes hold the key to the 'free' medicine cabinet, as had a newly government-trained so-called dai in Pangjur (Towghi 2012). Government dais are permitted to assist homebirths; only LMOs are authorized to assist facility-based childbirths. However, at least until the recent (NIPS 2019) report based only on the study of approximately 12,000 households in Pakistan, dais and LHVs had been attending a majority of the 10 to 20% of births taking place in government and private facilities—a point that also emerged in my own interviews of health professionals.

This context is consistent with my observations, wherein dhīnabogs often found themselves instructing newly matriculated and established LMOs and LHVs how to detect the proper stages of pregnancy and the status of a labouring woman's cervical dilation (Towghi 2018). This recognition and value afforded to dhīnabogs' skills and expertise is a contrast to the homogenizing and de-individualizing construction of the TBA/dai reflected in the colonial demonization of the dai, and the post-colonial Pakistan governments pejorative statement: 'the culture of homebirth', a common refrain in policy documents constructing the home as an unhygienic and risk-laden space for mother and the foetus (Lal 1994; Malhotra 2003; Towghi 2014). Unable to institutionalize most childbirths, in 2007 Pakistan initiated a policy towards creation of a new cadre of women health workers called skilled birth attendants (SBAs) or community midwives (CMWs) in the hope that they would compete with and eventually replace TBAs in homebirths (WHO 2010). While this initiative advances the cause of increasing women medical workers, programme evaluations demonstrate a replication of issues related to deployment of LHVs that still plagues the state (Baig et al. 2017). The failed idea, originating in 1951, that LHVs, who were then considered community midwives, would eventually replace or displace the traditional midwives (dai/TBA), itself a replication of colonial ideology regarding dais/TBAs, is now evident in the push for SBAs/CMWs (Bhutta 2004; Government of Pakistan 2012).

Disciplining the 'Culture' of Homebirths, Yet Again, Now with SBAs

In the 1970s, the dai was reinscribed as a 'TBA' due to WHO decisions to train and incorporate her into the biomedical system to advance primary health care until all women gave birth in a biomedical facility (Towghi 2004). As anthropologists have noted, the term TBA has produced a generic, universal figure to serve the 'shifting' requirements of national health care goals, thereby occluding the heterogeneity of female medicinal work within and across nations (Towghi 2004). Yet, such processes of reduction/categorization are by definition incomplete and not internalized by midwives themselves. In contexts where health facilities are also inaccessible, indigenous midwives actually save lives, as was evident in Panjgur and further delineated below (Chawla 2006; Matthews 2002; Towghi 2018).

In Pakistan, the state first recruited dais in 1948 to advance family planning, due to their substantive role in homebirths and trust afforded to them by women (Towghi 2004). Subsequently, according to the Pakistan Ministry of Health, the 'traditional culture of birthing, in most rural and urban areas of Pakistan, hinders utilization of available [allopathic] services', encouraging governmental and non-governmental programmes to provide 'cash incentives to women to give birth in hospitals . . . [a]nd cash incentives to TBAs to bring the women there' (Government of Pakistan 2005: 23; WHO 2007). Premised on the link between persistence of homebirths, high maternal mortality ratio (MMR), and absence of SBAs, the 2007 CMW initiative aimed to replace TBAs tacitly constructed to be the raison d'être for the persistence of maternal deaths in the country (Government of Pakistan 2012: 66). Akin to the LHVs, CMWs were trained for 18 months in antenatal, intrapartum, postnatal and newborn care, placed in communities to redirect women away from TBAs to them. In the selected districts of Punjab and Balochistan (excluding Panjgur) where CMWs were deployed, their utilization for delivery was very low—in Punjab about 1.8 deliveries per CMW in one year. Women sought the CMW for antenatal care and the TBA for delivery. Conducting deliveries in a health facility, the CMWs charged women from US$11 to US$66. As a new young cadre of women in their twenties, childbearing women viewed them as inexperienced and thus distrusted them (Government of Pakistan 2012). This was not an irrational response. Before their deployment, 16% of CMW graduates had never conducted a delivery independently in hospitals, whereas 46% had never conducted one independently in the community (Eycon Private Ltd. 2014; Government of Pakistan 2010: 8).

Subsequent studies note that CMWs are 'struggling for survival' in rural Panjab, having been deployed in communities without adequate training, hands-on practice or experience, sufficient resources, or integration into the district health system (Sarfraz and Hamid 2014: 1). Similar issues arose with CMWs in Sindh, whose assessment identified significant deficiencies in their maternal and neonatal healthcare knowledge and skills (Lakhani et al. 2016). Moreover, the deployment of the CMWs, whether in the Punjab or Balochistan, could not resolve the type of infrastructural issues that were evident obstacles for dhīnabogs and women's health in Panjgur. The absence of transport, ambulance services, and quality services in nearby BHUs and RHCs to address complicated pregnancies and childbirths challenged CMWs' referral services (Ur Rehman et al. 2015: 181).

However, as the government advocates SBAs as a means to also replace TBAs, its contradictory relationship with TBAs is evident in its simultaneous authorization of TBAs to administer misoprostol in all childbirth cases for the pre-emptive prevention of PPH, despite uncertainty about the pill's safety and efficacy and in the absence of EmOC (Towghi 2014; Millard et al. 2014). While the global rationale to recruit and involve TBAs into state health projects is continually revised, the TBA is simultaneously misrecognized, and treated as an object to be eradicated. Her particular knowledge, expertise, social status, and life-saving work are effaced (Pigg 1995). Yet, the fact that the dai remains a powerful resource for women is evident in the re-returns of TBA training programmes (Towghi 2004). The first government TBA or dai training in Panjgur began only in 2004, nearly half a century after it was made available in the rest of Pakistan. Many dhīnabogs refused to attend this training, critiquing also the emergence of inexperienced 'dais' and the push for hospital births. Mirroring the global problem of recruitment and selection of TBA trainees first noted by Jordan (1989), among the 120 TBAs on the government ledger provided to me by the DHO, there were women who were not dais or had little to no experience assisting childbirth. Yet, in my search for them throughout the district, I would meet more than 200 dhīnabogs, many not on the ledger.

What these policies overlook is the ongoing harmful effects on women of biomedical obstetrics. In Pakistan, LHVs are noted to be endangering women's lives, causing injuries from legal and illegal invasive dilation and curettage (D&C) and uterotonic injections (Ahmad 2018; Khaskheli et al. 2014; Sathar et al. 2013). The rise of life-threatening maternal morbidities due to medical error and widespread misuse of oxytocin in South Asia among authorized and unauthorized practitioners is well documented (Brhlikova et al. 2009; Karachiwala et al. 2012). In Pakistan, Khaskheli et al. (2014) studied women who were referred from a periphery facility to the intensive care unit of Liaquat University Hospital. The researchers identified oxytocin misuse by LHVs or doctors, and negligence in blood transfusions and anaesthesia, as the main factors behind the women's condition. Drawing on multi-country studies, Lovold et al. (2008) found that injudicious oxytocin administration caused a substantial proportion of ruptured uterus cases in a facility or at home. Their analysis identified the increased need for neonatal resuscitation, and the rise in stillbirths due to oxytocin use during normal labour.

Malpractice by LHVs emerged as a common issue in my discussions with the DHQH Medical Superintendent (MS), Pakistani doctors, Panjguri men, women, and dhīnabogs (Towghi 2018). The absence of government oversight over the private sector means LHV and LMO malpractice is overlooked. While no longer state workers in their private clinics, LMOs particularly retained the state power to exert force, for example, in conducting routine episiotomies. LMOs and LHVs would also force premature childbirth with artificial labour induction. Men and women doctors I interviewed tacitly acknowledged LHVs' routine and untimely labour induction. While LHVs did not conduct episiotomies, dhīnabogs stated that they *zabar dasth* (intensely, forcefully, and in great quantity) administered uterotonics to force labour and delivery, often leading to perineum tear or a more serious problem that the LHV would then refer to an LMO, who in turn might refer the woman to a tertiary hospital in Quetta or Karachi. Panjguri dhīnabogs and women agreed that the absence of doctors in the hospital constrained women to seek out the LHVs, whose management of women's condition often resulted in iatrogenesis that LMOs might later manage. But they also witnessed LMOs pressuring women to use uterotonics (Towghi 2018). One doctor's uterotonic administration resulted in the death of a baby, an incident dhīnabogs, women, and their kin narrated at various times and locations, suggesting that stories of biomedical related harm, debility, and neglect travelled far and wide in the district. Whether we see this as false rumour or not, that the incident was also confirmed to me by both women and men doctors as well as the DHO I interviewed, indicates that the link between misuse of uterotonics and the woman's death was not merely about the circulation of the story or rumours among Panjguri women, but rather a tacit acknowledgement among doctors of the iatrogenic related risks faced by childbearing women.

Demanding Injections

Yes, we tell them that it is up to them to get the *thāgath wālā gooli* [the strength-giving pill—referring to the glucose drip] but we don't allow the *garme'n sūch-chin* [hot injection—referring to a uterotonic]. *Thāgathe'n sūch-chin is marzī wālā* [the strengthening injection is the one they can choose to have administered]. The child will die with the *garmā-ishī sūch-chin* if injected when the child is too far up.

Khatija

Historically, women's strength to endure the labour of childbirth depended especially on boiled milk and *roghan* (clarified butter/ghee), among other foods—important dietary sources for childbearing women, access to which had been dramatically disrupted by the 7-year-long drought underway during my fieldwork (Towghi 2012, 2014). *Dalda*, the commercial ghee available in the market, though considered less nutritious than the traditional homemade ghee, was unaffordable to most families. Consequently, along with uterotonics, some families, might request the 'glucose' IVs to enable 'weakened' women to bear the labour of childbirth (Towghi 2018). Dhīnabogs, as Khatija noted above, were familiar with the term glucose, employing it interchangeably with the vernacular term *thāgath* (strength).

Although dhīnabogs recognized and generally cautioned women and their kin about the consequences of unnecessary sūch-chins, they might still demand it. A mother and daughter (Fatima), both dhīnabogs, were not the first or the last to tell me that younger women were becoming accustomed to the sūch-chin. In their words, 'They *ladyān* do it as a habit now'. Consequently, if women do not have the *sabr* (patience) required to labour through childbirth, they request the injection to speed up childbirth. Fatima shares that, while certain things have improved for birthing women, artificially quickening contractions to create labour pain has its own set of consequences. In her view, women must now confront new difficulties, by and large, absent in the past:

When we did not have the *sūch-chins*, the *zahg-dān* [uterus; lit. child's sac] would not spoil and the child would not rot/decay and decompose [macerated foetus due to intrauterine death]. If the birth does not occur today, then perhaps it will tomorrow. Now God will open the way. If it is in Allāh's plans to take her/him then she/he won't be born. But, she/he will be born the day she/he is to be born. Now, forcing the birth with *garme'n sūch-chins* [hot injections] is forcefulness that causes harm, damages the woman's *jān* [uterus and body]. Those who do not understand this, may they not exist.

Dhīnabogs were tactful in their response towards *ladyāns'* increasing state-sanctioned biomedical influence over young women and their kin, reshaping their expectation about the delivery process. Consequently, some of them might demand labour-inducing injections from a dhīnabog. Dhīnabogs managed these bio-cultural transformations explicitly with their words and implicitly via the respect earned as elders and from the reputation of their dhīnabogiri. Khatija, a dhīnabog who had introduced me to Fatima and her mother was sitting among us. She explained how she managed impatient women:

> We tell women the child is about to be born, and that it is in its place. 'And you yourself will deliver the baby, and the child will be born as it is supposed to, and it is in position as it is supposed to be'. We tell them that, *'Shumā-rā Allāh Talā Rahmat kanth* [God will have mercy on you]'. In the past women had patience, they would wait; now they are focused on getting the baby out, even when their labour is not long or difficult.

The three dhīnabogs were quick to assure me that the young women typically 'listen to our words', regarding proper and improper timings of injection administration. Occasionally, however, the labouring woman or her kin refuse to wait. Rather than succumb to the family pressure, as Fatima explains, 'We instructed them to go to a lady'. Sometimes they insist that the dhīnabog call a compounder and instruct him to administer the injection.

This seeming divergence between younger and older women's perceptions of best approaches to caring for women is partly related to the pressures exerted on women and dhīnabogs by the ladyān towards institutionalized childbirth, and the transformations of nomadic lifeways due to forces of modernity and a long-standing drought. This has resulted in younger women's decreasing exposure to familiar Balochi herbal remedies, reshaping some women's attitudes towards Balochi medicine. For example, on a different lilated, as she further explained. Khatija remarked that dhīnabogs should be taught to administer the injection.

In general, dhīnabogs I interviewed did not have a dualistic or hierarchical view about the past versus the present situation confronting childbearing women. While Khatija was pragmatic about the injection, Fatima's mother similarly did not hold an entirely romantic view of women's past conditions, nor was she enamoured with the modern biomedical technologies subjected upon women. She tells me,

> Yes, there were difficulties in the past. Now things are improving, it is better now. In those times *Khudhā* [God] herself brought them into the world. Things could be stressful in the past. Yet, now, when one is in difficulty, immediately she is sent to the doctor. Once they reach there, immediately the cord is *cut*. Those who are sent to Karachi get operated on [referring to hysterectomies]. Now days, this is the difficulty. In those days she would be in labour pains for two to three days. Allāh delivered the baby. Now women are not allowed much time to labour. Instead, as soon as she goes into labour, the child is forced to be born, if the child is not born, the woman is sent to the city [Chitkan]. If the birth occurs in *lady*'s hand in the *shahr* [Panjgur city], then okay. If not, she is sent to Karachi, Turbat, or Quetta, and immediately she is *cut*.[4]

Fatima's mother, whose own mother had taught her to understand labour pains and assess the baby's in-utero position among other dhīnabogiri skills, was mentoring Fatima in the dhīnabogiri craft, continued: 'We know when it is right and wrong to administer the injection.' Then, referring to the first-ever TBA training recently instituted in Panjgur, she stated rhetorically, 'Where was training in those days'?' followed by, 'I have always been *Baloch*'. Evidenced in Fatima's mother's statement is the ways dhīnabogiri is inherent to be being Baloch. What does it mean when a Panjguri says, 'I am a Baloch'? How is this related to dhīnabogs and their view of their dhīnabogiri praxis? While dhīnabogs consistently invoked Allāh when speaking of the benefits of their dhīnabogiri and Balochi dhawā, they typically linked these to their Baloch rather than religious identity. In conversations about matters not apparently about politics, nationality, ethnicity, or tribal identity, Panjguris variously articulated the meanings of Balochness, or being a Baloch, iterating, 'I am a Baloch' in reference to things they deemed positive, negative, humorous, and sad about their life-world. For them, being Baloch was signified by a life lived with camels, mountains, trees, dates, lamb, sheep, and goats;

occasion, as I observed Khatija examine several pregnant wc
home, soliciting prenatal care there, two other dhīnabogs sittin̨
explained that their daughters too refuse Balochi dhawā due to
sion to the odour of the cooked herbs. One daughter refused despi
encing infertility for nearly 7 years. The second daughter reasoned
herbs: *manā bazh-zhī, mani dhil-ā bazh-zhī* (make me nauseous, n
feels queasy). This expression would become a mantra to my ears, echc
common explanation among dhīnabogs regarding young women's att
towards Balochi dhawā—a perception predominating in villages clos
Chitkan (central town of Panjgur), where LMOs' and LHVs' private prac
are concentrated and the DHQH located. Indeed, the further I travelled ft
Chitkan, the greater the criticisms of injections, as in the rural region whc
I met Khatija.

Khatija was not wholly against the use of uterotonics, having observec
that they provide relief to some women when administered properly. In her
view, however, many gynaecological problems can be avoided if women used
Balochi dhawā rather than be subjected to the risks of 'bad injections,'—often
prematurely administered. Khatija, like many other dhīnabogs, did not seem
to require a TBA training programme to learn about the misuses of labour-
induction biotechnologies. They were well aware of cases of trauma inflicted
on childbearing women from these injections:

> Yes, there are problems with the *sūch-chin*, such as if the baby is far and you
> inject her in the absence of real labour pains. Or you inject before ensuring
> the delivery of the placenta, or avoid ensuring that the cord is not around
> the baby's neck; or you inject when the child is not ready to be born. The
> child will die. You can damage her uterus. All this has occurred, and too
> often with a *lady*, and sometimes with a dai.
>
> Khatija

Here the reference to 'dai' is a balluk (a grandmother)—not a dhīnabog. The
dai had called a compounder to administer the uterotonic. Ten days later the
woman was taken to an LMO who told the woman's kin, 'The child *sa'rithag*
[has spoiled] and now you have brought her to me, now what can I do with
her?' The patient was then referred to Karachi, where she died following a
hysterectomy later the same year. She had three separate operations to help
stop chronic bleeding and stomach pain. So, as Khatija stated, 'This is a huge
damage caused by the *sūch-chin*. This *balluk* did not check to see if the child
was far'. The child was not ready to be born because the cervix was not fully

gathering and using herbs and wild plants; harvesting onions and other crops; residing in a *gidhām* (nomadic tent); being a generous and kind host to visitors and weary travellers; respecting one's mother, and other mothers; and living a rural, nomadic life (Towghi 2012). They spoke nostalgically about how some positive rural ways are losing ground to negative and less-hospitable city sedentary ways that include the rise in cocaine and hashish use among young men, encountering strangers one cannot trust, and the new habit of offering water only rather than tea and food to visitors.

Dhīnabogs' sense of Balochness was also marked by how childbirth was managed and situations like *dhuzzay dhardh* (false pain) with *Balochi dharmān* (herbal medicines) that they themselves have prepared with a variety of different *dhārū* (raw herbs), which they may have gathered from the fields or purchased from a *pensār*:

> When the real labour pain does not arrive, I administer the *Balochi dharmān* vaginally. The pain subsides if she has *dhuzz* [false labour pains] or some other situation such as vaginal or internal itching. Then in three to four days or even ten days she could be ready to give birth. If she has [real] labour pains, then the pains will speed up after the *dharmān* is administered. *Allāh thalā Shafā kanth* [God the exalted will heal her].
>
> Fatima's mother

Shafā is to heal; *Shafā kanth* means the one who heals. Dhīnabogs iterated Shafā sparingly to mark the efficacious power of dhīnabogiri work, certain herbs, and herbal formulas. That is, if and when their dhīnabogiri techniques and skills evidently healed women's ailments, they viewed this not to be their doing but God's work; God's hand is always present. They consistently referred to the medicinal properties of plants and herbs in this way. If herbs help to achieve the desired results, it is because God's hands are present. Allāh is working through the plants and their hands.

The post-partum *chillag/chillagi* (noun and adjective) is a herbal remedy that also carries the positive valence of Balochness. For example, a Punjabi woman asks a dhīnabog, 'How do Baloch women keep their stomachs so flat, small, and prevent bloating and gas after childbirth?' Many of the dhīnabogs spoke about chillagi herbal formula with a pride formed by their and women's observation of its efficacy. Their reference to chillagi dhawā's efficaciousness in women's post-partum care and recovery was entwined with their view of childbirth as energy-consuming physical work. Also, the encounter between a Punjabi woman and Panjguri kawwās revealed how cross-ethnic exchanges have the power to validate the continued worthiness of herbal practices and dhīnabogiri. Such stories served to re-signify and de-emphasize the claims that 'new' biotechnologies are an improvement upon 'old' ways of protecting women's health and healing bodies; at the same time, they demonstrated to the young generation the corporeal consequence of giving up 'past' practices. For instance, Gul Bibi, in her mid-eighties and one of the oldest dhīnabogs I met in Pangjur, exclaimed rhetorically:

> Where were the *doctir* and *lady* in the past? How would we have administered the *sūch-chin*? . . . You see there is one problem with *sūch-chin janag* [injecting]. I observe, is the child far? If I see that there is no hope of the child's birth now, in this situation, I don't inject. Now, once it is clear that the child is getting closer to the *nukkī* [cervix], you know then the child is nearing his/her time of birth, but you think the child may slide back up, you tell the *doctir* to administer the *thāghathe'n sūch-chins* [strengthening injection] . . . As soon as she becomes alert and gains strength, then she gains life in her heart . . . when strength comes to her, she is then able to give in to the pain, bear and push through the pain. The *lady* tends to inject before the labour pain start, the child is far, and not ready to be born.

Just as dhīnabogs acknowledge the various forms of biomedical cutting and operating, they understood that not all sūch-chins are equal in their purpose and effect. They explained that the *tukka* (tetanus vaccine injection) prevents the pregnant woman from catching 'the *hisābī* sickness [eclampsia/hypertensive disease]. Her hands and feet will not become swollen. So that she will not get sick'. Dhīnabogs and pregnant women did not complain about receiving the tukka to prevent neonatal and maternal tetanus.

Clearly, the Katagiri kawwāsi dhīnabogs did not reduce their objections to the overuse of certain injections to allopathic drugs versus Balochi dharmān. Rather, their principal concern was the mother and child's safety and future health, which they felt was further jeopardized due to declining use of Balochi medicine and inappropriate and unnecessary administrations of a variety of biomedical techniques and technologies, including the sūch-chin. They acknowledged that allopathic drugs could quicken labour, reduce the duration of the pain, force out a stillborn or live baby obstructed in childbirth, or dislodge a stuck placenta. However, they also observed the consequences of biomedical technologies on the foetus and the women that, in their view, often could have been prevented if women had used Balochi dharmān. In this regard, many women and dhīnabogs bemoaned having to go to the hospital, given their experience of obstetric violations—expressed to me in the refrain: 'They inject and inject, they inject too much' (Towghi 2018: 679). In their view, what brought women to the DHQH were political and economic disruptions of their extant though declining nomadic rural life-worlds, and clinical excesses of modernity in the form of unnecessary labour induction with synthetic drugs (Towghi 2012, 2014). According to a woman whose daughter at risk of a miscarriage was admitted to the DHQH after visiting an LHV's private clinic, the 'government gives us pills when we and our livestock require water and food'.

Panjguri women and dhīnabog explained that during antenatal visits the lady terrifies women and their families with diagnoses of high blood pressure, 'that they have this or that sickness, that the baby's head is big or small [premature]; or *nindhok* (in sitting position),' warning them, 'if you don't deliver in the hospital/clinic, you will die otherwise; the child will die, your veins will burst'. Women described how LMOs frequently held back the newborn until obtaining the demanded cash payment. Ironically, such abuses by biomedical practitioners are largely overlooked, leading at times to deadly consequences that remain unaudited (Towghi 2018). As such, while MMR declines are credited to biomedicine—attributed to facility-based births—the negative effects sometimes include a rise in caesarean surgeries and unnecessary hysterectomies, and mortality is not given same the visibility (NIPS 2019; Towghi 2014). In this unjust context, we can see next how affect might materialize in and outside of biomedical settings, with the potential to 'prime' dinabogs and women 'into action' against 'obstetric violence' (Castro and Savage 2018; Thrift 2008: 221).

Dhīnabogs' Embodied Affective Labour and Ethics of Care

The Ladies charge two to four thousand rupees and turn them away. We feel for the women. They are near death; they are our country people, poor people. Each month I do fifteen or more cases. This month I have already done four cases, and several more to deliver. In a day usually five to six people see me. My fate is good. The Ladies complain: 'you are taking my case; telling women, come we will check your BP [blood pressure], you can deliver here, don't go to the *dai*. None of my daughters have BP. Seven kids were born in my hands recently, none of the women had BP. The *shakar wālā* [diabetes] cases too, we did not have this problem . . . Placenta is delayed or stuck, loose or too soon, none of this the *lady* will work with'.

Murad-Bibi

Murad-Bibi was one of many dhīnabogs frequently sought out by women's kin for childbirth cases refused or mismanaged by LHVs and LMOs. Murad-Bibi described numerous cases that LMOs turned away, including women in an obvious critical medical condition. Six days prior to my first interview with her, Murad-Bibi assisted a woman in delivering twins. The LMO had refused to assist—informing the kin that one twin was dead, thus to take her to Karachi or Quetta. Instead, the family approached Murad-Bibi, who assessed that both babies were alive and helped deliver two healthy girls in the birthing woman's home. A mother of three sons and six daughters, Murad-Bibi is one of the few dhīnabogs who travelled extensively within and outside of Panjgur, to Karachi, to Sarawan in Iran, as well as to Dubai and Bahrain because of family ties in these places. Unsurprisingly, then, women from these locations journeyed to Panjgur to see Murad-Bibi for a resolution to their ailments ranging from infertility to gynaecologic cysts and abnormal bleeding. As she told me, they sought her 'for any and every woman's problem'. Then, concurrently, as if to conjure her mother's dhīnabogiri voice, she states, 'my mother would say, Allāh is with us and would proceed to assist them'.

Moved by the circulating narratives regarding past pious, respected, and accomplished dhīnabogiri, dhīnabogs frequently remembered the affective quality embodied by their foremothers when they reflected on their own capabilities, stating that they knew very little in contrast with their grandmother, great-aunt, or *kawwāsi* (expert) dhīnabog from a prior generation, whose work demonstrated deeper knowledge and skills. As Mazzarella (2009: 292) contends, Massumi (2002) characterizes affect as a domain of intensity, indeterminacy, and above all potentiality. Affect is both embodied and impersonal, which for Massumi is not equated with emotion. Affect registers how society is inscribed on our nervous system and flesh before appearing in our consciousness: 'The affective body . . . preserves the traces of past actions and encounters and brings them into the present as potentials: "Intensity is asocial, but not pre-social. In it lie trace of past actions including a trace of their contexts conserved in the brain and in the flesh"' (Massumi 2002: 30).

Dhīnabogs also accompanied women and their kin to Quetta or Karachi due to an obstructed childbirth that LMOs refused to manage. Having attended hundreds of childbirths, Murad-Bibi was sufficiently experienced to recognize, for example, when a baby could appear shoulder first, in a sitting position, a hand or arm hanging out of the uterus, or in breach position. LMOs refuse to work with women with such a presenting foetus or twins. For example, a family was told by the LMO to take their daughter to Karachi. 'So, they come to me, frantic', to avoid taking the long journey, 'I am now in a quandary, I have no choice but to help them. I feel responsible. I massage her, instruct her to move this way and that way. *Allāh Talah* then does the work, protects the mother and child, the head of the baby moves to its proper position', explains Murad-Bibi—understating her own role in the materialization of her embodied knowledge or the traces of her past actions, pace Massumi (2002).

Dhīnabogs were often hailed to assist women who were diagnosed with type-2 diabetes and instructed by the LMO to deliver at the DHQH. Upon reaching the hospital, many women would find there was no LMO; in effect, they learn the hospital is not the safe place it was constructed to be. It is also possible that women's kin could not pay the private fees of the LMO, who then turned them away. In such situations, Murad-Bibi has been summoned to the DHQH at 2, 3, or 4 a.m. by women's kin. Murad-Bibi's reputation as a skilled dhīnabog also attracted the attention of LMOs and LHVs, who requested she work with them. She declined, stating resolutely, 'I will never work in the hospital. I am not a government person. I don't work in front of men', referring to compounders sometimes called upon to administer the injection at the instruction of a midwife. 'I use my mind and intelligence. Do you understand? I am not *hispitali* (one who works in the hospital)'. Yet, Murad-Bibi's affective and practical response has been to act, even if it requires going to the DHQH when no doctor is present there. Disturbed by the bodily effects of the cracks of biomedicine, she like other dhīnabogs, viewed assisting women in emergencies as an ethical responsibility and the successes of their healing less as their own doing, and more the labour of Allāh transmitted through their hands.

I ask Murad-Bibi what motivated her to do her work, she replies:

This work cannot be done without the aid of Allāh . . . It is Allāh who heals the sick. There is one God who prays for us, provides us strength and her blessings. What other reason and benefit can there be than this? It is Allāh who does the healing, not me. I pray that Allāh bless and protect the woman and her baby, I say Amen, what other benefit can there be but this?

Murad-Bibi's ethical disposition was not an uncommon characteristic of dhīnabogs, whose 'relational care' produced and informed vernacularized forms of truth, authority, and expectations (Waldby 2012). Dhīnabogs embodied their ethics of care in their interactions with women and their kin. Their authoritative influence in Baloch women's lives was gained by their respectful approach to the care of women's bodies as much as their skills managing complex and serious reproductive conditions.

Unlike Murad-Bibi, Mah-Jaan—who was called a dai or TBA by the government health personnel—was one of the few expert dhīnabogs recruited by DHQH to work in the attached MCH centre, one of the four in the district. Just like Murad-Bibi, Mah-Jaan did not rely on a compounder. She was trained and allowed to administer the injection herself. She did not refer to herself as a dai. She told me, 'Before I was a *nawkar* [servant, government employee], I would not administer the *sūch-chin*. My mother never did. I managed many childbirth cases before becoming a *nawkar* as I watched and learned from my mother'. Mah-Jaan explained her decision to become a dhīnabog thus:

> My mother said do it, I said I was scared, but then attended my sister's and aunt's cases, helping them to deliver their children. My mother told me, 'A time will arrive when you will have a peace of mind in your home in having this work. With your help, God will make lives of other Musalmāns better. Your work will be of support to others. This is a very good and right type of work. It is not only a livelihood, but also a service to humanity'.

In a classic Balochi expression: *hakkn jāghā hak dayanth; sawābī jāghā sawābe'n* (honest work returns honest results; pious work is a blessing), Mah-Jaan's mother expressed core moral and ethical principles embodied by dhīnabogs and associated with their self-imposed responsibility in caring for women. This phrase would be iterated by many dhīnabogs for whom doing dhīnabogiri was considered an honest, sacred duty that one must do without expectation of any material gain. They viewed such work a blessing for the one doing the work. This was work that required them to be attuned to women's contingent individual conditions and biomedical experiences that were increasingly being shaped by infrastructural failures that also constrained biomedicine and medical doctors' capacity to provide the care women in an obstetric emergency require (Towghi 2018).

Conclusion

Dhīnabogs confront and contain the lingering violence of colonial medical ideology that the hospital is the proper place of childbirth, the home and dais dangerous, reflecting the persistent failure of the state to relegate them to the past. Thus, with their continued presence, they not only offer a powerful critique of women's iatrogenic suffering but save women's lives from iatrogenically-induced emergencies. The dhīnabogs inform and produce localized forms of truth, authority as well as ethics of care, that contest biomedical hegemony. The state cannot ignore them, and nor can women ignore them, despite state pressures to produce the contrary. In Panjgur, 'the time of the lady', as dhīnabogs would often say, is not a triumphant arrival. How the ethical self is fashioned, embodied, articulated in the everyday is reflected in choices dhīnabogs made regarding the care of childbearing women. Dhīnabogs' commitment to their craft was a value passed on from one generation to another, less through any clearly defined social structures of inheritance or customary hierarchy, but rather through their understanding of ethical imperatives shaped by women's need for care and the exigencies of childbirth. For them, this time of the lady is suggestive of an era that is 'out of joint' from another time when safe and healthy pregnancy, childbirth, and post-partum were a norm rather than an exception (Ram 2013: 101). In *Fertile Disorder*, Ram describes the way spirit 'possession, located by performance traditions as the culmination of a *repeated process of retelling* and reliving the life and death of a murdered hero, dramatizes . . . a human capacity' to act in the face of injustice and suffering (2013: 102; emphasis mine). Following Deleuze and Guattari (1987), she calls this the capacity to be affected by the violent death of another human being.

Dhīnabogs too are affected, but also affect the techno-medicalized experiences of childbearing women. Ram (2013: 102) describes the spirit possession of women in Tamil Nadu as a heightened attunement to women's suffering. Deleuze and Guattari (1987: 278), she notes, emphasize the mobile flow of energies and intensities not only between human subjects but also between human subjects and all that the world contains. Affect in this sense is intimately connected with the body's capacity to act, the capacity to be affected by others and to affect others in turn. This is the sense in which I understand dhīnabogs' actions. Of course, unlike the experience of women that Ram is writing about, dhīnabogs are not possessed by spirits, rather they witness the repeated and increasing numbers of women's physical suffering and the iatrogenic reproductive traumas experienced by them. Dhīnabogs are moved to act from a place of ethics, a virtue that they viewed, at times consciously, to be a sacred action that mattered because it pleased Allāh.

Notes

1. Western biomedicine was brought to India by the British, vernacularly known, variously, as 'allopathy', 'Ingrezy' (English medicine), or 'Doctiri' (Arnold 1993). In Pakistan, the use of 'allopathy' or simply 'medicine' persists in lieu of 'biomedicine'.
2. All names have been anonymized.
3. Women's Health Project Baseline Survey (2004), District Panjgur. Unpublished Report for Save the Children @USA.
4. Here Fatima uses 'cut' in multiple senses: cutting the umbilical cord, cutting the abdomen and uterus for a C-section, the episiotomy cut, and cutting out the uterus. Her reference to an operation refers to a C-section, the surgical removal of the uterus, or a hysterectomy—all types of cutting and operating that women can end up experiencing in a biomedical institution.

References

Ahmad, Israr. 2018. 'Ill-Trained LHV Endangers Women's Life'. *The Nation*, 25 January. Accessed 23 March 2020. https://nation.com.pk/25-Jan-2018/ill-trained-lhv-endangers-woman-s-life

Arnold, David. 1993. *Colonizing the Body*. Berkeley & Los Angeles: University of California Press.

Arshad, Maha, Mohammad Ahmed Arif, Sadia Riaz, Kashaf Naz, Mohammad Haseeb, Maryam Nazir, and Fatima Mukhtar. 2017. 'Medical Students' Preferences for Working in Rural Areas after Graduation: Results of a Cross-Sectional Study'. *Pakistan Journal of Medical & Health Sciences* 11 (3): 1032–7.

Baig, Marina, Rafat Jan, Arusa Lakhani, Sadia Abbas Ali, Kiran Mubeen, Shahnaz Shahid Ali, and Farzana Adnan. 2017. 'Knowledge, Attitude, and Practices of Mid-Level Providers Regarding Post Abortion Care in Sindh, Pakistan'. *Journal of Asian Midwives* 4 (1): 21–34.

Bhutta, Zulfiqar Ahmed, ed. 2004. *Maternal and Child Health in Pakistan: Challenges and Opportunities*. Karachi: Oxford University Press.

Brhlikova, Petra, Patricia Jeffery, Gitanjali Priti Bhatia, and Sakshi Khurana. 2009. 'Intrapartum Oxytocin (Mis)use in South Asia'. *Journal of Health Studies* 2: 33–50.

Castro, Arachu, and Virginia Savage. 2019. 'Obstetric Violence as Reproductive Governance in the Dominican Republic'. *Medical Anthropology* 38 (2): 123–36. doi: 10.1080/01459740.2018.1512984.

Chawla, Janet. 2006. *Birth and Birthgivers: The Power behind the Shame*. New Delhi: Har-Anand Publications.

Deleuze, Gilles, and Félix Guattari. 1987. *A Thousand Plateaus: Capitalism and Schizophrenia*. London: Bloomsbury Publishing.

Eycon Private Ltd. 2014. *Baseline Survey Report: Integrated Maternal, Newborn and Child Healthcare Project, Districts Gwadar, Lasbela & Ziarat of Balochistan Province*. Pakistan: Save the Children & the Australian Agency for International Development.

Ghaffar, Abdul, Shehla Zaidi, Huma Qureshi, and Assad Hafeez. 2013. 'Medical Education and Research in Pakistan'. *The Lancet* 381 (9885): 2234–6. doi: 10.1016/S0140-6736(13)60146-4.

Government of Pakistan. 2005. *The Roadmap for Action: Millennium Development Goals in Pakistan. National Maternal and Child Health Policy and Strategic Framework (2005–2015)*. Islamabad, Pakistan: Ministry of Health.

Government of Pakistan. 2010. *Assessment of the Quality of Training of Community midwives in Pakistan*. Islamabad: Technical Resource Facility.

Government of Pakistan. 2012. *Midterm Evaluation of the Maternal Child Health Program*. Islamabad, Pakistan: Technical Resource Facility.

Hezekiah, Jocelyn. 1993. 'The Pioneers of Rural Pakistan: The Lady Health Visitors'. *Health Care for Women International* 14 (6): 493–502.

International Federation of Gynecology Obstetrics. 2012. 'Prevention of Postpartum Hemorrhage with Misoprostol'. *International Journal of Gynecology & Obstetrics* 119 (3): 213–14. doi: 10.1016/j.ijgo.2012.09.002.

Jeffery, Patricia, Roger Jeffery, and Andrew Lyon. 1989. *Labour Pains and Labour Power: Women and Childbearing in India*. London: Zed Books.

Jeffery, Roger, Patricia Jeffery, and Andrew Lyon. 1984. 'Only Cord-Cutters? Midwifery and Childbirth in Rural North India'. *Social Action* 34 (3): 229–50.

Jordan, Brigitte. 1989. 'Cosmopolitical Obstetrics: Some Insights from the Training of Traditional Midwives'. *Social Science & Medicine* 28 (9): 925–37. doi: 10.1016/0277-9536(89)90317-1.

Karachiwala, Baneen, Zoe Matthews, and Asha Kilaru. 2012. 'The use and Misuse of Oxytocin: A Study in Rural Karnataka, India'. *BMC Proceedings* 6 (S1): P12. doi: 10.1186/1753-6561-6-S1-P12.

Khaskheli, Meharun-nissa, Shahla Baloch, and Aneela Sheeba. 2014. 'Iatrogenic Risks and Maternal Health: Issues and Outcomes'. *Pakistan Journal of Medical Sciences* 30 (1): 111. doi: 10.12669/pjms.301.4062.

Lakhani, Arusa, Rafat Jan, Kiran Mubeen, Sadia Karimi, Shahnaz Shahid, Rozina Sewani, Marina Baig, and Farzana Adnan. 2016. 'Strengthening the Knowledge and Skills of Community Midwives in Pakistan through Clinical Practice Internships'. *Journal of Asian Midwives* 3 (2): 26–38.

Lal, Maneesha. 1994. 'The Politics of Gender and Medicine in Colonial India: The Countess of Dufferin's Fund, 1885–1888'. *Bulletin of the History of Medicine* 68 (1): 29–66. doi: https://www.jstor.org/stable/44451545

Lovold, Ann, Cynthia Stanton, and Deborah Armbruster. 2008. 'How to Avoid Iatrogenic Morbidity and Mortality While Increasing Availability of Oxytocin and Misoprostol for PPH Prevention?' *International Journal of Gynecology & Obstetrics* 103 (3): 276–82. doi: 10.1016/j.ijgo.2008.08.009.

Malhotra, Anshu. 2003. 'Of Dais and Midwives: "Middle-class" Interventions in the Management of Women's Reproductive Health—A Study from Colonial Punjab'. *Indian Journal of Gender Studies* 10 (2): 229–59. doi: 10.1177/097152150301000203.

Massumi, Brian. 2002. *Parables for the Virtual: Movement, Affect, Sensation.* Durham, NC: Duke University Press.

Matthews, Zoe. 2002. *Maternal Mortality and Poverty.* London: DFID Resource Centre for Sexual and Reproductive Health.

Mazzarella, William. 2009. 'Affect: What Is It Good For?' In *Enchantments of Modernity: Empire, Nation, Globalization,* edited by Saurabh Dube, 291–309. London, New York, and New Delhi: Routledge India.

Millard, Colin, Petra Brhlikova, Allyson M. Pollock. 2014 'Commentary: Evidence versus Influence in the WHO Procedure for Approving Essential Medicines: Misoprostol for Maternal Health'. *British Medical Journal* 349: g4823.

National Institute of Population Studies (NIPS). 2008. *Pakistan Demographic and Health Survey 2006–07.* Islamabad & Calverton, MD: National Institute of Population Studies and Macro International.

National Institute of Population Studies (NIPS). 2013. *Pakistan Demographic and Health Survey 2012–13.* Islamabad & Calverton, MD: National Institute of Population Studies and ICF International.

National Institute of Population Studies (NIPS). 2019. *Pakistan Demographic Health Survey key findings 2017–18.* Islamabad & Rockville, MD: National Institute of Population Studies and ICF International.

Pigg, Stacy Leigh. 1995. 'Acronyms and Effacement: Traditional Medical Practitioners (TMP) in International Health Development'. *Social Science & Medicine* 41 (1): 47–68.

Pinto, Sarah. 2008. *Where There Is No Midwife: Birth and Loss in Rural India.* New York & Oxford: Berghahn Books.

Ram, Kalpana. 2013. *Fertile Disorder: Spirit Possession and Its Provocation of the Modern.* Honolulu: University of Hawai'i Press.

Ram, Kalpana, and Margaret Jolly, eds. 1998. *Maternities and Modernities: Colonial and Postcolonial Experiences in Asia and the Pacific.* Cambridge: Cambridge University Press.

Renfrew, Mary J., Alison McFadden, Maria Helena Bastos, James Campbell, Andrew Amos Channon, Ngai Fen Cheung, Deborah Rachel, Audebert Delage Silva, Soo Downe, Holly Powell Kennedy, and Address Malata. 2014. 'Midwifery and Quality Care: Findings from a New Evidence-Informed Framework for Maternal and Newborn Care'. *The Lancet* 384 (9948): 1129–45. doi: 10.1016/S0140-6736(14)60789-3.

Rozario, Santi. 1998. 'The Dai and the Doctor: Discourses on Women's Reproductive Health in Rural Bangladesh'. In *Maternities and Modernities: Colonial and Postcolonial Experiences in Asia and the Pacific,* edited by Kalpana Ram and Margaret Jolly, 144–76. Cambridge & New York: Cambridge University Press.

Sarfraz, Mariyam, and Saima Hamid. 2014. 'Challenges in Delivery of Skilled Maternal Care: Experiences of Community Midwives in Pakistan'. *BMC Pregnancy and Childbirth* 14 (1):59.

Sathar, Zeba, Susheela Singh, Zakir Hussain Shah, Gul Rashida, Iram Kamran, and Kanwal Eshai. 2013. *Post-abortion Care in Pakistan: A National Study.*

Islamabad: Population Council, National Committee for Maternal and Neonatal Health, Guttmacher Institute, and Research and Advocacy Fund.

Shah, Sayed Masoom, Shehla Zaidi, Jamil Ahmed, and Shafiq Ur Rehman. 2016. 'Motivation and Retention of Physicians in Primary Healthcare Facilities: A Qualitative Study from Abbottabad, Pakistan'. *International Journal of Health Policy and Management* 5 (8): 467. doi: 10.15171/ijhpm.2016.38.

Society of Obstetricians and Gynaecologists of Canada. 2004. 'FIGO/ICM Global Initiative to Prevent Post-partum Hemorrhage'. *Journal of Obstetrics and Gynaecology Canada* 26 (12): 1100–2. doi: 10.1016/s1701-2163(16)30440-6.

Tanner, Jeffery, Ana M. Aguilar Rivera, Tara L. Candland, Virgilio Galdo, Fredrick E. Manang, Rachel B. Trichler, and Ritsuko Yamagata. 2013. *Delivering the Millennium Development Goals to Reduce Maternal and Child Mortality: A Systematic Review of Impact Evaluation Evidence*. Washington DC: Independent Evaluation Group (IEG), World Bank.

Thrift, Nigel. 2008. *Non-representational Theory: Space, Politics, Affect*. London: Routledge.

Towghi, Fouzieyha. 2004. 'Shifting Policies toward Traditional Midwives: Implications for Reproductive Health Care in Pakistan'. In *Unhealthy Health Policy: A Critical Anthropological Examination*, edited by Arachu Castro and Merrill Singer, 79–95. Walnut Creek, CA: Altamira.

Towghi, Fouzieyha. 2012. 'Cutting Inoperable Bodies: Particularizing Rural Sociality to Normalize Hysterectomies in Balochistan, Pakistan'. *Medical Anthropology* 31 (3): 229–48. doi: 10.1080/01459740.2011.623488.

Towghi, Fouzieyha. 2014. 'Normalizing Off-Label Experiments and the Pharmaceuticalization of Homebirths in Pakistan'. *Ethnos: Journal of Anthropology* 79 (1): 108–37. doi: 10.1080/00141844.2013.821511.

Towghi, Fouzieyha. 2018. 'Haunting Expectations of Hospital Births Challenged by Traditional Midwives'. *Medical Anthropology* 37 (8): 674–87. doi: 10.1080/01459740.2018.1520709.

Towghi, Fouzieyha, Farid Midhet, and Iain Aitken. 2000. Women's Perceptions of Causes and Consequences of Obstetric Bleeding in Khuzdar, Balochistan. In *Working Paper Series 10(8)*. Cambridge, MA: Harvard Center for Population and Development Studies, and Harvard School of Public Health.

Ur Rehman, Shafiq, Jamil Ahmed, Sher Bahadur, Amber Ferdoos, Muhammad Shahab, and Nazish Masud. 2015. 'Exploring Operational Barriers Encountered by Community Midwives When Delivering Services in Two Provinces of Pakistan: A Qualitative Study'. *Midwifery* 31 (1): 177–83. doi: 10.1016/j.midw.2014.08.006.

Waldby, Catherine. 2012. 'Medicine: The Ethics of Care, the Subject of Experiment'. *Body & Society* 18 (3–4): 179–92. doi: 10.1177/1357034X12451778.

WHO Health and Life Sciences Partnership & National Maternal Newborn and Child Health Programme. 2010. *Guidelines for the Deployment of Community Midwives*. Islamabad: Government of Pakistan.

WHO. 2007. *Health Systems Profile: Pakistan*. Cairo: EMRO Regional Health Systems Observatory.

4

Training Birth Attendants in India

Authoritative Knowledge Social Forms, Practices, and Paradoxes

Pascale Hancart Petitet

Unlike many mammals, human females have many problems in giving birth: they have a small pelvic outlet and bear infants having large heads. Post-partum haemorrhage, one of the main causes of maternal death, may be a consequence of human placental biology and also related to the shift towards bipedal locomotion approximately 7 million years ago and its consequences for pelvic anatomy (Rockwell et al. 2003, cited in Abrams and Rutherford 2011). When nothing is done to avert maternal death, natural mortality is estimated at 1,500/100,000 live births.[1]

From the last decades of the 19th century, training of traditional birth attendants (TBAs) was one strategy implemented in various colonies in order to reduce maternal mortality. As described in Samiksha Sehrawat's chapter in this volume, India was no exception in the mobilization of TBAs in attempts to introduce safe childbirth practices. The issue of TBA mobilization offers a lens to observe the social construction and the social production of the hierarchy of knowledge in the field of maternal health and childbirth. This chapter interrogates the local and global processes of construction, legitimization and delegitimization, and political use of the knowledge of TBAs in the Indian context. The issue also offers a prism to analyse the long-running division between two conceptions of the body. One, reflecting World Health Organization (WHO) policies, sees the physical body as an essentially uniform construction across time and cultures, allowing biomedical obstetric knowledge to be applied everywhere. The second conception acknowledges that various determinants shape the variability of birthing systems. The issue of mobilizing TBAs offers a starting point for analysing how the authoritative knowledge (Jordan 1978) surrounding birth is channelled, experienced, and enacted. Here we use the theoretical concept of authoritative knowledge in two ways. Firstly, to examine how the Western biomedical system imposes

Pascale Hancart Petitet, *Training Birth Attendants in India* In: *Childbirth in South Asia.*
Edited by: Clémence Jullien and Roger Jeffery, Oxford University Press. © Oxford University Press 2021.
DOI: 10.1093/oso/9780190130718.003.0004

its authority in discrediting 'alternative' home-based healthcare practices. Secondly, to understand how recent Indian policies with respect to the location of birth have interacted with these alternative systems. More specifically we will observe to what extent the knowledge of rural women in India acquired through their lived experience is marginalized, challenged, and sometimes reinvented.

I draw on the analysis of the literature on TBAs, on my own experience of designing and implementing programmes aiming at reducing maternal mortality, as well as on my intensive ethnography conducted from 2003 to 2006, in Tamil Nadu, South India. My research involved observation and interviews with rural women of ex-untouchable castes (mainly Paraiyar, Arundhatyar, and Vannan) in villages neighbouring Pondicherry and Namakkal cities. Additional data from TBAs and biomedical caregivers were collected in a public district hospital, in a rural healthcare centre, and in a private nursing home (Hancart Petitet 2008). The chapter is organized in four sections. The first approaches briefly the different roles that trained TBAs have played in successive health policies. The second section aims to examine the plurality of discourses produced on TBAs. The third section provides ethnographical insights to document TBA training from the point of view of TBAs in Tamil Nadu. The last section describes the local interpretations of TBAs as a biomedical concept. Then it sheds light on the processes and the local forms of the reappropriation of TBAs' training by themselves and by their users. Here my aim is to show the heterogeneity of TBAs' social power, the eclectic modes of their practices, and their strategic use of training to enhance their positions.

Historical Facts and Health Justifications

With the assumption that biomedicine was capable of preventing the majority of maternal deaths, one of three WHO recommendations was to train TBAs in the basic principles of obstetrics and in the recognition of complicated delivery cases to be referred to health centres.[2] In 2004, after years of debates among the scientific and developmentalist communities related to the role of TBAs in the reduction of maternal mortality rates, WHO recommended stopping training activities targeting TBAs and gradually replacing them by training so-called skilled birth attendants (World Health Organization 2006). Until then TBAs were the targets of various development programmes and the subject of various social sciences research projects. But what were the representations and roles attributed to TBAs in the social history of the medicalization of childbirth in India?

In India, the first services involving the provision of healthcare during childbirth date from the beginning of the 19th century. In those days most deliveries took place at home with the assistance of a TBA or a member of the family and birth was described as a very welcome event for the pregnant woman and her family while also being considered a polluting and impure moment (Good 1991; Jeffery and Jeffery 1993). Scholars have analysed the medicalization of childbirth as interrelated to various social movements: first the social reform movement in the 19th century and then the nationalist politics and colonial public health policies of the 20th century (Guha 2017). In Tamil Nadu, the Madras Lying-in Hospital played a pioneering role in maternity provision and midwifery training in India (Lang 2005). As in the other Indian states, TBA training also took place within the National Dai Training Scheme initiated during the sixth Five-Year Plan (1980–85). The training had the objective to shape TBA practices during pregnancy and childbirth according to biomedical principles. As in numerous Southern countries, the training of TBAs has been centred mainly on the promotion of so-called safe practices (washing the hands, cutting the umbilical cord with a sterilized razor blade etc.) and the abandonment of practices deemed to be harmful (such as repeated vaginal examination, uterine massages during labour). The training proved to be mostly effective in reducing harmful practices and in raising positive post training practices. However, it had a very limited impact on maternal mortality because of the absence of any connection with a referral system by which complicated deliveries could be speedily transferred to healthcare facilities (Saravanan et al. 2011). The 1994 report, 'Action Plan for Revamping the Family Welfare Programme in India', brought out by the Ministry of Health and Family Affairs (Government of India 1994), also mentions the insufficient number of instructors, the lack of pedagogic materials, the maladapted, too technical, and too lengthy teaching courses, and the fact that TBAs' knowledge and skills were not taken into account in the training modules. However, in India and as in other Southern countries, it might have contributed to reducing the rates of perinatal death, stillbirth, and neonatal death (Sibley et al. 2012). Within the National Rural Health Mission (NRHM) (2005–12) various reforms were implemented in maternal healthcare provision (Srivastava et al. 2018) including a new module for TBA training. This measure, mostly taken in order to supplement the unavailability of health workers in remote rural areas (Sengupta

2019), also aimed to improve the referral system between birth attendants and obstetric care centres.

Plurality of Discourses Pertaining to TBAs

The literature produced by public health experts and social scientists in India on the role given to TBAs in the establishment of public health services is abundant, not always based on scientific facts and, as elsewhere, contradictory. Two major opinions can be distinguished. Some support the benefits of the involvement of TBAs in the implementation of health programmes. Others assume a position favouring the disappearance of them and their practices.

TBAs and Public Health Policymakers

What has been called 'the failure of the training of TBAs' regarding the objective of reducing maternal mortality rate is commonly acknowledged by decision-makers in international public health institutions, some researchers and some representatives of non-governmental organizations (Berer 2003) who agree that when human resources of a level of medical competence higher than that of the TBAs are available, TBAs should be 'consigned to history and that is where they belong'. Some authors argue that investment in the training of TBAs may have had as its sole effect to delay, in countries with 'limited resources', the establishment of adequate emergency obstetric services. TBAs do not have the ability to apply the measures required for the care of obstetric complication. Also, any TBA training has to be supported by the establishment of a referral system between 'the community' and the biomedical care services, which was rarely the case. By around 2000, the adopted consensus was that the proportion of deliveries made by 'skilled birth attendants' was the only reliable indicator to measure programme effectiveness. This term, from which even 'trained' TBAs are excluded, refers to the midwife, the doctor, or the nurse who has benefited from a theoretical and practical training (Abouzahr and Wardlaw 2001).

Parallel to these points of view, a fair number of those who are in favour of TBAs continue to believe strongly in the major role they play in the improvement of the health of mothers and children (Ray and Salihu 2004). When and where the access to obstetrical services is limited, TBAs appear as relays of biomedical health services. Some years ago, the transnational WHO recommendations envisaged the use of TBAs to reduce neonatal hypothermia and to prevent chlamydial ophthalmologic infection (World Health Organization. Maternal Health and Safe Motherhood Programme.1996). In the context of the spread of the HIV/AID epidemic many initiatives have also been taken to involve TBAs in the prevention of mother to child transmission of HIV including giving to HIV infected mothers the short course treatment with nevirapine (Hamela et al. 2014).[3] Recently TBAs have been mobilized to use misoprostol to treat post-partum haemorrhage in home deliveries (Abbas et al. 2019).[4] In India, TBAs were sometimes designated as the ideal actors for improving the perception and acceptability of contraceptive methods in rural areas (Singh and Kaur 1993), or for the screening of pulmonary infections in their village and the administering of anti-tuberculosis treatment at the patient's home (Balasubramanian 1997). Several studies have demonstrated positive health outcomes among mothers and infants after training of TBAs (Saravanan 2012), for example, the positive effects of neonatal resuscitation training on the survival of newborn babies (Bang et al. 1999).

Some authors (Pigg 1997) have also shown the obvious complexity of the limitation of the training of TBAs by underscoring the mistakes made during the implementation of the training: the lack of awareness of the social and cultural context of the birth as well as the employment of inappropriate pedagogic practices based mainly on didactic methods of instruction. The other deficiencies mentioned are the TBA's lack of social power (when, for example, she is supposed to make the decision to send a woman giving birth to the hospital) and the economic limitation of the referral decision (payment for transport and medicines). The limitations of the biomedical services may also stand as a determinant of the failure of the training of TBAs, given the lack of personnel, equipment, organization, and medicines (Pendse 1999). Lastly, the applicability of the practices that women have been taught is also questioned.

Outside this sphere, circumscribed by biomedicine, TBAs are also at the centre of discussions related to the social production of hierarchy among medical systems. The protagonists of the movements in favour of TBAs tend to emphasize to representatives of the biomedical system the idea according to which the manners of treatment do not depend only on biomedical competence but also have to do with other forms of knowledge in which TBAs are judged to be skilful and experienced (Chawla 2006). At first, we propose a focus on the 'Natural Childbirth' promoters. Then some positions formulated by the 'Traditional system of medicine' defenders will be examined.

TBAs and 'the Traditions'

The 'Natural Birth' Promoters

The issue of training of TBAs must also be analysed in considering the criticisms of the biomedicalization of childbirth made by the defenders of natural childbirth. These positions come within a perspective of Western feminist movements stating that childbirth carried out in the biomedical milieu is a form of alienation of the female body by technologies (Davis-Floyd and Sargent 1997). In this context, systematized care practices (such as the utilization of oxytocic drugs, electronic surveillance of foetal heart rate, uterine activity, and epidural analgesia) are perceived as making the woman an 'object to give birth' (Jordan in Davis-Floyd and Sargent 1997). Notwithstanding a certain idealization of 'traditions', this ideological interest has made it possible to shed light on the major drawbacks of the biomedicalization of birth.

In India from 2005, the programme Janani Suraksha Yojana (JSY) aiming to reduce the maternal mortality ratio (MMR) has contributed to an increase in the proportion of institutional births from 20% to 49% in 5 years (Sabde et al. 2018). Alongside the biomedicalization of birth, and mostly among the urban high and middle class, an increasing number of voices and initiatives have been raised to promote natural childbirth. For example, Mira and Bajpai (1996) studied the TBAs' practices (use of medicinal plants, massages, food prescriptions, fumigations, etc.) in various states in India. Some activists suggest that childbirth should be understood as an everyday event for which the contribution of technology would not be justified. Gulati (1999) notes, in substance, that childbirth is an ancient event and that its process is 'as simple as breathing'. Nutan Pandit, who directs a birth centre in Delhi, has no training in obstetrics and introduces herself as a pioneering natural childbirth expert. She started teaching childbirth preparation in 1978, after experiencing two easy, normal deliveries herself. She asserts that 'Surely if nature has gifted fertility to women, it has also gifted the power of birthing. All women should have faith in their body's ability to birth a baby naturally'.[5]

The organization MATRIKA (Motherhood and Traditional, Resources, Information, Knowledge and Action), led by Janet Chawla, a medical anthropologist, aims to index and to promote traditional delivery care, particularly in the states of Rajasthan, Bihar, Punjab, and Delhi (Chawla 2006).[6] Chawla assumes that TBAs are an homogenous group of people and practices, and that the TBA, always seen as a sympathetic caregiver, takes into consideration the desires of the woman giving birth. Doctors, midwives, and nurses overuse technologies (foetal monitoring, episiotomy, forceps, caesarean section); they do not care about obtaining the consent of their patients for the decisions they make, and they give them no choice regarding the care received (Van Hollen 1998), or disrespect and abuse women during institutional childbirth Chattopadhyay et al. 2018) By contrast, a TBA is seen as facilitating the birth event by allowing the female body to express itself freely (Gulati 1999). According to this current of thought, issues related to TBA training are off the subject: their 'traditional' know-how is sufficient to manage a 'natural' birth.

The Defenders of Indigenous Medicine

Numerous Indian organizations have established programmes with the objective of preserving and revitalizing indigenous medicine. In the 2000s, their stated aim was to fill the gap of the biomedical system and provide care accessible for vulnerable communities.[7] Among the multitude of projects and organizations, I will mention here the two largest. The Centre for Indian Knowledge Systems (CIKS) had the objective of 'exploring and developing the contemporary relevance and application of traditional Indian systems of medicine'.[8] Based in Chennai since 1995 and initially involved in Vrkshayurveda promotion (the ancient Indian plant science), CIKS has also developed activities in the field of organic agriculture and biodiversity conservation. Based in Bangalore since 1991, the Foundation for Revitalization of Local Health Traditions (FRLHT) is at the origin of the Institute of Ayurveda and Integrative Medicine (I-AIM) and of the University of Transdisciplinary Health Sciences and Technology (TDU).[9]

The representatives of the two organizations cited above put forward the benefits of the traditional system of medicines. They also argue that indigenous medical knowledge can compensate for the deficiencies of the Indian biomedical system and offset the endemic shortcomings of biomedical care. According to Hafeel and Suma (2000), the recognition by international organizations of the interest in training TBAs, at that time, speaks in favour of the relevance of preserving the 'monumental heritage' of ancient medicines.

Since 2000, both CIKS and FRLHT have widely developed their activities respectively in organic agriculture/biodiversity and for the institutionalization of the AYUSH systems of medicine.[10] Similarly to the position taken by international organizations, integrating TBAs into biomedical services is no longer a claim. This issue illustrates the various social forms of interrelations between the medical systems existing in both India and the West since the colonial period. As described by scholars (Harrison 2001), the impact of Western medicine on existing health systems in India has indeed to be analysed as an agency, a complex interface that produced adaptation, assimilation, reinterpretation, or resistance.

To resume, the training of TBAs was seen as a special leitmotiv suited to satisfy, on the one hand, the obligations of international institutions in need of low-cost services favouring the health of mothers and children. For other organizations that defended tradition, the training of TBAs provided a good opportunity for recognition and access to national and international funding. TBA training was proposed in regions such as Ladakh, in Himalayan India, where TBAs 'traditionally' do not exist. In such a context, training TBAs has been seen as a cost-effective relevant strategy to provide healthcare to poor and remote villages.

After this exploration of the plurality of representations and discourses on TBAs in India from an 'etic perspective', the second section of this chapter is dedicated to its examination on our field site, Tamil Nadu. Our aim is to question the construction of the authoritative knowledge in the sphere of childbirth by giving voice to TBAs themselves.

TBA Practices in Tamil Nadu: An Emic Perspective

In Tamil Nadu, TBAs or *maruttuvacci*,[11] have long been the main actors in the care of pregnancy and childbirth, mainly in the rural areas. In the context of the generalization of biomedical services, the continuation of their activities was linked to several factors: the social role, sometimes very important, that the community attributes to them; the meagre recourse to biomedical care among certain populations; and the absence of generalized distribution of these services in isolated rural areas.[12] Spouses of barbers (Ambattan) are often practising as TBAs. Other TBAs belong to untouchable castes such as Paraiyar, Arundhathiyar, or Vannan.[13] Mostly, those women came to occupy the role of TBA from one generation to the next, or more recently due to economic difficulties. Indeed, TBA used to be a hereditary occupational position but in a context of poverty the lack of job opportunities also led women to become TBAs, even if nobody in their family was involved in this field (see, for example, Jeffery et al. 1989). Moreover, the practices of TBAs are not always limited to care given during pregnancy and normal delivery. Some of them also provide treatment for infertility, obstructed labour, post-partum haemorrhage, or genital infections (see Hancart Petitet 2011b). Some TBAs occupy a prominent place during ceremonies celebrating the events connected with reproduction. This is the case of the puberty rite of a girl, the *mañcanīr*, the rite of the seventh month of pregnancy, the *valaikāppu* (Hancart Petitet and Vellore 2007), and the *tiṭṭukkaṛittal*, the bath of purification given to the delivered mother and the newborn. Other TBAs know how to prepare the *naṭṭu maruntu*, local remedies. Lastly, some TBAs from the Ambattan caste are able to recite the *manrāṭṭam*, ritual formulae used in order to move aside demons and bad spirits (Hancart Petitet 2009). Other TBAs also occupy broader roles in providing healthcare. The TBA Angelai, about 60 years old from the caste of Vannan paria, the untouchable caste of whiteners, told me: 'From the conjuration of the evil eye (*drsti*) during funeral, to the ritual where the *tali* is removed, I am present. It is not just that. I healed the foot strains, hip strains, neck strains, shoulder strains' (Hancart Petitet 2011a).

The low social status awarded to TBAs in India has often been described. The variability of this status exists and is not unrelated to the ambivalence of childbirth as both an auspicious and an impure event. Birth is also considered to be a good omen as it comes along with a change in the status of the delivered woman and of her relatives, especially if the newborn is a boy. Also, the tasks, the social status, and the decision-making power of TBAs vary according to geographic location, social position, and requirements of the family of the labouring woman (Jeffery and Jeffery 1993; Pinto 2008).

According to my observations in Tamil Nadu, TBAs mostly operate only inside their caste, or in castes of similar or lower rank. The blood and the products of excretion of the childbirth (amniotic liquid, stool, urine) are certainly considered as polluting. If certain TBAs are relegated to the world of the impure, others are respected and worshipped. One of the most reputed TBAs in the surrounding area was called a *kula deivam* (family deity). She was seen as very brave as she had no fear of performing very sensitive acts such as touching the blood of delivery, which used to be considered highly polluted: 'Contrary to the doctor at the hospital, who uses gloves, she is courageous. She makes the delivery with her bare hands. If she has to search for the placenta, she does not use an aspirator, she puts her hand directly inside' (Villager woman, near Pondicherry).

We now need to pay closer attention to the preference of villagers to use TBA services rather than to go to health centres and hospitals at the time of delivery. Those arguments, formulated by the women and their families and ignored by the detractors of the TBAs, plead in favour of a preference for home delivery. Home delivery indeed requires no preliminary preparation, prenatal consultation, blood test, or examinations, which multiply the visits to the centre of care and the expenses associated with this mode of therapeutic recourse. In Tamil Nadu, Ram (1994) and Van Hollen (1998) pointed out reasons why women do not go to the hospital even if the TBA does recommend it. Indeed, people preferred not to go to the hospital because of previous bad experiences (delay in being attended by health staff, not receiving care at all, bad behaviour of staff). I observed that women would go to the primary healthcare centre for delivery only if they knew and trusted the caregivers posted there. Many women also spoke about the isolation and the solitude felt during childbirth in a biomedical environment. Very often, according to them, the nurses visit them only at the last moment of birth or sometimes even 'when everything is done and when the baby is already out!' About childbirth at home, on the other hand, the birth attendant Angelai recalled: 'Her relatives such as her aunts, sisters-in-law, sisters, mother and mother-in-law will stay with her. They will play tricks and mockeries to lead to forget her labour pain. They will say: "when you were happy with my brother, you said nothing, but you had pain isn't it? then you cannot bear this pain? eh!"' (Hancart Petitet 2011b).

With the implementation of local strategies aiming to reduce the maternal mortality rate, new health actors appeared in villages: the auxiliary nurse midwife (ANM). ANMs, occupy the lowest rank in the Indian public health bureaucracy. They are young women recruited after the end of their tenth year of schooling and they receive 18-month's training. They oversee encouraging women from rural areas to go to hospital for the follow-up of their pregnancy and childbirth. Furthermore, they are expected to be responsible for the birth itself. The ANMs are posted in primary healthcare centres where they are supposed to live and to be on duty 6 days per week. However, absenteeism is common and ANMs operate various strategies to be able to justify it. In Rajasthan, Banerjee et al. (2008) observed that ANMs overused the term 'exempt days', which stands for any absence that is the result of a government-mandated meeting, survey, or other authorized health work. Let us give an example from our fieldwork. The TBA Palavankodie explained the modalities of her collaboration with the young ANM recently posted in her village: 'She [the ANM] asked me to record my home deliveries under her name. So I recorded fifty cases under her name. She told me that she would pay me 50 rupees for each one, but she still did not give the money to me'. Besides, as an economy measure, the villagers preferred to request the help of Palavankodie, despite the latter being forbidden to assist home births.

In order to bypass this ban, Palavankodie is called only at the last stage of the labour when the time of expulsion is imminent. Such practice appears dangerous: no care is given to the woman during labour—while it is likely that certain remedies given by Palavankodie could be effective. Also, no one is present to diagnose obstetrical complications—while Palavankodie could identify some signs of the danger (Hancart Petitet 2013).

Numerous variations exist among TBAs. They are mainly related to the various circumstances that led them to take on this role (caste origin, social events, economical need, etc.), to their social networks, and to their contacts with the biomedical system—many factors that determine the heterogeneity of their practices (see further below). However, TBAs are often perceived as constituting a homogeneous group of 'traditional' practitioners. Scientific, 'developmentalist',[14] or ideological discourses regarding them are always constructed and developed based on this presupposition.

'Traditional Birth Attendants'

Local Interpretations of a Biomedical Concept

In the 19th century, colonial administrators, missionaries, and medical professionals had already grouped all the Indian TBAs under the appellation 'dai' (Van Hollen 2003). Such assumption leading to the invisibilization of plurality for the benefit of a normative homogeneity has been analysed by anthropologists. In the 1980s, and following Brigitte Jordan (1978), various researchers raised issues related to the construction of biomedical power as an imposition of normative values on birth. For example, they investigated popular versus biomedical birthing practices: position during labour and delivery; childbearing and newborn care, etc. They described how the implementation of the biomedical model of childbirth produced various coercive forms of control of the targeted population. It also shaped the subordination of indigenous medical practitioners to biomedical representatives (Ginsburg and Rapp 1991). Consequently, TBAs appeared on the scene of international public health as an invented, supposedly homogeneous category. The purpose of the appellation 'TBA' was to respond to a need for generalization required to transcribe international organizations' objectives in the language of transnational expertise (Pigg 1997: 233–362).

In international public health institutions, transnational expertise is exercised mostly without any sensitivity to local distinctions. The institutional need to find women to train as TBAs led to grouping together women who had quite different functions under a single generic term. Consequently, three categories of practitioners were presented as similar. The first included women whose social role in the community consists not only in the regular practice of childbirths at home, but also in providing treatments for diverse bodily afflictions as well as the performance of rites marking the different stages of life. The second category was represented by women who occasionally assist at their relatives' and friends' childbirths. The last group consists of women who never practised childbirth, but who were recruited in the training framework based on criteria such as age or level of education. At the end of common training, these women were supposed to carry out deliveries. All in all, they did not necessarily see themselves as 'TBAs'. They mostly saw the TBA training as an opportunity to learn new practices, to legitimize their own ones, to get social recognition or financial gain. In Tamil Nadu, criteria used in order to recruit TBAs vary according to districts. In a village near Pondicherry, a nurse responsible for the recruitment of TBAs for training told me:

> We give training to the birth attendants of the village by taking their experience into account. It is necessary to have worked at least five years as birth attendant to take part in this training. If we come to know that the mother or child die during the childbirth attended by a birth attendant, we do not take this birth attendant who caused these deaths.

This quote illuminates one viewpoint of representatives of the biomedical system regarding the practices of TBAs. Those practices are mainly decontextualized from the social and economic realities underlying health practices. I observed, as did Davis-Floyd earlier, that TBAs are perceived by authorities and public health stakeholders as responsible for the high maternal and child mortality rates in their village. This attitude allows them to provide politically correct explanations on maternal mortality issues. Firstly, it minimizes the deficiency of infrastructure, such as the absence or bad condition of roads suitable for motor vehicles, the lack of transport and/or resources. Secondly, such an explanation overlooks the previous bad experiences of women at hospital and their underlying causes, such as the lack of resources, poor training, and recognition of the staff.[15] Finally, the imputation of the responsibility for maternal mortality rates to TBAs leads to various difficulties when recruiting candidates to be trained. As the nurse cited above explains, the solution to recruiting TBA candidates is as follows: 'Finally, we train the girls who want to be trained. That is how birth attendants without experience take part in this training. After the training, they are called traditional birth attendants'.

The social construction of the role of the TBAs is sometimes related to their previous training in the biomedical system. Indeed, that training may have provided benefits for women expecting upward social mobility. However, their role and status were also shaped by other factors such as the social function attributed to them by their respective communities before the training. In some regions of North India, the birth attendants would be of inferior social standing. Their tasks are perceived as limited to the handling of waste matter from the delivery—blood, umbilical cord, placenta—which are deemed to be impure (Jeffery and Jeffery 1993). However, such a statement that the dai's functions during childbirth are limited to the practice of dirty work needs to be revisited. As Pinto (2006) suggests: 'While all of these acts can be understood through the idiom of "pollution taboo", to think of Dalit women's labour solely in those terms is to undermine its symbolic, physical and social value'. According to the peasant women I have met in South India, the removal of polluting matter was never presented as an essential act of the delivery, nor seen as the major function of the TBAs.

I now wish to draw attention to what remains after the training of TBAs. In this last section, training will be examined first as the acquisition of new knowledge and skills whether or not put into practice. Training also needs to be analysed as a form of social capital.

The Traces of TBAs' Training and Their Mode of Reappropriation

My long-term ethnography in Tamil Nadu gave me various opportunities to explore the various aspects of the traces of TBAs' training. My purpose here is to present the TBAs' intimate perceptions and experiences of this training. I propose to examine the contradictions they encountered in implementing the learned practices as well as their modes of reappropriation of these practices. We found that mostly TBA training had limited impact on the functions and practices of the maruttuvacci, who already benefit from a good social status in their community. However, some maruttuvacci were disappointed after the training, as villagers thinking that they were already paid by the government were not willing to pay for their services anymore. This policy had another unintended consequence. In Tamil Nadu, for example, the term maruttuvacci, designating the Hindu TBAs of this region, received a negative connotation after the implementation of the government TBA training. It brought about the distinction between the dai 'trained' in the biomedical framework and the untrained maruttuvacci (van Hollen 2003).

Numerous training programmes concluded with the awarding of a small metal valise to those newly trained TBAs. This valise contained diverse materials and consumable products that were supposed to be appropriate for establishing the new status of the 'trained' women and the application of the good practices that have been learned. However, few of these programmes foresee the implementation of follow-up activities and the renewal of the materials distributed. For example, I met Panchalie, an old village birth attendant in a deserved area surrounding Pondicherry. She said: 'Yes, since the training I always use gloves to make a delivery. But now only one remains as the other was taken by a crow'.

In some cases, the main objective of TBA training implemented in this area in the 2000s was simply to increase the number of delivering women sent to the hospital. TBAs were supposed to recognize obstetrical complications and to encourage and accompany these women to deliver in health institutions. Those complications were said to be easy to identify (bleeding during pregnancy, haemorrhage during or after delivery, fever, headache, oedema of member and face, duration of labour over 12 hours). However, the absence of recognition of obstetrical complications by TBAs was frequently reported by the nurses and midwives I met in village health centres. They understood that the abundance of bleeding was, for example, not interpreted by TBAs and villagers as a retention of the placenta or a uterine rupture, but as the proof of the ejection of impure blood and of the good functioning of nature. Much remains hidden from the view of the evaluators of TBA training.

For some of my informants in Tamil Nadu, placental retention was not seen as a dangerous and unpredictable obstetric anomaly but as a voluntary action effected by the woman who gives birth. It is said in this case that this woman is *pisani* (stingy). 'She hides her placenta and eats it in secret, without telling it to her stepmother', says Angelai. This was a commonly shared perception among our informants. The symbolic significance of this retention was seen as an act of rebellion against the hierarchical order established in the marital home. In everyday life the young wife, subject to the authority of her mother-in-law, is required to take her meals in the kitchen, only after having served at table members of her family (Hancart Petitet 2011b). Moreover, other reasons stand behind the non-application of good learned practices. Social and commercial logics also led some TBAs to shape their practices according to the desire of their patients and not according to the biomedical technique they are supposed to implement after the training. Satchadie, a 'trained' TBA in the town of Pondicherry remarked: 'If I do as they do in the hospital, why would the women prefer to give birth with me?'

As rightly remarked by Satchadic in the previous sentence, there is a need to understand why women choose to deliver with her help rather than to go to the hospital. How and why did Satchadie recompose episiotomy,[16] a very well-known obstetrical practice? This practice is the object of numerous controversies within the biomedical environment. In South India, the episiotomy seems widely practised in public or private maternities. At home, as well as in the campaign in urban areas, numerous TBAs also resort to its use in cases of complicated childbirth. Satchadie, trained in the biomedical practice of the episiotomy in a hospital, justified her refusal to apply the learned cutting and suturing practices when performing an episiotomy:[17] 'During my training they gave me all the equipment: scissors, thread and a thin needle, but I do not use them. I apply my former method, I make the cut by knocking'. Applied in the last phase of the expulsion when 'the baby is stuck', the 'cut by knocking' consists in applying a jerking twisting motion with the index and major fingers, joined and tightened on the low and median part of the vulva. The immediate, obtained, and wished effect is a vertical tear of the perineum. This tear will not be sewn up again and will need specific and repeated medical care:

> If the baby does not go out it means that the mouth [the vulva] is too small. At the hospital they open it with scissors, but I do it this way, and it will open. Then, when the baby is outside, I wipe the body of the woman. I wet a tissue with brandy and I apply it on the cut. I ask the lady to hold the joined legs and the bandage will stick to it. After the third day, I apply *Dettol* and I do the bandage once again. But I do not make the suture.
>
> Satchadie

As explained by Satchadie, the methods of the repair of the cut are a determining factor in the acceptance of episiotomy by the patients:

> People call me at their home because they are afraid of the cut and of the suture at the hospital. If I make it as they do at the hospital, what they will do? The women cannot bear the pain of the suture. Thus they refuse. Sometimes I tell them, that it will not hurt, that we can do it, but they say no. They want me to apply my method as usual.

This quote illustrates how the learned practices within the biomedical system are reinterpreted and incorporated into the construction of new practices. This issue has been discussed, for example, by Jordan (1989) and Pigg (1997). They highlight that, contrary to the presuppositions of the biomedical trainers, a learned practice is rarely applied. In our example the gap proceeds at another order. If the argument 'they do not want' makes sense within the problem of the relations of caste, class, and power governing social relationships between Satchadie and the woman giving birth, it also illustrates a form of equal sharing power between Satchadie and the women she assists. It is true that scholars widely highlight the correlation between power and use of technology in the biomedical arena of the birth (Davis-Floyd and Sargent 1997). However, the example of Satchadie shows that within a 'traditional' system the use of technology does not reduce the space of negotiation of care practices.

Contrary to what Stephens (1992) found in Andhra Pradesh, in a survey of urban TBAs who trained in the biomedical field and who got improved status after the training, the status of Satchadie remains unchanged before and after the training. Her status did not improve (which could be the case because of a recognition gained as a health professional or using new equipment). Nor is it devalued (for example, because of a lack of remuneration for home-based acts that users would consider from now as paid by the government). The status of Satchadie is not linked to the rate of remuneration for her care services, nor to her low caste, but to her knowledge and skills guided by her spiritual power acquired as *kula deivam* (Hancart Petitet 2009).

According to biomedical instructors, only the knowledge learned during the training is to be integrated and applied by the TBAs. Nevertheless, the ethnography of their practices teaches us that 'trained' TBAs recompose this new knowledge. This knowledge and the apparent advantages that its dispensation involves (an allowance for daily expenses, association with the hospital and its actors) can be at the root of familial, social, and economic emancipation of the TBAs. They favour the invention of new practices. Far from being the major influence in the transformation of the practices of TBAs, the biomedical system training represents only one of several factors determining TBA practices. Some TBAs integrate different components of the act of caring—the context, the choice of medicine used, the earlier practice exercised, the practice learned, or the request of the patient—in order to recompose a practice of caring that is better adapted to a given situation and patient at a given time. These practitioners opt for a legitimization that no longer depends on their rank in the hierarchy of the biomedical system. This legitimization is built according to their capacity to produce and to spread new forms of care, forms of theory and practice borrowed from the register of biomedical knowledge *and* from the corpus of popular knowledge regarding childbirth.

The Emergence of New TBAs?

Jordan observed that during TBA training, biomedicine, which she terms 'cosmopolitan medicine', presents itself as a form of authoritative knowledge. This training relegates indigenous knowledge to the benches of illegitimacy and does not accord any consideration of the 'traditional' modes of apprenticeship. It favours the acquisition of knowledge through biomedical instructors in a system in which all traditional practices are absent or devalued. Jordan concludes that in spurning indigenous knowledge, 'cosmopolitan' obstetrics becomes 'Cosmo-political' obstetrics, that is, a system that reinforces a particular distribution of power among different social and cultural strata (Jordan 1978). Nevertheless, the supposed monolithic hegemony of biomedicine on indigenous medical systems has been widely dismantled (Harrison 2001), and the encounters between Western medicine and traditional childbirth practices are much more complex than a vertical imposition of the values of one system on the other. As far as TBAs are concerned, they are still very active in many places as the biomedical obstetric services are far from covering the needs of the entire Indian population and they mostly reinterpreted and transformed the practices learned during the teaching received in the biomedical system. Public health actors also perceived, reinterpreted, and used the knowledge of TBAs in different ways. Once TBAs were perceived as wicked mothers whose archaic practices must be controlled. Later, TBAs brought together ideal elements of any development activity—locality (with a rural, local character), community, and low cost—and were also seen as the emblematic ambassadors of traditional knowledge. Then, following the new global strategy to reduce maternal mortality, TBAs have been gradually replaced by ANMs. In early 2000, a large proportion of the population still had no access to maternal healthcare and delivered at home with a TBA (Hogan et al. 2010). Since 2000, under India's National Population Policy and the Reproductive and Child Health programme (RCH-II) and its commitment to achieving Millennium Development Goal 5 (MDG5), various initiatives have been introduced in order to promote and implement institutional birth services.[18]

Despite this recent and unprecedented commitment of donors in the field of maternal health in the Southern countries, various questions remain in uncertainty. Given the persistent inequalities in access to healthcare and the interrelated collapse of the market economy, the universal biomedicalization of childbirth may remain limited. We talked to the daughters of Angelai,

Palavankodie, Satchadie, and others. None of them was willing to be trained by their mother or take over their tasks and responsibilities. TBA work was seen as 'too difficult' because they have to be available day and night, 'too dirty', and 'too badly recognized and paid'. Nevertheless, many non-biomedically trained birth attendants continue to take care of women's childbearing in India and in many other parts of the world (Sarker et al. 2016). In India, many activists are raising their voices (Sadgopal 2009) and acting to continue to promote traditional birth practices in deserved areas.[19] Also, various initiatives offer alternative natural birth options for upper- and middle-class women.[20] Therefore, a careful reading of contemporary reconfigurations of the knowledge and practices mobilized in the field of human reproduction remains relevant: What are the emerging social forms of 'authoritative knowledge' when the 'biomedical things' (Hardon and Moyer 2014) are not available, or when people do not want to interact with it?

Notes

1. Between 1990 and 2015, maternal mortality worldwide dropped by about 44%. Today 99% of all maternal deaths occur in developing countries (World Health Organization 2015).
2. The two other recommendations were: (1) to inform pregnant women regarding risks and possibilities of recourse should an obstetric complication arise; (2) to establish medical institutions for obstetric emergencies as well as a service providing medical care for abortions.
3. Nevirapine is the antiretroviral treatment specific to the reduction of the vertical transmission of HIV at childbirth. On issues related to TBAs and HIV in India, see Hancart Petitet in Hancart Petitet 2011a: 199–226.
4. During the second half of the 1980s, Misoprostol was registered, under the name Cytotec, for the treatment of peptic ulcers in many countries. Since then, it has also been used to start labour, treat post-partum bleeding, or induce an abortion.
5. 'See http://ncbchildbirth.com/about/, accessed 10 March 2021, devoted to the Nutan Pandit Natural Childbirth Centre, based in Delhi.
6. See chapters by Chawla and by Mehrotra in Chawla (2006).
7. The unstated goal can be a personal desire for social, political, and/or economic emancipation. But this is not specific to these organizations. On the social and political stakes in the 'revitalization' of the so-called traditional medicines, see Pordié (2005).
8. See the website: http://ciks.org/, accessed 10 March 2021.
9. See the website: http://www.frlht.org/, accessed 10 March 2021.

10. AYUSH is the acronym of the medical systems that are being practised in India such as Ayurdeva, Yoga, Unani, Siddha, and Homeopathy.

11. Tamil vernacular term: *maruttu*: local remedies, *vacci*: woman. The vernacular terms noted in italics are transliterated according to the rules adopted by the Tamil Lexicon (1924–36).

12. Because of lack of knowledge regarding the factors of obstetric complications or because of lack of trust in biomedical service. See, for example, the works of Ram (1994).

13. Paraiyars: Traditionally, peasants and drums players. Arundhathiyars: Contemporary term used to define the leather worker caste speaking Telugu, also named Sakkili. Vannan: Washerman. Responsible for ceremony of birth, puberty, wedding, and death. The schematic elements are indicative. For a contemporary treatment of the caste system see Deliège (2004).

14. That is to say, the discourse of experts in development activities.

15. See the analysis of Jaffré (2009) related to the structural determinants of maternal mortality in West Africa.

16. The episiotomy is a median cutting of the perineum during the last phase of childbirth to quickly enlarge the opening for the baby to pass through.

17. Generally, the practice of episiotomy is not included in TBA training.

18. See Chapter 1 of this volume.

19. For example, Jan Swasthya Sahyog in Madhya Pradesh organizes dai training on a regular basis: see http://www.jssbilaspur.org/dai-training, accessed 10 March 2021.

20. For example, the Natural Birthing Centre in Kerala, http://birthvillage.in accessed 10 March 2021.

References

Abbas, Dina F., Nusrat Jehan, Ayisha Diop, Jill Durocher, Meagan E. Byrne, Nadeem Zuberi, Zafar Ahmed, Gijs Walraven, and Beverly Winikoff. 2019. 'Using Misoprostol to Treat Postpartum Hemorrhage in Home Deliveries Attended by Traditional Birth Attendants'. *International Journal of Gynecology & Obstetrics* 144 (3): 290–6.

AbouZahr, Carla, and Tessa Wardlaw. 2001. 'Maternal Mortality at the End of a Decade: Signs of Progress?' *Bulletin of the World Health Organization* 79 (6): 561–73.

Abrams, Elizabeth T., and Julienne N. Rutherford. 2011. 'Framing Postpartum Hemorrhage as a Consequence of Human Placental Biology: An Evolutionary and Comparative Perspective'. *American Anthropologist* 113 (3): 417–30.

Balasubramanian, Rani. 1997. 'Feasibility of Utilising Traditional Birth Attendants in DTP'. *Indian Journal of Tuberculosis* 44 (3): 133–5.

Banerjee, Abhijit V., Esther Duflo, and Rachel Glennerster. 2008. 'Putting a Band-Aid on a Corpse: Incentives for Nurses in the Indian Public Health-Care System'. *Journal of the European Economic Association* 6 (2–3): 487–500.

Bang, Abhay T., Rani A. Bang, Sanjay B. Baitule, M. Hanimi Reddy, and Mahesh D. Deshmukh. 1999. 'Effect of Home-Based Neonatal Care and Management of Sepsis on Neonatal Mortality: Field Trial in Rural India'. *The Lancet* 354 (9194): 1955–61.

Berer, Marge. 2003. 'Tbas Cannot Be Expected to Carry Out HIV/AIDS Prevention Activities for Women Giving Birth at Home'. *Reproductive Health Matters* 11 (22): 36–9.

Chattopadhyay, Sreeparna, Arima Mishra, and Suraj Jacob. 2018. ' "Safe", Yet Violent? Women's Experiences with Obstetric Violence during Hospital Births in Rural Northeast India'. *Culture, Health & Sexuality* 20 (7): 815–29.

Chawla, Janet. 2006. *Birth and Birthgivers: The Power Behind the Shame.* New Delhi: Har-Anand Publications.

Davis-Floyd, Robbie E., and Carolyn Fishel Sargent. 1997. *Childbirth and Authoritative Knowledge: Cross-Cultural Perspectives.* Berkeley: University of California Press.

Deliège Robert. 2004. *Les castes en Inde aujourd'hui.* Paris: Presses Universitaires de France.

Ginsburg, Faye, and Rayna Rapp. 1991. 'The Politics of Reproduction'. *Annual Review of Anthropology* 20 (1): 311–43.

Good, Anthony. 1991. *The Female Bridegroom: A Comparative Study of Life-Crisis Rituals in South India and Sri Lanka.* Oxford: Clarendon Press.

Government of India. 1994. *Plan for Revamping the Family Welfare Programme in India.* New Delhi: Ministry of Health and Welfare.

Gulati Ambica. 1999. *Birth: In Whose Hands?* Lifepositive. Accessed 8 March 2021. https://www.lifepositive.com/birth-in-whose-hands/

Hafeel, Abdul, and T.S. Suma. 2000. 'Monumental Heritage'. *The Hindu*, 8 October, Folio: Indian Health Traditions.

Hamela, Gloria, Charity Kabondo, Tapiwa Tembo, Chifundo Zimba, Esmie Kamanga, Innocent Mofolo, Bertha Bulla, Christopher Sellers, R.C. Nakanga, and Clara Lee. 2014. 'Evaluating the Benefits of Incorporating Traditional Birth Attendants in HIV Prevention of Mother to Child Transmission Service Delivery in Lilongwe, Malawi'. *African Journal of Reproductive Health* 18 (1): 27–34.

Hancart Petitet, Pascale, and Vellore Pragathi. 2007. 'Ethnographie Views on the "valaikāppu": A Pregnancy Rite in Tamil Nadu'. *Indian Anthropologist* 37 (1): 117–45. Accessed 8 March 2021. http://www.jstor.org/stable/41920031.

Hancart Petitet, Pascale. 2008. *Maternités en Inde du Sud. Des savoirs autour de la naissance au temps du sida.* Paris: Edilivre

Hancart Petitet, Pascale. 2009. 'Transformations contemporaines des pouvoirs, des savoirs et des pratiques de Satchadie, matrone à Pondichéry'. In *Figures contemporaines de la santé en Inde*, edited by Patrice Cohen, 195–214. Paris: L'Harmattan.

Hancart Petitet, Pascale 2011a. *L'art des matrones revisité : Naissances contemporaines en question.* Paris: Éditions Faustroll.

Hancart Petitet, Pascale. 2011b. 'Les mots d'Angelai: Figures de discours et pratiques de soins d'une matrone en Inde du Sud'. In *Dire les maux: Les médecines traditionnelles en paroles, études, témoignages et documents*, edited by Rémi Bordes, 189–210. Paris: Karthala.

Hancart Petitet, Pascale. 2013. 'Les derniers jours de Palavankodie. Transformations et effacement de la pratique de matrone en Inde méridionale'. In *Les nouveaux guérisseurs. Biographies de thérapeutes au temps de la globalisation*, edited by Laurent Pordié and Emmanuelle Simon, 99–107. Paris: Edition EHESS.

Hardon, Anita, and Eileen Moyer. 2014. 'Medical Technologies: Flows, Frictions and New Socialities'. *Anthropology & Medicine* 21 (2): 107–12.

Harrison, Mark. 2001. 'Medicine and Orientalism: Perspectives on Europe's Encounter with Indian Medical Systems'. In *Health, Medicine and Empire: Perspectives on Colonial India*, edited by Biswamoy Pati and Mark Harrison, 37–87. London: Sangam.

Hogan M.C., K.J. Foreman, M. Naghavi, S.Y. Ahn, M. Wang, S.M. Makela, A.D. Lopez, R. Lozano et C.J.L. Murray. 2010. 'Maternal Mortality for 181 Countries, 1980–2008: A Systematic Analysis of Progress towards Millennium Development Goal 5'. *The Lancet* 375 (9726): 1609–23.

Hours, Bernard. 2003. 'Coopérations, conflits et concurrences dans le système international de santé'. In Coopérations, conflits et concurrences dans le système de santé, edited by Geneviève Cresson, Marcel Drulhe, and François-Xavier Schweyer, 21–30. Rennes, EHESP : Presses de l'Ecole des hautes études en santé publique.

Jaffré, Yannick, ed. 2009. *La bataille des femmes: Analyse anthropologique de la mortalité maternelle dans quelques services d'obstétrique d'Afrique de l'Ouest*. Paris: Éditions Faustroll.

Jeffery, Patricia, Roger Jeffery, and Andrew Lyon. 1989. *Labour Pains and Labour Power: Women and Childbearing in India*. London: Zed Books.

Jeffery, Roger, and Patricia Jeffery. 1993. 'Traditional Birth Attendants in Rural North India: The Social Organization of Childbearing'. In *Knowledge, Power and Practice: The Anthropology of Medicine and Everyday Life*, edited by Shirley Lindenbaum and Margaret Lock, 7–31. Berkeley: University of California Press.

Jordan, Brigitte. 1978. *Birth in Four Cultures: A Crosscultural Investigation of Childbirth in Yucatan, Holland, Sweden and the United States*. Montreal, Canada: Eden Press Women's Publications.

Jordan, Brigitte. 1989. 'Cosmopolitical Obstetrics: Some Insights from the Training of Traditional Midwives'. *Social Science and Medicine* 28 (9): 925–37.

Lang, Sean. 2005. 'Drop the Demon Dai: Maternal Mortality and the State in Colonial Madras, 1840–1875'. *Social History of Medicine* 18 (3): 357–78.

Mira, Sadgopal, and Smita Bajpai. 1996. *Her Healing Heritage: Local Beliefs and Practices Concerning the Health of Women and Children: A Multistate Study in India*. Chetna Publication.

Pendse, Vinaya. 1999. 'Maternal Deaths in an Indian Hospital: A Decade of (No) Change'. In *Safe Motherhood Initiatives: Critical Issues*, edited by Marge Berer and T. K. Sundari Ravindran, 119–26. Oxford, England: Blackwell Science.

Pigg, Stacy Leigh. 1997. 'Authority in Translation: Finding, Knowing, Naming, and Training "Traditional Birth Attendants" in Nepal'. In *Childbirth and Authoritative Knowledge: Cross-Cultural Perspectives*, edited by Robbie E. Davis-Floyd and Carolyn Fishel Sargent, 233–62. Berkeley: University of California Press.

Pinto, Sarah. 2006. '*More Than a Dai: Birth, Work and Rural Dalit Women's Perspectives*'. In Seminar: Special Issue, Dalit Perspectives, Delhi, February 2006.

Accessed 8 March 2021. https://www.india-seminar.com/2006/558/588%20 sarah%20pinto.htm.

Pinto, Sarah. 2008. *Where There Is No Midwife: Birth and Loss in Rural India.* New York & Oxford: Berghahn Books.

Pordié Laurent (Dir.). 2005. *Panser le monde, penser les médecines. Traditions médicales et développement sanitaire.* Paris : Karthala.

Ram, Kalpana.1994. 'Medical Management and Giving Birth: Responses of Coastal Women in Tamil Nadu'. *Reproductive Health Matter* 2 (4): 20–22.

Ray, Alison M., and H.M. Salihu. 2004. 'The Impact of Maternal Mortality Interventions Using Traditional Birth Attendants and Village Midwives'. *Journal of Obstetrics and Gynaecology* 24 (1): 5–11.

Sabde, Yogesh, Sarika Chaturvedi, Bharat Randive, Kristi Sidney, Mariano Salazar, Ayesha De Costa, and Vishal Diwan. 2018. 'Bypassing Health Facilities for Childbirth in the Context of the JSY Cash Transfer Program to Promote Institutional Birth: A Cross-Sectional Study from Madhya Pradesh, India'. *Plos One* 13 (1):1–16.

Sadgopal, Mira. 2009. 'Can Maternity Services Open Up to the Indigenous Traditions of Midwifery?' *Economic and Political Weekly* 44 (16): 52–9.

Saravanan, Sheela, Gavin Turrell, Helen Johnson, Jenny Fraser, and Carla Patterson. 2011. 'Traditional Birth Attendant Training and Local Birthing Practices in India'. *Evaluation and Program Planning* 34 (3): 254–65.

Saravanan, Sheela, Gavin Turrell, Helen Johnson, Jennifer Fraser, and Carla Maree Patterson. 2012. 'Re-examining Authoritative Knowledge in the Design and Content of a TBA Training in India'. *Midwifery* 28 (1): 120–30.

Sarker, Bidhan Krishna, Musfikur Rahman, Tawhidur Rahman, Jahangir Hossain, Laura Reichenbach, and Dipak Kumar Mitra. 2016. 'Reasons for Preference of Home Delivery with Traditional Birth Attendants (Tbas) in Rural Bangladesh: A Qualitative Exploration'. *Plos One* 11 (1): e0146161.

Sengupta, Nirmal. 2019. *Traditional Knowledge in Modern India: Preservation, Promotion, Ethical Access and Benefit Sharing Mechanisms.* New Delhi: Springer.

Sibley, Lynn M., Theresa Ann Sipe, and Danika Barry. 2012. 'Traditional Birth Attendant Training for Improving Health Behaviours and Pregnancy Outcomes'. *Cochrane Database of Systematic Reviews* (8). doi: 10.1002/14651858.CD005460. Pub3.

Singh, Amarjeet, and A. Kaur. 1993. 'Perceptions of Traditional Birth Attendants Regarding Contraceptive Methods'. *Journal of Family Welfare* 39 (1): 6–39.

Srivastava, Aradhana, Devaki Singh, Dominic Montagu, and Sanghita Bhattacharyya. 2018. 'Putting Women At the Center: A Review of Indian Policy to Address Person-centered Care in Maternal and Newborn Health, Family Planning and Abortion'. *BMC Public Health* 18 (20): 1–10.

Stephens, Carolyn. 1992. 'Training Urban Traditional Birth Attendants: Balancing International Policy and Local Reality: Preliminary Evidence from the Slums of India on the Attitudes and Practice of Clients and Practitioners'. *Social Science & Medicine* 35 (6): 811–17.

Van Hollen, Cecilia. 1998. 'Moving Targets: Routine IUD Insertion in Maternity Wards in Tamil Nadu, India'. *Reproductive Health Matters* 6 (11): 98–106.

Van Hollen, Cecilia. 2003. *Birth on the Threshold: Childbirth and Modernity in South India*. Berkeley: University of California Press.

World Health Organization. Maternal Health and Safe Motherhood Programme. 1996. Mother-baby package: implementing safe motherhood in countries: Practical guide. World Health Organization. Accessed 8 March 2021. https://apps.who.int/iris/handle/10665/63268

World Health Organization. 2006. *Skilled Attendant at Birth: 2006 Updates*. Geneva: World Health Organization.

World Health Organization. 2015. *Trends in Maternal Mortality: 1990–2015: Estimates from WHO, UNICEF, UNFPA, World Bank Group and the United Nations Population Division: Executive Summary*. Geneva: World Health Organization.

SECTION 3

CONTESTED CATEGORIES

5

'Since It's a Pleasure to Save Somebody's Life, I Do This'

Midwifery and Safe Motherhood Practices in Urban India

Helen Vallianatos

Motherhood in India has long been reified, evident in the respected status of the Hindu goddess Parvati, of mothers in the Qur'an, and the depiction of the modern nation-state as Mother India. Since independence, a series of health policies and programmes have worked to address the health needs of mothers. And yet, mothers in India continue to suffer high rates of morbidity and mortality; despite significant improvements in maternal health, with a decrease in the maternal mortality ratio from 570 per 100,000 live births in 1990 to 230 in 2008 due to population size, the death of Indian mothers still contributes between 15 and 20% of annual global maternal deaths (UNICEF-India n.d; World Health Organization 2015). Maternal mortality rates are not uniform within India; significant variations are evident between states in the North and the South, with lowest maternal deaths reported in Kerala and Tamil Nadu and the highest in Assam, Uttar Pradesh, and Rajasthan (Rai and Tulchinsky 2015). One challenge for the Indian context has been providing quality healthcare to rural communities, where two-thirds of the population continues to reside (World Bank 2017), while simultaneously addressing the needs of the growing urban poor. The urbanization of poverty has led to an increase in slum populations, where high population density combined with minimal access to basic services, including sanitation, water, and health, negatively affects the health and wellness of mothers (Ministry of Housing and Urban Poverty Alleviation 2009).

Giving birth is not done in isolation. The care of mothers during pregnancy and the perinatal period has long been the domain of 'women's work', particularly by female kin and midwives. The need to be with others during the birthing process has deep roots, originating at the time when human brain size

Helen Vallianatos, *'Since It's a Pleasure to Save Somebody's Life, I Do This'* In: *Childbirth in South Asia.* Edited by: Clémence Jullien and Roger Jeffery, Oxford University Press. © Oxford University Press 2021. DOI: 10.1093/oso/9780190130718.003.0005 increased significantly. Concomitant with these biological changes was a so-cial shift, where birthing mothers typically were assisted by a familiar member of their social group (Rosenberg and Trevathan 2002). The familiarity of the person providing assistance is hypothesized to help the birthing mother cope with fear and other emotions during labour, and in turn, reduce the produc-tion of hormones like adrenaline that cause a delay in the labour process via hormonal inter-orchestration (Buckley 2015). Across cultural contexts, the person providing assistance during birth typically was a midwife, who often had other healing knowledge such as uses of medicinal plants in addition to experiential knowledge (Ehrenreich and English 2010; Jordan 1992). Since the mid-20th century, a shift in birthing personnel, from midwives to biomedical practitioners (that is, doctors, obstetricians), and in birthing places, from home to hospitals, has occurred to varying degrees throughout the world (Burst and Thompson 2015; Fahy 2007; Plummer 2000; Relyea 1992; van Teijlingen et al. 2004). The shift in birthing places resulted from a privileging of scientific tech-nology and accompanying authoritative knowledge grounded in a modern, bi-omedical system, as opposed to the embodied, traditional knowledge common among midwives. This medicalization of pregnancy and birth has been cri-tiqued, in part, due to the equation of reproduction with illness, which in turn requires management by physicians and other biomedical health providers (Davis-Floyd 1992). In other words, medicalization of reproduction involves a shift from embodied knowledge and practices that were located in homes to authoritative knowledge grounded in scientific biomedical systems taught in formal schools and practised in hospitals. It should also be noted that in some locales, physicians and midwives partner, combining the strengths of both approaches in order to serve the interests of birthing mothers. This medicaliza-tion process is ongoing globally, albeit to different degrees in diverse locations, thus further work is needed on understanding how medicalization of child-birth continues to evolve.

Unpacking the medicalization of birth and recent historical trends in maternal morbidity and mortality in India requires problematizing what constitutes authoritative knowledge and how embodied or experiential knowledge may intersect with authoritative knowledge. As pointed out by Roger Jeffery and Patricia Jeffery (2010), midwifery is not a homogenous practice, for how women give birth and how they are supported by midwives varies cross-culturally; reproduction is very much a product of specific social, cultural, economic, and political contexts. In India, dais (midwives) have his-torically been important in supporting underserved women, both in remote and rural contexts, as well as urban poor communities.[1] This is illustrated by governmental strategies prioritizing training for dais and incorporating them into the healthcare system, from the Bhore Committee (1946) recommendation to have one midwife per 100 births, to the reliance on auxiliary nurse midwives in post-independence 5-year National Plans until the 1970s (Mavalankar et al. 2011). However, governmental recognition and support for dais is not consistent, and training may target not only dais but also other women who are then called 'traditional birth attendants'. Thus, in this chapter I distinguish between dais—women who have learned midwifery through apprenticeship (typically with female relatives) and who earn income through their midwifery work—and traditional birth attendants—women who have learned basic midwifery skills and knowledge at specific training provided by governmental or non-governmental organizations. How experiences may differ between these two categories of midwives, dais' and traditional birth attendants' thoughts on training and the practice of midwifery, and how dais' and traditional birth attendants' practices foster improvements in maternal healthcare requires further attention.

The objective of this chapter is to examine an ethnographic case study of maternal health services in one urban poor community, from the perspective of trained birth attendants and traditional dais at a moment of noteworthy shifts in governmental funding and support for health services. These findings were part of a larger ethnographic study focused on women's food practices during pregnancy, conducted over a period of 14.5 months in a squatter settlement in New Delhi, India (Vallianatos 2010, 2011) at a significant moment of philosophical shifts in government political and economic policies, as neoliberal ideologies became integrated in 1999 and 2001. In this chapter, the sociocultural contexts of birthing are framed, followed by an exploration of how medicalization of birth and reproduction of authoritative knowledge were propagated in this locale, ending with a discussion on the implications for the contemporary role of dais, both trained and traditional, in ongoing efforts to promote safe motherhood in India.

Midwifery Knowledge and Practices within Social Margins

This chapter is based on the experiences and perspectives of six women who 'caught babies' in a *jhuggi-jhopri* (squatter) settlement in New Delhi. I first provide a snapshot of the community in order to situate the context within which the dais worked.[2]

As previously noted, universal health coverage has been a long-standing commitment by the Government of India, but funding for health services changed to align with funders' goals and priorities as India embraced neoliberalism in 1991.[3] Note that implementation of neoliberal economic policies is not undertaken by an individual nation-state unilaterally but is connected to their place in the world order and indebtedness to the World Bank and other global lenders. India's commitment to universal health coverage is unattainable when neoliberal economic policies limit spending on social welfare: in 2001, national government expenditure on public health services accounted for only 0.8% of GDP. This has not significantly changed in recent years, with government health expenditure hovering around 0.9% of GDP in 2014–16.[4] Private and voluntary health sectors have flourished in order to fill gaps in health services since 1991, while successive national governments between 1991 and throughout my fieldwork maintained a token towards universal healthcare by legislating low user fees (which does not equate with universal access).

The closest public (government) hospital providing care to the poor was more than 10 kilometres away from the community, translating to at least a 30-minute drive in a rickshaw, or much longer, depending on traffic—for those that could afford a rickshaw. The mothers with whom I worked preferred to give birth at home, under the care of a dai. Those who had some experience of hospitals described traumatic experiences of being mistreated by hospital staff, or worse, being turned away because of a lack of beds (see Vallianatos 2010, ch. 7). Other healthcare options did exist. On the outskirts of the community where I worked, several non-governmental organizations and a few private hospitals could be found. The private hospitals were economically out of reach for jhuggi-jhopri residents, for even the small costs to receive healthcare at some of the non-governmental organizations were widely critiqued.

The community itself had a number of public health issues including overcrowding (50,000 people lived within 4 square kilometres); limitations in water quality and quantity (water was only available at block handpumps that, if working, were only available twice per day); lack of toilet facilities; garbage was disposed of in 'parks' (that is, open areas within the community); and animals, including goats, pigs, chickens, cows and dogs, wandered freely throughout the settlement, foraging in the garbage and the drains that were found on either side of the pathways between homes, which flooded with regularity during the monsoon. While the public health issues were many, it should be noted that not all jhuggi-jhopri communities are equivalent; this was an older community, having been in existence for about 25 years (Ali 1990). The majority of residents and participants in the research had originated from Uttar Pradesh and Rajasthan, maintaining ties to natal villages through visits, housing new arrivals, and returning to fulfil familial obligations as necessary (for example, to assist with harvests, participate in ceremonial occasions, etc.).[5] Nevertheless, their community and lives were stable in New Delhi. Consequently, many families had invested in their homes, using concrete or stone for the floors and walls, and metal roofing. While some homes consisted of only one small room measuring approximately 6 feet square, others were a bit more spacious, or the family had two rooms. Fears of further resettlement or demolition were minimal for the residents, despite my observations of demolitions of business and housing on the outskirts of the community and in other parts of New Delhi.

As suggested by the differences in the quality of the housing, there were economic differences among residents, despite all being poor. Among the families with whom I worked, household incomes averaged Rs. 2,564 (about USD 60) per month, or an annual income of Rs. 30,775 (about USD 700), slightly higher than the monetary poverty line of Rs. 24,200 (about USD 540) in 2001.[6] These were estimated based on household members' economic activities, but note the precariousness of earnings, which depended on husbands' finding employment (most were daily labourers, working in construction sites or markets). Some women also completed 'piece-work' within their homes, including sewing or creating paper bags. As I describe elsewhere (Vallianatos 2010), these economic differences affected the health and well-being of residents; women described networks of support, sharing food and other resources with friends and neighbours. This sharing network was a critical means of navigating financial and food insecurity.

It was in these conditions that the six dais worked and lived. Catching babies was a source of income for these six women, four of whom were elderly widows.[7] One of these women, Adhira, was a trained birth attendant, someone who had been approached by one of the non-governmental organizations (NGOs) working in the area to do this work.[8] All of the other women were traditional dais. The traditional dais were older, four significantly older than Adhira, who was still of childbearing age (my estimate is late thirties). The most experienced was Charu, who seemed to be the most active of the six women, at least according to the mothers I interviewed. One of the traditional dais, Basanti, had also pursued and received training at one of the local NGOs. I visited these women in their homes, accompanied by a woman research assistant who helped to translate as required. Semi-structured interviews were undertaken, with open-ended questions allowing for dais to share what issues, concerns, and stories they felt were important. Particularly with the older traditional midwives, my prior knowledge of what could be considered 'typical' midwifery knowledge led to increased openness and sharing of their knowledge and wisdom. Interviews were transcribed and translated in the field by a different research assistant, and a third research assistant checked translations. Thematic data analysis was conducted, with four key aspects of midwifery care emerging: training, toolkit, types of knowledge, and managing complications. A final theme focused on dais' social locations and competition among local dais and trained birth attendants. In analysing these themes, I examine how various kinds of authoritative and embodied knowledge intertwine, in order to assess how medicalization of birth and reproduction of authoritative knowledge were propagated in this locale in the midwifery work of Adhira versus the other five dais. Findings have implication for ongoing efforts to improve gaps in maternal healthcare through midwives, both trained and traditional.

Training

Apprenticeship models were the primary means of building midwifery knowledge and skills for all five traditional dais. Working with women to provide support during pregnancy and labour, traditional dais' primary role, I was told by Charu, was to 'calm [the mother] and takes away the pain'. Charu was well respected in the jhuggi-jhopri settlement, the preferred dai, and this was reflected in the number of babies she had caught: 'I delivered one thousand children, with my own hands'. While Charu did not keep track of the exact number of babies she had personally caught, this statement functions to highlight her experience. Charu had six children of her own, all born in her village, and all of her births were assisted by a dai who was also her mother-in-law. She emphasized the importance of learning from elders: 'You should understand and listen to what I have to say. Let me tell you, from older people you learn'. All the traditional dais had learned their craft from their mothers or mothers-in-law in their villages, often as teenagers. This was often a family trade, with knowledge passed down through women in the family, as another dai, Esha, noted:

My grandmother did this work, my mother is a dai, my father's sister is a dai, my whole family is dai. My mother took me with her. I went with my mother to a birth and my mother showed me the umbilical cord. She said to thread the belly button very tightly closed. Some others loosely thread them. I did this work in childhood. My mother told me to do this work.

Thus, traditional dais began their training by accompanying their elders to care for pregnant and birthing women, and then assisting in the births, before moving to New Delhi. Their training, and eventually their own birthing experiences, were grounded in experiential learning, relying on their cumulative embodied knowledge to care for mothers. Dais' hands were critical tools; in their hand movements, as dais told their stories, they illustrated how they would move to touch a pregnant or labouring mother explicitly, to make sure I understood, while at other moments their hand movements seemed an unconscious action, part of the recollection of a birth story.

The legitimacy of traditional dais' embodied knowledge is arguably questioned, as I heard over the course of my fieldwork from doctors and other healthcare providers, as well as higher-status women, for dais are frequently viewed as problematic, unskilled, in need of training. A recent news article speaks to ongoing stereotypes of traditional dais: 'India has an irrational fear of midwives. To some, it is a reminder of the village dais of yore—who were untrained, unlike proper midwives—with their unhygienic practices and unscientific opinions' (Kumbhar 2016). This statement highlights the low value of embodied knowledge versus the authoritarian knowledge embedded in biomedical practices that are grounded in a scientific system. The embodied knowledge of village dais is unacknowledged; while there is no question that the skills and knowledge of dais are not uniform, as seen with mothers' preference to have Charu attend their births, the assumption that lack of formal training means lack of knowledge is also problematic—as is the lack of consideration of the role of poverty, chronic undernourishment, and other factors affecting the well-being of mothers. In other words, poor outcomes are not solely due to 'untrained' dais.

One traditional dai recognized the social value of receiving training, of engaging with the hegemonic biomedical system. Basanti participated in the training offered by a local NGO:

I learned myself and then when I came to Delhi, then the dispensary [NGO] people called me and gave me more knowledge . . . I [first] learned from my elder cousin, brother-in-law's wife and from her mother-in-law. Dispensary people taught me new things about cleanliness and gave good knowledge. I started doing this practice in a much better manner . . . when

> I [attend the birth] I have clean room, clean cloths, and for twenty minutes boil our blade, scissors, thread and then use this for the delivery of the child.

Interestingly, Basanti's words speak to the same concerns around stereotypes of the unhygienic nature of traditional dai practices. When she described the knowledge she had gained in catching babies, hygiene was emphasized, not other particulars of how to support and encourage the mother, how to catch the baby, or the like. Her emphasis on hygienic practices is notable, especially since in this community, boiling water was a rare occurrence. People knew that boiling water for 20 minutes would kill disease-bearing germs, as all training emphasized, but noted that the fuel costs to do so was prohibitive. Among the pregnant women I interviewed, if water was boiled at all it was only when a family member suffered from an illness accompanied with diarrheal symptoms. Upon recovery, this practice ended. Thus, Basanti's words share her positionality as modernizing, as participating in and acquiring authoritative knowledge; however, in reality, the translation of the knowledge to practice was mitigated by the poverty and the limited water resources in the community.

Adhira's experiences with midwifery training illustrate the model of recruiting women to serve as traditional birth attendants. Since 1947, providing some basic health training to women was one strategy to improve frontline community health services, including midwifery care. However, training shifted over time to focus on the health priorities of the era, and in the late 20th century (1970s onwards), this focus was on disease control via immunizations and family planning. Vora and colleagues (2009: 190) argue that these shifts resulted in a 'drastic decline in the quality of [their] midwifery training and practice'. In the early 1990s, the Child Survival and Safe Motherhood (CSSM) initiative launched to address gaps in maternal health, quickly followed by a revised model called Reproductive and Child Health 1 (RCH 1). This was the programme in place between 1997 and 2004, overlapping with my 14 months of data collection in 1999 and 2001. RCH 1 aimed to provide essential obstetric care and improve quality of services, in part by training community birth attendants. Adhira shared her experiences of recruitment and training:

> I learnt this work, *dai* is very much needed. I was scared, how touch that, how will cut the cord of baby? This is not good, I thought it's dirtiness. I don't eat meat how can I touch that? . . . Then they [NGO recruiters] said

it is not vulgarity . . . it is not dirtiness it is blood of lady. I was scared very much, how know that baby is coming? I had no knowledge. They [NGO recruiters] said we'll teach you. I used to go to the centre, I was taught about pregnant ladies, how look after them, how to do a check up. [Describes some details] Doctor said . . . 'don't be afraid, when you work with us fear is gone since you're taught in our centre' . . . Now I give injections also, check the pregnant woman, now I have much knowledge.

Recruitment was an issue for Adhira, for midwifery was not part of her family's history, and following the normative ideas described above, where dais are viewed as lower on the social stratum, Adhira's family resisted her recruitment: 'My home thinks it is a dirty work, they don't want me to do this'. Her husband had told her this work was 'rubbish work, nobody is doing this work in my house'. But she noted that 'when doctor can do [this work], why don't we?' Perhaps because of the power of the local NGO centres and workers, as well as her own motivation, Adhira was able to persist. At another point, Adhira spoke of how she thought her *sas* (mother-in-law) was jealous of her acquiring new knowledge, knowledge that was taboo or dangerous, for in her training with the NGOs, she not only acquired knowledge of childbirth but also 'every type of knowledge about AIDS, secret diseases, I know how these happen'. Note that disease prevention continues to be an important component of the training.

While Adhira spoke of her growth in knowledge and comfort in assisting birthing mothers, Vora and colleagues (2009) noted that training was too short to allow for skill development. Without skill development and appropriate supervision, the ability to foster safe motherhood goals is questionable. Adhira had shared how training was delivered in her community: 'There was training every two to three months. In the past a different NGO gave training, but now they said you have all learnt. Now you are a complete dai, you know everything. No, I don't, I tell them I have to learn more'. This limitation in training highlights one benefit of the training traditional dais received through apprenticeship—experiential learning allowed these women to cultivate their sensory and embodied skills, such as to be able to massage a pregnant mother's belly to attempt to turn a breech-positioned foetus, and learning these skills requires practice, supervised practice. Arguably, learning the concepts in an office or centre is a necessary first step, but even Adhira wanted further support and training. Of the six women I interviewed, she was the least comfortable catching babies.

Toolkit

An emblem of modern training was the toolkit. The toolkit functioned as a symbol of having undergone biomedical training at a local NGO, of having knowledge on birthing best practices, especially hygiene, and incorporating these into one's daily midwifery work. Basanti explained how she had received tools 'to weigh the child, to check the heartbeat, Dettol [antiseptic], soap and these gloves, this all [she] got from the dispensary', all the while showing the tools while talking. However, it was Adhira who spent the most time explaining each tool and the role of that tool, as exemplified by her description of the gloves:

> [I received] gloves from one NGO, but other NGOs also give. Gloves prevent infection, never spread dirt. Should use [gloves] for cleaning, should use a room with a window [for the birth], your bed should also be clean. Any cloths should be washed and clean. If bleeding during birth, wipe with the cloth . . . when [gloves are] used they [NGOs] give again.

The key here was that by wearing gloves, she was also protecting herself as well as the mother, and using new pairs after each use was a critical component in using this object in her toolkit.

In contrast, the traditional dais spoke of how the tools are given to the mothers directly at the dispensary, relying on the tools provided by the mother in their midwifery work. The traditional dais typically used their own tools only if necessary, as this would increase their costs. Not attending the training at the local NGOs also meant they had fewer opportunities to gather elements of the toolkit, but it could also be seen as resistance to the hegemony of the biomedical system (discussed further below, as dais discuss perceptions of the cleanliness of themselves and their work).

Traditional Knowledge: Blurring Embodied/Authoritative Knowledge Boundaries

Thus far, I have presented the findings as a contrast between the experiential, embodied knowledge of dais with the authoritative knowledge of modern scientific medical systems. In this section, a blurring between these polarities begins, to incorporate other types of authoritative knowledge grounded in Ayurvedic medical systems.

Traditional knowledge was based on the lessons and experiences learned as young women, when first learning midwifery skills, but this knowledge also included localized interpretations of knowledge from Ayurvedic medicine. Passed on through family lines, this information could affect not only the quality of maternal care any dai provided but also the kinds of help provided. For instance, traditional dais had some awareness of the use of foods or herbs during labour to manage the pain. While some elements were shared, such as the use of milk, the components that were added to the beverage varied. Charu shared that one ought to use

> fenugreek and almonds, mix within milk, if she eats then the pain can subside. Other things may cause further pain, but these don't, they don't cause damage. If she wants to have the child at home, the *dai* must know if the house is full [of the herbs and foods required] to make the medication and give it to her to drink. Then the pain will subside and the child will come easily.

Another dai, Deepa, also used milk, but instead added ghee and sugar and then boiled the milk because 'it gives warmness to the body . . . gives some energy. Many don't eat or drink, deliver on an empty stomach. Then have to give tea or milk'.

Other knowledge was more secretive, not widely shared. For instance, Charu shared specific knowledge on herbs that could cause miscarriage, as did Basanti, but only after I had volunteered some knowledge and examples of how this is done in a different cultural context. Charu, in particular, was very interested in what I knew about other cultural practices, and then shared specific knowledge of particular seeds and herbs—which I was not supposed to widely disseminate. Other participants disavowed any knowledge, repeatedly stating that pregnancy and birth are in God's hands; of course, this could have been due to not wishing to share such dangerous knowledge, of risking being judged by community members, which in turn could affect whether community members would choose to use the dais' services. There is power in knowledge, and as such, it is with great care that knowledge is transferred, especially when there are potential social risks, thus it is also possible these participants did not wish to divulge to me what they knew. Many of the mothers with whom I worked had experienced miscarriages. In private discussions with approximately a dozen of these mothers, it became evident that a particular tea had been drunk prior to the miscarriage, although the mothers did not admit or necessarily know the components of the tea.

Much of the understanding of how particular herbs and medicines affected a pregnant woman's body was grounded in Ayurvedic traditions, as were more general food and diet recommendations. Simply put, Ayurveda is a humoral medical system, where the body can, at any moment in time, be on a 'hot' to 'cold' spectrum, and bodily states, like pregnancy, can shift where one's body sits on this spectrum. Pregnancy is a 'hot' condition, thus to maintain health, a balance of humoral elements is required (Jeffery et al. 1989). One way to manage this is through daily food practices, by avoiding 'hot' foods (see, for example, Nichter and Nichter 1996; Rao 1985). Among my study participants, these foods consistently included meat, egg, tea, potato, and garlic, while fruits like mango, and vegetables like eggplant, were labelled 'hot' by the majority of participants (Vallianatos 2010: 121). The avoidance of hot foods is to ensure that too much heat does not build in the body, because this can lead to health problems and/or miscarriage. This advice was uniformly shared by traditional dais such as Deepa, who said 'after eating hot food she will be in trouble', and Basanti, who noted that 'we advise to abstain from hot things like potato, pulses'. Charu gave a fuller list of foods to avoid: 'don't eat red masala (spices), fried food, ghee', elsewhere noting not to 'eat things that give off heat'. However, consuming milk, green vegetables, and rice was highly recommended during pregnancy.

In contrast, Adhira's dietary advice corresponded to typical biomedical recommendations: 'Fresh things, fruits, juice, and whatever have should eat until full belly. Dal, rice, roti, daliya, sabji, then baby will be healthy. Iron pills, they should eat that'. She continued that Ayurvedic recommendations were unnecessary: 'Every thing she should eat during pregnancy. Whatever she desires she should eat. She desire eggs, meat, she should eat'. This woman also challenged traditional ideas around causes of miscarriage, instead noting 'when womb is weak it can't bear a baby. So hot and cold is nothing, womb is weak'.

Farha, a dai not much younger than Charu, vented her frustration with younger women not following her advice: 'The thing is harmful today is that today's daughter-in-law and [pregnant] ladies do not agree. I tell them you are not to eat these things, but she eats'. Deepa echoed this, noting 'today nobody wants to eat green veg, green veg is always good'. This creates a challenge for traditional dai's practice, when their expertise and wisdom is only selectively applied. Arguably, the same could be said for biomedically-grounded health advice, as people simultaneously adopt some recommendations while resisting others, but in a societal context where dais are considered uneducated and unclean, the dismissal of their advice has affective consequences for these women.

Managing Complications

All six women spoke of the need to rely on biomedical care, specifically hospitals, when complications arose. Charu explained, 'If the women and the pain is manageable, and if she wants the child at home, if the road is clean and the child is able to be seen, then the child will be born at home. If the child is unable to be seen and the road is blocked then she will go to the hospital'. At another point in time, Charu added that people 'prefer not to go to the hospital and rather have it at home. The rich and the poor both do this. When there is a problem with the pregnancy the midwife will send the patient to the hospital'. Her statement that all people, regardless of social class, prefer home births has recently shifted with government maternal health programme strategies (RCH 1) that included providing honoraria to primary health centre and community health centre staff for attending births after hours, to provide 24-hour deliveries at both aforementioned centres. Assistance by doctors during birth rose from 22% in 1993 to 35% in 2006, and institutional deliveries increased from 26% to 40% in the same time frame (Vora et al. 2009). The shift in personnel and places of birth are not uniformly experienced across society, but vary by social class, as noted by Vora and colleagues (2009), who add that the institutional increase represented an increase in private facilities, not government or public establishments. Recognizing that the poor could not afford health facilities, the Government of India introduced a new programme, 'Janani Suraksha Yojana (JSY; translated as safe motherhood scheme)—a national conditional cash transfer scheme—to incentivise women of low socioeconomic status to give birth in a health facility' (Lim et al. 2010: 2009). Women living below the poverty line in urban areas would receive 600 rupees, although this programme did provide 500 rupees to women living below the poverty line who gave birth at home, for their first two children. Early analysis indicated that more women were giving birth in health facilities (albeit with large variations across India), although concerns were raised that workloads for health practitioners were increasing and quality of care needed to be addressed (Lim et al. 2010). More recent analysis suggests that the shifts to birthing in health facilities has not been accompanied by improved maternal mortality rates, probably due to ongoing quality of care issues, such as infrastructure and staffing limitations (Montagu et al.

2017). In other words, the financial incentives may lead to more mothers living in poverty giving birth in facilities,[9] but this shift might be mitigated by poor experiences that in turn can affect maternal (and neonatal) health outcomes. More research is needed to understand how caste, social class, and other aspects of social status affect women's experiences of giving birth in a variety of facilities across India.

It became clear that the dais assessed each pregnant woman, referring some to biomedical care before birth, while others have complications that arise during the birthing process, requiring emergency transport. Dais spoke of the need to transfer to hospital during birth, explaining, in Deepa's words, that this occurs when 'the womb's mouth is not open or the baby will not be born, we say for hospital'. It was better to transfer care earlier. Charu assessed each mother, early in pregnancy and once labour commenced. She shared:

> If a dai feels that something is wrong then she should tell the truth to the mother. Don't lie. If you want to hold the child in the womb due to certain circumstances, then you should give her medication that would allow her to stop the child. We can tell a month before [if there will be problems] and we can tell when the child is ready [for birth] . . . I don't touch the case that I'm unable to handle. I tell them to take her to the hospital. I don't touch them if I feel that I cannot handle it. If I touch then my hands are going to be ruined. Why would I touch them?

Defining potential problems was variable between the six women, based on their own levels of expertise and knowledge. Basanti, who also pursued training from local NGOs, had clear choices:

> No, the dangerous cases I don't take into my hands. When I see there is danger, then I don't take that case in my hands . . . [when] the heartbeat of mother and child is less then I don't do it, I directly send her to the hospital . . . when the child is reversed [a breech], the child goes to the latrine during the pains [labour], poison spreads, then I don't take it in my hands. [Later she continues to explain] Whatever is fit for my knowledge I do, [otherwise] I have to deny. Think, if I look after two lives, then why is there hospital? Those are built for that type of work. So we do only as much as we have knowledge. Don't do anymore. When everything is okay then we take the case after praying to God. After all, lady is alive, and it is very difficult to save a mother and child.

However, note that some of the traditional dais described breech and twin cases with successful outcomes. Farha shared one such case: 'a baby was born in the opposite direction. First came leg. I was alone. I was alone, her husband was there, I said please call anybody, baby is in opposite direction, so an elder lady who lived nearby, she came and sat. Her whole body then came out, then I dragged out the head easily, then cut the cord'. In other cases, Farha was able to massage the mother's belly in order to turn the baby, but she was not too worried by challenges of breech births: 'change baby's direction if can, if not take birth in opposite direction is absolutely okay'. Yet, later she also spoke of how she was not able to relax until after the placenta was delivered. It is not always possible to transfer to the hospital in a timely fashion, plus the dais that had been practising for decades had trained in their villages where bio-medical care would not have been nearby (see Jeffery et al. 1989 for detailed descriptions of rural contexts of birth).

A striking difference was Adhira's perspectives on when to transfer care to biomedical contexts:

[If the foetus] is weak and sticks, don't deliver at home, this is dangerous. Any sick lady with tuberculosis, sugar [gestational diabetes] or any other heart problem her delivery will not be at home, should be in hospital. When woman is healthy then delivery in the home. If pregnant woman is under eighteen years, then there is difficulty in delivery and above forty years, that also is dangerous. Young and old both have difficulty, their delivery shouldn't be at home. Doctor said we'll tell you, you have to do this.

As the least experienced, Adhira once again emphasized the knowledge she had been taught, echoing the advice, even the language used in training to describe her knowledge and practices.

Thus, the concept of complications was influenced by dais' experiences, but also by pragmatic concerns on how their reputations—and in turn, income—would be affected. Deepa noted that in contrast to normative understandings of health in the recent historical past (that is, maternal health was poor in the early to mid-20th century), in 'past times, women were healthy, were brave ladies, we did work [without troubles]; as facilities increase, disease increases'. Admittedly nostalgic for a past where women were active, therefore healthy, strong, and capable of birthing with minimal complications, this idealism is echoed in other post-colonial contexts (for example, Vallianatos and Willows 2016). This idyllic past for birthing mothers is also contrasted with modern health infrastructure, such as the public, government hospital, which faced chronic human and material shortages (Vallianatos 2010: 69–72). This was the hospital where women in the throes of complications were sent. Mothers, as well as dais, shared a series of concerns, including: a) locating a rickshaw, which was a problem since rickshaws did not come near the jhuggi-jhopri area—and this was exacerbated if the transport occurred in the night; b) the cost of transport; c) the need to bring one's own supplies, including blood, to the hospital; d) the probability of being turned away due to overcrowding at the hospital; e) if admitted, the probability of maltreatment by hospital staff. Thus, hospital transfers were fitting only in the most severe cases.

Social Location and Competition

Most dais stated there was no competition among them, yet further discussions suggested some differences of opinions or judgements about another's expertise. For example, Esha said 'I don't talk about another dai', and then proceeded to explain how many other dais 'do not correctly solve a problem, like the birth canal not opening'. She was critical of the use of injections to speed labour, seeing their use also linked to problems for the mother and infant, as illustrated with a case study of a mother in her mid-thirties who was given four injections by another dai. Afterwards, people came to Esha to ask her advice. After checking the mother, Esha told the family 'it was not correct time for delivery, wait a month, and after a month this woman's baby was born safely. I advised her to not go to another *dai*, sometimes this creates problems, but I saved the baby, I solved the problem'. Trained birth attendants who have no experience, who have not put in the years of apprenticeship to gain an embodied knowledge, troubled Esha. Like Charu and other elderly, experienced dais, Esha spoke of the use of her hands, how through her 'experienced, touching hand' she could assess the needs of mothers.

While Basanti had been practising for 20 years, first learning through observation and accompanying her female relatives in their work in the village, she highly valued modern education and knowledge, and pursued any training opportunities offered by the local NGOs, as well as attending meetings organized by the NGO workers. This was an astute decision on her part, recognizing that uptake of the training may manage perceptions of cleanliness, and also held economic consequences, for 'it will be good for my fame if I learn more'. While linking her pursuit of training with economic benefits, Bashanti claimed to not be bothered 'if someone earns more than me ... it is her good luck', but then noted that others could be irritated, not wanting to share information or knowledge with her.

The one who spoke most openly about differences in status among the dais was Adhira, once again focusing on the stereotypes of cleanliness underlying dais' status. She spoke out quite clearly on the differences between her work and that of traditional dais, noting 'this difference: they haven't got this knowledge that room should be clean. They are called and they make the delivery, but they don't attend to cleanliness'. She further elaborated on some differences in their methods, such as when to cut the cord (Adhira did it before traditional dais, who waited until the birth of the placenta). Another time, Adhira spoke of how her care of mothers was more restricted compared with dais who do the 'cleaning, throw dirt out [after birth, the dirty cloths and the like] I don't do. I care only for the baby and mother. Other dais they do all the work, clean them, throw garbage out, I don't do all this. I deny ... only [care of mother and baby] I do'. This contrasts with Farha, who said 'we do the [cleaning] work ... after taking bath and changing clothes nobody thinks she is dirty ... nobody is thinking this'.

Adhira was also younger than the other dais, which complicated her standing with others. She felt that if she 'told them something, since mostly aged compared to me, if I told them something then I am wicked'. Interestingly, she was the only one who had not given birth to her own children at home with a dai, but instead had utilized a health centre.

Lessons from the Past: Implications for Current Maternal Care

Safe motherhood global initiatives are now 30 years old, yet challenges remain in ensuring that mothers, and their infants, are healthy. In India, significant declines in maternal mortality have been made, but more remains to be done. The ethnographic case study presented here highlights childbirth experiences and practices among the urban poor at the turn of the 21st century. Government initiatives since the mid-2000s have continued to attempt to address ongoing gaps in maternal healthcare. In addition to the National Health Mission (NHM) and JSY programmes mentioned earlier, the Government of India, in 2016, launched a new programme, Pradhan Mantri Surakshit Matritva Abhiyan, part of the Reproductive Maternal Neonatal Child and Adolescent Health (RMNCH+A) strategy. The primary objective of this new programme is to improve antenatal care by ensuring all pregnant women are seen by a physician or obstetrician at least once during the second or third trimesters. This visit aims to identify high-risk pregnancies, to provide early diagnosis and intervention for issues related to malnutrition, and to improve the quality of care during antenatal visits. Building on gaps from preceding programmes, the following challenges must be considered:

a) this national initiative is complicated because health programmes are state-run; for success, the initiative must also be a priority for state governments (Shiffman and Ved 2007).

b) gaps in public infrastructure have been noted across India, and this includes lack of quality services for the urban poor—the women living in this jhuggi-jhopri community were no different (see, for example, Lim et al. 2010; Srivastava et al. 2014; Vallianatos 2010; Vora et al. 2009).

c) the ill-treatment of birthing mothers in health institutions, or obstetric violence, has been a documented challenge in India and elsewhere (see, for example, Bohren et al. 2015; Jeffery and Jeffery 2010; Sudhinaraset et al. 2016; Vallianatos 2010, ch. 7); to improve women's health experiences in facilities, and in turn their own (and their infants') health and well-being, they must be treated with dignity and respect, regardless of their social status, education level, and the like (Montagu et al. 2017; Srivastava et al. 2014).[10]

d) the recent government initiative relies on physicians and obstetricians for antenatal care. However, numbers and distribution of obstetrical services have been a problem in past programmes (Shiffman and Ved 2007); a call for volunteers was made at the launch of this programme, and assessment on the availability of these personnel must be part of this programme's evaluation.

e) this new initiative includes non-specialist members of the healthcare landscape in India, such as auxiliary nurse midwives and community workers (for example, ASHA), however they are seen as having a key role in communication of the programme and mobilization of the community, by identifying and connecting with pregnant women, encouraging them to participate in the programme. Traditional dais' knowledge and experience could be incorporated to improve antenatal care;[11] past programmes were critiqued for not training non-specialist healthcare providers with life-saving obstetric skills (Shiffman and Ved 2007), and this appears to continue in the new programme.

f) the majority of maternal deaths occur in the post-partum period (Islam 2007) and it appears the new programme's emphasis is on the antenatal period; midwifery care models include care during this period, and the dais in this study did check in on the new mother for 8–9 days post-birth, thus utilizing these women by building on their current knowledge, skills, and practices could assist with in-home post-partum care.

All women who caught babies were proud of the work they did, including Adhira, who began this work against the wishes of her family, and who eloquently noted, 'Dais are everywhere. Without dais, how will people [society] go on? Dais helps to give birth to a baby; without dais, how will births happen?' None of these women thought of retirement, of stopping their work, instead saying they would do this work 'as long as I have energy' in Adhira's words, or as Farrah said, 'as long as I have power in my body'. They took their roles seriously in supporting maternal care, recognizing the links between maternal and infant well-being, as Basanti noted: 'Suppose there is a healthy woman, she has no disease, so her baby will be healthy and mother is also healthy. If another woman is ill, so baby will be ill, then she has to go to the hospital [to deliver] and bear the difficulties of treatment'. However, there were challenges for some of the traditional dais, with no junior family members exhibiting interest in undertaking the years of effort required for apprenticeship modes of learning (for example, Deepa's three daughters-in-law 'don't want [to learn], don't like the dirtiness').

The concept of dirtiness speaks to both the hygiene (or lack thereof) among traditional dais and to a more ephemeral concept of pollution that accompanies exposure with bodily fluids, and connects dais to unclean, lower-status work and social status. The assumption that lack of formal education means dais are unknowledgeable must continue to be challenged, while simultaneously working with dais to improve knowledge and skills; for, of course, not all dais are equally skilled. Addressing limitations while acknowledging the strengths of traditional experiential knowledge systems may (finally) lead to better maternal care for all. Continued support for ongoing experiential learning of newer midwives, community health workers, or traditional birth attendants is crucial, to ensure that women can apply their knowledge so that their hands are comfortable doing the work of catching babies. I end with the words of Adhira: 'For help at birth time a dai should be'.

Notes

1. 'Midwife' and 'dai' are heterogeneous categories. Midwives are frequently understood to be 'expert[s] who comes equipped to provide both the practical help and the emotional support that a woman needs . . . on the basis of a bond of empathy already built up over a series of encounters for ante-natal care' (Van Teijlingen et al. 2004: 1). However, across cultures, women who attend births have different degrees of knowledge and expertise. In north India, the birthing process is typically managed by the senior attendant, who is often the mother-in-law or other older woman—it is this woman who will send for a dai and usually remains in control over decisions in the management of labour and birth. The dai herself is often regarded as 'a low status menial necessary for removing defilement' (Jeffery et al. 1989:108).

2. For further in-depth descriptions of the historic, political-economic contexts of this community and residents' access to healthcare, see Vallianatos 2010 and 2011.

3. See Ahmed et al. (2010) and Münster and Strümpell (2014) for analyses of the emergence and implementation of neoliberalism in India.

4. https://data.worldbank.org/indicator/SH.XPD.GHED.GD.ZS?locations=IN. This is not to suggest that efforts have not been made since 2001, for a major initiative was launched in 2005 aimed at strengthening primary healthcare and maternal health in particular, called the National Rural Health Mission (NRHM), renamed National Health Mission (NHM) in 2013. This programme improved antenatal service use and institutional delivery (Vellakkal et al. 2017). Also in 2013, a National Urban Health Mission launched, focusing on meeting the healthcare needs of the urban poor. In 2017, a universal healthcare initiative, focused on reducing the financial costs of healthcare for the poor was implemented: the Pradhan Mantri Jan Arogya Yojana (PM-JAY).

5. Residents were predominantly Hindu, with a large minority Muslim (~20%) and a few Christians and Sikhs. Study participants echoed this distribution. While particular caste group memberships varied, all were classified by the government as 'scheduled castes'.

6. Surveys of jhuggi-jhompi settlements in India's cities indicate that 40–50% of residents live below the poverty line, whereas 11% have an income just above the poverty line and the remaining households are even financially better off (Barrett and Beardmore 2009). Thus, this jhuggi-jhompi community follows the financial configuration of urban poverty observed throughout India.

7. While I was able to obtain ages for mothers that had participated in the research, it was difficult to estimate actual ages of the dais; the four 'elderly' dais were grandmothers, with grey hair, and through conversations on life experiences, were at least over the age of 65, with the eldest being in her seventies.

8. All names are pseudonyms, to protect the anonymity of participants.

9. Although this assumption must be interrogated; for example, see Sidney and colleagues' (2016) research that suggests the financial incentive plays a relatively small role in women's choices to use facilities.

10. Obstetric violence emerged out of frameworks holistically examining violence against women. An example is an Argentinian law passed in 2009 that states '[v]iolence exercised by health personnel on the body and reproductive processes of pregnant women, expressed through dehumanizing treatment, medicalization abuse, and the conversion of natural processes of reproduction into pathological ones' (Vacaflor 2016).

11. While past failures at incorporating dais' knowledge has been noted, it worth re-examining this prospect, for it is possible that what was considered 'knowledge' was not inclusive of the embodied knowledge or was dismissive of this kind of knowledge. Successful incorporation of non-biomedical carers requires mutual respect, as has been noted for other cultural contexts (Kruske and Barclay 2004). It must also be recognized that significant time must be invested in not only building these relationships and training across medical systems (for example, building on the referral processes that are already in practice) but also ensuring there are enough people and facilities to support mothers through the reproduction journey.

References

Ahmed, Waquar, Amitabh Kundu, and Richard Peet. 2010. *India's New Economic Policy: A Critical Analysis*. London: Routledge.

Ali, Sabir. 1990. *Slums within Slums: A Study of Resettlement Colonies in Delhi*. New Delhi: Har-Anand.

Barrett, Alison J., and Richard M. Beardmore. 2009. 'Poverty Reduction in India: Towards Building Successful Slum-Upgrading Strategies.' In *Human Settlement Development Volume 1*, edited by Saskia Sassen, 326–33. Oxford, UK: EOLSS Publishers.

Bohren, Meghan A., Joshua P. Vogel, Erin C. Hunter, Olha Lutsiv, Suprita K. Makh, João Paulo Souza, Carolina Aguiar, Fernando Saraiva Coneglian, Alex Luíz Araújo Diniz, and Özge Tunçalp. 2015. 'The Mistreatment of Women During Childbirth in Health Facilities Globally: A Mixed-Methods Systematic Review.' *PLoS Medicine* 12 (6): 1–32. doi: 10.1371/journal.pmed.1001847.

Buckley, Sarah J. 2015. 'Executive Summary of Hormonal Physiology of Childbearing: Evidence and Implications for Women, Babies, and Maternity Care.' *The Journal of Perinatal Education* 24 (3): 145–53.

Davis-Floyd, Robbie. 1992. *Birth as an American Rite of Passage*. Berkeley: University of California Press.

Ehrenreich, Barbara, and Deirdre English. 2010. *Witches, Midwives, & Nurses: A History of Women Healers*. 2nd ed. The Feminist Press at CUNY.

Fahy, Kathleen. 2007. 'An Australian History of the Subordination of Midwifery'. *Women and Birth* 20 (1): 25–9.

Islam, Monir. 2007. 'The Safe Motherhood Initiative and Beyond'. *Bulletin of the World Health Organization* 85 (10): 735.

Jeffery, Patricia, and Roger Jeffery. 2010. 'Only When the Boat Has Started Sinking: A Maternal Death in Rural North India'. *Social Science & Medicine* 71 (10): 1711–18.

Jeffery, Patricia, Roger Jeffery, and Andrew Lyon. 1989. *Labour Pains and Labour Power: Women and Childbearing in India*. London: Zed Books.

Jordan, Brigitte. 1992. *Birth in Four Cultures: A Crosscultural Investigation of Childbirth in Yucatan, Holland, Sweden, and the United States*. 4th ed. Long Grove, IL: Waveland Press.

Kruske, Sue, and Lesley Barclay. 2004. 'Effect of Shifting Policies On Traditional Birth Attendant Training'. *The Journal of Midwifery & Women's Health* 49 (4): 306–11.

Kumbhar, Kiran. 2016. 'Shunned for Years, Can Trained Midwives Fix India's Maternity Mess'. *Quartz India*, 1 March.

Lim, Stephen S., Lalit Dandona, Joseph A. Hoisington, Spencer L. James, Margaret C. Hogan, and Emmanuela Gakidou. 2010. 'India's Janani Suraksha Yojana, a Conditional Cash Transfer Programme to Increase Births in Health Facilities: An Impact Evaluation'. *The Lancet* 375 (9730): 2009–23.

Mavalankar, Dileep, Parvathy Sankara Raman, and Kranti Vora. 2011. 'Midwives of India: Missing in Action'. *Midwifery* 27 (5): 700–6.

Ministry of Housing and Urban Poverty Alleviation. 2009. *India, Urban Poverty Report 2009*. New Delhi: Oxford University Press.

Montagu, Dominic, May Sudhinaraset, Nadia Diamond-Smith, Oona Campbell, Sabine Gabrysch, Lynn Freedman, Margaret E. Kruk, and France Donnay. 2017. 'Where Women Go to Deliver: Understanding the Changing Landscape of Childbirth in Africa and Asia'. *Health Policy and Planning* 32 (8): 1146–52.

Münster, Daniel, and Christian Strümpell. 2014. 'The Anthropology of Neoliberal India: An Introduction'. *Contributions to Indian Sociology* 48 (1): 1–16.

Nichter, Mark, and Mimi Nichter. 1996. 'The Ethnophysiology and Folk Dietetics of Pregnancy: A Case Study from South India'. In *Anthropology and International Health*, 2nd edition, edited by Mark Nichter and Mimi Nichter, 35–69. New York: Routledge.

Plummer, Kate. 2000. 'From Nursing Outposts to Contemporary Midwifery in 20th Century Canada'. *Journal of Midwifery & Women's Health* 45 (2): 169–75.

Rai, Rajesh Kumar, and Theodore Herzl Tulchinsky. 2015. 'Addressing the Sluggish Progress in Reducing Maternal Mortality in India'. *Asia Pacific Journal of Public Health* 27 (2): NP1161–NP1169.

Rao, Meera. 1985. 'Food Beliefs of Rural Women during the Reproductive Years in Dharwad, India'. *Ecology of Food and Nutrition* 16 (2): 93–103.

Relyea, M. Joyce. 1992. 'The Rebirth of Midwifery in Canada: An Historical Perspective'. *Midwifery* 8 (4): 159–69.

Rosenberg, Karen, and Wenda Trevathan. 2002. 'Birth, Obstetrics and Human Evolution'. *BJOG: An International Journal of Obstetrics & Gynaecology* 109 (11): 1199–206.

Shiffman, Jeremy, and Rajani R. Ved. 2007. 'The State of Political Priority for Safe Motherhood in India'. *BJOG: An International Journal of Obstetrics & Gynaecology* 114 (7): 785–90.

Sidney, Kristi, Rachel Tolhurst, Kate Jehan, Vishal Diwan, and Ayesha De Costa. 2016. '"The Money Is Important but All Women Anyway Go to Hospital for Childbirth Nowadays": A Qualitative Exploration of Why Women Participate in a Conditional Cash Transfer Program to Promote Institutional Deliveries in Madhya Pradesh, India'. *BMC Pregnancy and Childbirth* 16 (1): 47.

Srivastava, Aradhana, Sanghita Bhattacharyya, Christine Clar, and Bilal I. Avan. 2014. 'Evolution of Quality in Maternal Health in India: Lessons and Priorities'. *International Journal of Medicine and Public Health* 4 (1): 33–9.

Sudhinaraset, May, Emily Treleaven, Jason Melo, Kanksha Singh, and Nadia Diamond-Smith. 2016. 'Women's Status and Experiences of Mistreatment during Childbirth in Uttar Pradesh: A Mixed Methods Study Using Cultural Health Capital Theory'. *BMC Pregnancy and Childbirth* 16 (332): 1–12.

UNICEF-India. n.d. 'Maternal Health: Introduction'. Accessed 19 February 2020. http://unicef.in/Whatwedo/1/Maternal-Health

Vacaflor, Carlos Herrera. 2016. 'Obstetric Violence: A New Framework for Identifying Challenges to Maternal Healthcare in Argentina'. *Reproductive Health Matters* 24 (47): 65–73.

Vallianatos, Helen. 2010. *Poor and Pregnant in New Delhi, India*. New Delhi: Munshiram Manoharlal.

Vallianatos, Helen. 2011. 'Placing Maternal Health in India'. In *Locating Health*, edited by Erika Dyck and Christopher Fletcher, 11–27. London: Pickering & Chatto.

Vallianatos, Helen, and Noreen D. Willows. 2016. 'Tradition and Transformation of Eastern James Bay Eeyou (Cree) Foodways in Pregnancy: Implications for Health Care'. In *Indigenous Peoples: Perspectives, Cultural Roles and Health Care Disparities*, edited by Jessica Morton, 71–106. Hauppauge, NY: Nova Science Publishers.

Van Teijlingen, Edwin R., George W. Lowis, Peter McCaffery, and Maureen Porter, eds. 2004. *Midwifery and the Medicalization of Childbirth: Comparative Perspectives*. New York: Nova Publishers.

Vellakkal, Sukumar, Adyya Gupta, Zaky Khan, David Stuckler, Aaron Reeves, Shah Ebrahim, Ann Bowling, and Pat Doyle. 2017. 'Has India's National Rural Health Mission Reduced Inequities in Maternal Health Services? A Pre-post Repeated Cross-sectional Study'. *Health Policy and Planning* 32 (1): 79–90.

Vora, Kranti S., Dileep V. Mavalankar, K.V. Ramani, Mudita Upadhyaya, Bharati Sharma, Sharad Iyengar, Vikram Gupta, and Kirti Iyengar. 2009. 'Maternal Health Situation in India: A Case Study'. *Journal of Health, Population, and Nutrition* 27 (2): 184–201.

World Bank. 2017. 'World Bank DataBank: Rural Population'. The World Bank. Accessed 19 February. https://data.worldbank.org/indicator/SP.RUR.TOTL.ZS

World Health Organization. 2015. *Trends in Maternal Mortality: 1990–2015: Estimates from WHO, UNICEF, UNFPA, World Bank Group and the United Nations Population Division: Executive Summary*. Geneva: World Health Organization.

6

Childbirth in Transit

Motherhood and Migration at Taljai, a Slum in Pune

Deepra Dandekar

This chapter ethnographically explores childbirth practices at Taljai, a large urban slum on the southern outskirts of Pune city, India. Based on women's recounting of their personal experiences and social relationships surrounding birth-giving at home, this chapter describes childbirth at Taljai as unstable, mirroring the migrant lives of women. Women's migrant lives at Taljai are precarious and subject to material paucity and systemic violence, defined by strong internal negotiation and sociability surrounding their birth-giving practices at home. While homebirths are predicated on friendship networks among women, clinical births either indicate individual exclusion from women's groups at Taljai or women's active choice to avoid being controlled by other women. This chapter explores the tight gendered sociability surrounding homebirth at Taljai, demonstrating how women amalgamate experiences of self-birthing at home with home-birthing at the slum, instrumentalizing childbirth rituals as a means of social bonding.

As the primary thrust of my argument, I suggest that childbirth practices are inseparable from women's socio-economic, family, and life conditions. More specifically, I propose that childbirth practices can be understood as a mirror or staging arena that reflects birthing women's economic status, social networks, and relationships. In this chapter, I will outline how childbirth practices among lower-caste women at a large slum (Taljai), located on the southern outskirts of Pune city, reflect the transitory lives of rural migrant women within urbanized slums (see Pinto 2008). I argue that women's birthing practices at Taljai reflect transformations in their family and caste relationships, anchored in an imagined past associated with village life that they juxtapose to their present-day impermanent and migrant lives within the urban slum.[1] The women I interviewed and worked with in Taljai defined themselves in ambivalent ways. On the one hand, they were negatively

Deepra Dandekar, *Childbirth in Transit* In: *Childbirth in South Asia*. Edited by: Clémence Jullien and Roger Jeffery, Oxford University Press. © Oxford University Press 2021. DOI: 10.1093/oso/9780190130718.003.0006 affected by their impermanent and slum life conditions that involved sharing small and unclean neighbourhoods characterized by paucity, and the lack of affordable quality medical care. This created an artificial community among some of them, who felt nostalgic about an imagined and glorified village life from the past, characterized by helpful and supportive relationships that transcended clan and caste barriers, and regional differences. On the other hand, despite such privations, women in the slum enjoyed greater access to clinical amenities (if not expensive private clinics) and transport facilities in comparison to villages located in the rural interior, since Taljai has increasingly become part of Pune's growing urbanism in the last four decades. At the same time, the slum's semi-urbanized milieu formed an unmarked domain for childbirth for women that was neither strictly relegated to clinics nor located at home. Instead, childbirth in the slum was defined by a sense of mobility, wherein women had babies wherever labour pains overtook them, sometimes at work and even in vehicles on their way to clinics. They often juxtaposed the insecurity of this mobility and impermanence of childbirth in the slum with the alleged security enjoyed by their parental generations in villages, recounting stories about mothers and aunts giving birth in the safety of ritually prepared birthing-corners, ensconced within traditional rural homes. I have termed this unmarked domain for childbirth at Taljai, which is reflective of women's impermanence and migration backgrounds, 'transitory'.

Birth attendants at Taljai were mostly of an informal variety and did not include specially trained midwives (*sooin* in Marathi) either. Any neighbourhood women, present at the time of labour and delivery, who helped in various capacities like massaging and baby catching, were considered midwives. Childbirth in Taljai, took place impromptu, as helping women and midwives made curtains out of saris at the nearest available shelter, to shield women giving birth from the public gaze. Slum inhabitations and homes clustered together, therefore, produced a permeable context that merged individual homes and neighbourhood homes within the locality. People streamed in and out of homes, simultaneously busy with other activities, as childbirth took place in a cordoned-off corner of the same room. Women's mobile slum lives, therefore, produced childbirth as transitory and mobile too, merging the location of birth in the slum, family, caste groups, their village background, and modern clinics, together with neighbourhoods, women's friendship networks, their work outside home, and their individual birth-giving body.

Research Method and Context at Taljai

I conducted research on home-birthing at Taljai during the two monsoon seasons of 2009 and 2010. Though I initially meant to triangulate the main body of my doctoral fieldwork on childbirth and goddess rituals in rural areas outside Pune (that I conducted in 2006 and 2008), research at Taljai soon developed its own, individual ethnographic character that proved to be different from my doctoral research. Childbirth at Taljai was not as deeply marked by traditional family rituals associated with birth pollution, as it was with everyday practices of childbirth that were deeply embroiled with the mobile status of women in the slum and their social networks.[2] While I presented some of my initial findings at a conference on nursing in Thailand in 2010, I included only a small description of Taljai in my published thesis (Dandekar 2016b). The contrast between rural and urban Marathi women turned out to be unhelpful, an untenable and constructed binary between village women and migrant slum life. Since rural women were not outside experiences of urbanization, and urbanized women from the slum at Taljai were not without rural roots, my women respondents in Taljai considered themselves simultaneously rural and urban. On the other hand, my respondents in the villages where I collected data for my doctoral research also considered themselves semi-rural: a group that frequently visited nearby towns for shopping, meeting relatives, and attending family functions and festivals.

And yet, there were differences between them. While my village respondents at the time had limited access to ready cash, means of transportation, especially required during reproductive emergencies, and urban amenities like electricity and water, they were more grounded in agrarian activities that gained them access to village-rights—traditional clan and caste residence and inheritance, in contrast to Taljai women. But an agrarian background was not completely missing among my Taljai respondents either. Many women at Taljai returned to their villages during the harvesting season to help out and partake of farm produce. But this agrarian addition to their income was already different from the wealth that their rural counterparts enjoyed, since their share contributed to smaller nuclear families and friendship networks at Taljai, and not to the larger clan network back home in the village. Contrasted to childbirth in the village, where each bride was an individual migrant, their migration being considered part of the marriage institution itself, migrant women in Taljai were different.[3] Women's transitory condition in Taljai was familial, supported by local, spatialized networks that became an elemental part of their individual-family lives, straddling neighbourhood relationships and locality friendships. Therefore, while childbirth rituals in the village served to integrate new mothers with their marital families and villages, marriages in Taljai were often (though not always) located within the slum itself, producing childbirth practices as part of the slum's impermanent sociality and spatiality that included entire families, reflecting the precarity of their everyday life.

Taljai was a large artificial community in Pune, made up of rural, migrant, and small family groups from all over Western Maharashtra that were too poor to depend completely on agriculture. As small agricultural ventures failed, nuclear parts of village clans disengaged from their joint village property and moved to urban slums such as Taljai, taking on menial jobs in Pune city. According to my women respondents, the slum had increased manifold in its demographic size after the 1990s, as an increasing number of migrants in Maharashtra and from all over India were attracted to Pune. In terms of its prehistory, however, my women respondents remembered the slum settlement to be as old as 1980, a place consisting mostly of bramble forests and occasional wild animals in a time when it was far from Pune. The Pune Municipal Corporation had allotted the area at the base of the thickly forested hillock on the Pune outskirts at the time, mainly to migrants from Marathwada, a region that had been cleaved away from Hyderabad (Nizam's province) and merged with Maharashtra in the 1960s. Poorer families from Marathwada that migrated to urban centres in Western Maharashtra, like Pune, were relocated to Taljai in 1985. Many of my respondents possessed land deeds for their tenements at Taljai and said they had even paid the government property tax for these small one-room establishments. The increasing urbanism of Pune had, however, attracted other migrants over time, and this had gradually marginalized the Marathwada substratum within Taljai, which had also diminished in size due to the rise of other urban centres within Marathwada like Aurangabad, Usmanabad, Latur, Jalna, and so on. While many of the older generation of women at Taljai belonged to different villages from Marathwada, they had continued to live on, at the fringes of urbanized Pune for more than 30 years now. They were, moreover, angry with the Pune Municipality for their marginalization that treated them as illegal criminals and squatters. They wanted, instead, to be credited for Pune's urbanism and modernity, and viewed themselves as deserving of reward. They aspired for recognition: political, social, and economic inclusion within Pune, and the removal of the unjust 'encroacher' label that enabled demolition drives, especially before every election. Though associating Marathwada migrants to Taljai may seem predicated on women's personal histories of migrating from Marathwada and being allotted land in Pune in the 1980s, this process of internal migration in Maharashtra is also central to the political formation of the state as a federal unit in the 1960s, which demarcated itself from Gujarat, Karnataka, and the Nizam's Hyderabad state. The migration of poorer Marathi families from the outlying parts of the Deccan beyond the erstwhile region of Bombay Presidency is, hence, integral to the history of Indian federalism in the Deccan, and the formation of the Maharashtra state that dissolved the colonial unit of Bombay Presidency (Godsmark 2019). However, many older families that had lived in Taljai for several years continued to 'feel' like outsiders and transitory groups in Pune city. They were subject to regular police harassment whenever a robbery or crime took place in a 10 km radius of Taljai. And their households, sometimes smaller than 10 square metres, were often subject to demolition. During demolition, no one considered their property documents valid, procured with great difficulty under the constant threat of eviction.

The anti-migrant and anti-poor politics of elite and urban Pune was, moreover, a thinly veiled garb, aimed at evacuating Taljai, that outwardly lamented the loss of environment-friendly zones in Pune's natural habitat. This garb of environmentalism held Taljai responsible for rising crime and increasing pollution encountered in Pune. While environmentalism is not an unworthy cause, in the case of Taljai it is politically deployed against slum dwellers in ways that undermine their role in providing Pune city with cheaply available labour utilized for urban planning and development in the last four decades.[4] The *Pune Mirror,* for example, published an article on 6 March 2011 (Chavan 2011) pronouncing Taljai unsafe and infested with criminal slum goons, who harassed and robbed Pune citizens taking morning and evening walks in the nearby forested hills. It further assured its readers that the police continue to comb nearby slums for assailants. A report about slum demolition in Taljai, published in the *Pune Mirror* on 16 November 2017 (Patil 2017), however, remains comparatively sympathetic, as it documents how a bulldozer led by a local police team demolished parts of the Taljai slum that had encroached onto forest department lands. Using an interview with one Taljai slum inhabitant, whose house had been razed in the demolition, the article documented that inhabitants had no forewarning about the demolition. The interviewee, a maid working in one of the nearby housing colonies, went on record describing how she was born and brought up in Taljai and was married in Taljai too. The family had been paying property tax to the government for many years and even owned their now-bulldozed tenement, for which they could also show ownership papers. However, they could not even salvage their utensils, belongings, and appliances, for which they had paid hard-earned money when demolition-time came. The Pune Municipal Corporation has in recent years, tried to 'reform' and develop the Taljai slum by evacuating it and relocating populations to low-income housing schemes, further away from the city (Pune Municipal Corporation 2019a). This government slum-development scheme in Pune has additionally seen the generation of raw data, especially as a result of a rapid household survey carried out between November 2015 and February 2016 across Pune slums under the 'Swachh Bharat Mission', aimed at providing individual tenements at Taljai with toilets (Pune Municipal Corporation 2019b). According to the survey, Taljai suffered from nearly a total absence of toilets and sewage drainage facilities—an important issue I return to, in the section on Taljai mothers and midwives.

At the time of my fieldwork, Taljai houses were precarious, single-brick, one-roomed shanty structures, covered with asbestos tin-sheets and tarpaulin. Hardly anyone had a toilet at home. They had only bathrooms with an open drainage system that, according to my respondents, served women as spaces for delivery during home-birthing. Nearly a total percentage of Marathi women at Taljai belonged to the *matang* caste (considered the lowest among Hindus) making their living from scrap collection, the resale of materials salvaged from the city's garbage dumps, temporary/permanent construction activities in Pune city, and domestic work in nearby housing societies. Women at Taljai were deeply susceptible and vulnerable to tetanus, along with the associated damage entailed, in their constant contact with dirt, pollutants, toxic materials, and fumes, commonly encountered while cleaning drains and collecting scrap from rubbish dumps. None of the women I worked with used protective gloves, helmets, or footwear while scaling and sifting through large dunes of rotting garbage. Needless to say, a few childbirths took place at work too, when women were outside the home. Some women recounted stories of birthing at garbage dumps, when they were either alone or accompanied by a couple of other neighbourhood women. This situation was said to be extremely dangerous, since not only were garbage dumps unclean and toxic, but they were infested with rodents, dogs, and other scavenging birds and animals that attacked easily. Although slum households at Taljai had stabilized enough over the last three generations to protect pregnant women from incurring the danger of 'birth at work', the inception period for the first generation of migrant women at Taljai was said to have been difficult. At that time, I was told that everyone had to work every day, to earn enough money to eat every day, pregnant or not. Older women said that it was in fact their experiences of self-birthing in those early years spent at Taljai that taught them midwifery skills and the ability to help other women in childbirth emergencies.

My decision to use the monsoons for fieldwork in Taljai, was somewhat deliberate, since monsoons usually generated very little work within Maharashtra's and Pune's urban informal sector, as well as agrarian sectors within rural areas. This is not just because of the disruption caused by the monsoon to scrap collection, though that too, but because of the ritual period of *chaturmasa* (four months) in Hinduism, when the Gods were said to sleep and withdraw from the world. No occasion or celebration was ever planned in Pune during chaturmasa with the exception of *Krishna Janmashtami*, occasions that were usually managed by locality groups within the city. In terms of small employment opportunities at Taljai, therefore, monsoons (June-end to mid-September) were considered fallow months, where working at domestic chores in nearby housing societies was the only source of women's family income. According to my women respondents, childbirth at Taljai was typically planned for the beginning of the monsoons, though conception did not always go according to plan. For those who managed to effectively plan conception during the *Navratri* (the autumn harvest festival of 'Nine Nights') in October, having babies at the beginning of the monsoons was ideal, since the child was already weaned and about 3 months old before the employment cycle began. It was convenient for new mothers to leave their babies at home with the older generation and other neighbourhood friends as they restarted work in Pune with the beginning of the *Ganpati* festival. As many of my respondents half-ironically said, the impermanence and precarity of women's lives at Taljai even resulted in limiting and restricting their childbirth to an annual calendar. They were not free to have children whenever they wanted.

However, doing individual interviews with women at Taljai, even during the monsoons, was next to impossible. Each household practically teemed with women and children, and everyone was curious about a city-bred researcher asking questions about childbirth. They first peeped in through the doors and windows and then just joined the discussion. Group discussions, moreover, did not have a constant number of women from start to finish. Some women sat for a while and then left, losing interest, and becoming busy elsewhere. Older women often tried to dominate larger group discussions, wanting the voice of morality to prevail, while younger women spoke about experiences of midwifery and homebirths, comparing it with clinics. I received small snippets from each of my respondents during group discussions, as interviews became extended afternoon chats, involving changing groups of women.

Though the whole of Taljai was considered a slum, most among my first-generation migrant respondents at Taljai, resisted the idea of a 'united' community here. Families had originally arrived here from different regions of Marathwada and Maharashtra. These regional communities had their own distinct identity and living areas within the slum, with the slum in its inception years being strictly divided on regional lines that was subject to internal infighting. This rivalry had, however, lessened in recent years, with some of the newer migrant families here belonging not only to other regions of India, but also to Bangladesh. Apart from micro-specificities, Taljai was not very different from a diaspora made up of migrants. On the one hand, women felt they belonged to a unified artificial community, simply because they were grouped together and 'othered' as one migrant group, unfairly discriminated against by outsiders. On the other hand, while their internal solidarity enabled their existence as migrants on the margins of Pune, they also contested and challenged the ontology of this unified 'othered' existence by upholding the internal segregations of the artificial community. Birthing and midwifing women supported each other at the slum and mimicked an imaginary, glorified village life combined with cheaper modern amenities. It was a place where they transcended differences despite the segregated parts of the slum, while at the same time upholding these segregations, in ways that were functional, and mutually competitive. Despite what seemed like a paradox, childbirth practices at Taljai sought to integrate and amalgamate the village past and semi-urban slum present, segregated by women's friendship networks within its segments, which mirrored and counterbalanced the crisis of precarious, poor, and impermanent circumstances of their everyday lives.

While members of a diaspora are known to keep their roots in their home-country/village intact, they also entrench themselves in individual relationships with other diaspora members, producing a mutually supportive bulwark of migrants living abroad and on the margins of an alien social mainstream. As Çaglar and Glick Schiller point out (2018), not all migrant diasporas are uniform social structures, without internal rivalry, differentiation, or segregations between groups that form an artificial community. It is well known that migrant diasporas are, in fact, rife with difference: differences born out of discrimination meted out by 'host' communities, who 'other' migrants as poor and parasitic dependents, disconnected from the enhancement of the social mainstream.[5] This is borne out well by Taljai, as my respondents pointed to segregations within the slum, especially economically better-off sections with permanent structures that challenged the discrimination meted out by Pune environmentalists, who 'othered' Taljai as uniformly disruptive, poor, unhygienic, backward, and criminal. The poverty and impermanence of women's slum lives, however permanent some of its one-roomed structures were, produced a fluid neighbourhood network among women, who simultaneously contested and endorsed their artificial micro-groups, using imagined ideals of both clinical birth and childbirth at home, to combat the hostile mainstream and the precarity of their childbirth emergencies. The exigency of women's childbirth experiences was, hence, ambivalently linked with their opinions about ideal birthing. While some of my women respondents at Taljai privileged a pristine image of homebirth that presented them as women with strong rural roots, others privileged the shining technology of modern clinics that presented them as modern and urban Pune citizens.[6] And their opinions, which were part of their self-representation, were deeply in contrast to how the emergency and exigency of labour was actually managed in their individual cases—exceptions that my women respondents often referred to as a 'compromise' (*tadajod*).

Taljai Mothers and Midwives

While many women accommodated medical facilities within home-birthing, depending on a trained nurse living in or nearby Taljai, they also introduced ritual traditions learned from an older generation within clinical births, often making small offerings to deity shrines, commonly encountered outside clinics and hospitals. And the second and third generation of women at Taljai usually said that they felt trapped between home-birthing, situated in a familiar environment that was lacking in hygiene on the one hand, and clinical birth, considered safe, hygienic but also unfamiliar on the other. Many felt apprehensive about home-birthing and midwives, while others felt apprehensive about untrustworthy and unaccountable doctors making mistakes, and then forcing women into dangerous and expensive C-section surgeries. Many younger women at Taljai considered the extolling of home-birthing 'superstitious' (*andhashraddha*), a remnant of ancestral rural life, even as they themselves ended up giving birth at home, due to the exigency of untimely labour. Also, what constituted a familiar environment was subjective, based on women's interpersonal relationships with other women and family members in the slum. While some preferred husbands to be present, others did not want any men lurking around. Some preferred midwives who were already personal friends to be present, even if they only served to accompany labouring women to the nearby clinic. Others depended on trained nurses and midwives who would come home to help in the delivery, at an extra charge, providing women with medicines if required. While many women considered traditional postures of home-birthing helpful (that involved squatting on their hind legs, while holding on to a rope suspended from the ceiling for support), they feared the lying down position that they said did not allow them to gain any purchase over their contractions. Others considered the lying down posture easier.[7] The youngest generation of women at Taljai were strong exponents of clinical birth. Many of my younger respondents associated clinical birth with personal prestige in their marital family, often reading it as a sign of their husband's love and care. This was a sore point, as older women accused the younger ones of being too individualistic, selfish, and focused on personal relationships, rather than on family and duty. 'Did our husbands never love us?', they asked rhetorically!

Exigent childbirth at home, often described by women as a 'compromise', resulted from the sudden onset of labour and breaking waters. However much women planned, my respondents said that the suddenness of their labour was inevitable in more than 50% cases of childbirth in Taljai, transforming their image of ideal childbirth into an exigent one often expressed rhetorically as 'what-all we had imagined—and what really happened' (*kai vichaar kelaa hotaa- aani kai jhaala*)! This process of transformation constituted a kind of a transit zone for women that reflected their impermanent lives as migrant women. Hence, women, who considered home-birthing ideal, often ended up with clinical births when the bleeding became uncontrollable or when midwives could no longer repair breach situations with massage and vaginal manipulation. On the other hand, those endorsing clinical births often ended up giving birth at home, while getting ready to go to the hospital. One of my respondents recounted having her baby in an auto-rickshaw, while on her way to the clinic. She was lucky that the rickshaw was being driven by her husband, and that her sister-in-law was accompanying them to the hospital. The sister-in-law and husband immediately lowered the rickshaw seat, curtained the back of the rickshaw with saris that were already packed into the night-bag for the hospital, and helped her give birth. Nearby vendors at a late-night roadside stall that sold omelettes to passers-by helped the family by providing them fresh food and water. By the time the other family members arrived, the baby was already born.

The bathroom played an important role in home-birthing at Taljai. As already mentioned, Taljai homes at the time I was working there did not have private toilets. Each home, however small, nevertheless had a bathroom with a tap encircled by a semi-circular half-wall, cordoned off by curtains in one corner of the room, useful during baths. Since Taljai lacked a drainage system at the time, water from these bathrooms poured out of holes in the wall, directly into gutters adjoining the streets. These bathroom holes were mostly protected by a wire-mesh on the inside, to stop rodents from climbing into the house through chutes. Women washed clothes and utensils in the bathroom, and the whole family bathed there.

Women who faced labour exigencies or decided to give birth at home also chose bathrooms to squat, once their contractions began. The mother was usually supported by a sling made from a sari, passed around her back and under her arms, and knotted to a ring or hook suspended from the ceiling. The birthing mother rested her shoulder blades and upper arms on the sling, while women helpers from the neighbourhood supported her lower back from behind, with every contraction, as she squatted, waited, and allowed the contractions to wash over her. They led her around, encouraging her to walk between contractions, till these came faster. And they continued to massage her lower back, till the baby's crown was glimpsed. Home-birthing could be a long and drawn-out process, especially since the many helping women or midwives refused to cut the cord before the placenta dislodged itself naturally. While women believed that breastfeeding the newborn immediately helped to dislodge the placenta, others stuffed a pinch of snuff into the mother's nose, hoping that a sudden spate of sneezes would help the placenta to come out. Still others tried to induce retching or laughing to dislodge the placenta, while some tugged gently at the cord. Tugging was however, considered risky since the cord could tear, the placenta torn prematurely from the uterus lining resulting often, in bleeding. The older generation of women at Taljai considered the placenta to be the child's actual mother, and the cord was kept intact till the placenta emerged. If the cord was cut too soon, older women believed that the placenta would travel upwards and get lost in the woman's body, finally touching her heart and killing her.[8] They recounted the importance of the empty space left behind by the baby (*vayu-gola*) that caused the new mother pain, unless childbirth goddesses were properly appeased and propitiated.[9] Others considered this association between goddesses and vayu-gola superstitious and declared that the pain was nothing more than the uterus contracting and returning to its normal size after childbirth. Still others considered the placenta to contain healing properties that had the capacity of resuscitating stillborn babies if it were massaged and heated (see also Sadgopal 2009).

Women who had spent more than four hours in labour at home were said to be in danger. None among the younger generation of my respondents who opted for homebirths waited for more than 4 or 5 hours, especially if contractions grew faster without adequate dilation, accompanied by bleeding. It was not like earlier times, bemoaned older women at Taljai, when women had the stamina to remain in labour for 15 hours at a stretch. Older women were, however, often cut short in such discussions by younger women, who were quick to point out that they were no longer living in villages. The small bathrooms of their slum homes were communal and for the use of other family members as well. These could not be occupied for 15 hours at a stretch by women in labour, slung to the ceiling and surrounded by other women huddled behind an impromptu curtain. While neighbours and helpers checked for developments during the first 3 hours of labour, calling for a trained nurse or midwife in the meanwhile, the obstructed woman was rushed to a nearby clinic for delivery if this did not help. According to my respondents, a prolonged delivery and a last-minute decision to take the birthing woman to a clinic often resulted in C-section surgeries.

Older women recounted some earlier rituals to ease obstructed childbirth that they had learned in their villages before coming to Taljai, which they practised during their initial years as migrants here.[10] According to this ritual, neighbourly midwives would form a chain with a young man, who was as yet unmarried at their helm. He would draw water from a well or a tap, and this water would be passed down the chain of women and given to the obstructed woman to drink. Drinking this water was said to release the woman in labour from childbirth obstruction, since the water contained the undiluted power of the man's moral purity and virtue. While the assumption behind this ritual indicated to women's sexual immorality as a cause for obstructed childbirth and the death of their children, these rituals had largely been discarded at the time I did fieldwork in Taljai. The focus of homebirth for women at Taljai had shifted to their facilitating of social networks and their access to clinics. Childbirth at Taljai, hence, consisted of a potent and hybrid amalgamation that mirrored the impermanent and precarious lives of migrant women, battling poverty here. Every woman who gained experience in helping with birthing at home, either by assisting others or by self-birthing, functioned as a midwife and helper at Taljai, operating in a larger social network of women.[11]

Women at Taljai formed competitive cohorts against other newcomer women, their personal enmity with these newcomers often garbed in ideological terms. For example, they often justified their personal dislike by accusing other women of foolishness, manipulativeness, wastefulness, and so on. Women and their friendship networks, therefore, arbitrarily 'out-casted' disliked newcomers based on their personal likes and dislikes, about which most powerful women in the group demanded consensus. Those who were accepted but not too powerful in the group kept quiet so as not to endanger their own acceptance. This segregated bonding within tightly woven friendship networks became manifest in women's childbirth support extended to each other during homebirth emergencies, making their delicately balanced multilateral web of gendered surveillance and exchange central to safe home-birthing in Taljai. Women watched, observed, and evaluated each other, based on everyday decisions and relationships with family and neighbours, all the while exchanging small favours and gifts with newcomers to test them. They decided whether they accepted or rejected a newcomer, based on their arbitrary liking for her, justified through ideological arguments. For instance, if a newcomer made too lavish a gift, then a group could either consider her boastful or generous, depending on whether they liked her. On the other hand, if a newcomer's gift was inadequate, then the group could either elect to feel unappreciated for the friendship they had extended her, denouncing her as miserly, or consider her as confident enough to not be needlessly obsequious to them.[12]

Opting for clinical birth for many women was, hence, more than aspiring to be urban and modern Pune citizens, since clinical birth also constituted an escape from group and neighbourhood politics and interpersonal dynamics between women and friendship groups. While, of course, women never openly admitted to excluding newcomers, this exclusion was obliquely indicated by not inviting a newcomer to help and support other women in the group during emergencies, explained away later as remiss, an easy mistake in the panic of an emergency. Not being invited meant breaking mutuality within network circles, disallowing newcomers from asking for any help in return. My women respondents considered the organizing of childbirth rituals an ideal way of soldering social networks between locality women, even though many families simply did not have the financial means to organize relatively expensive celebrations. Therefore, even those women who considered home-birthing superstitious, and extolled clinical birth, continued to celebrate childbirth at home, however small-scale, especially if it was their first delivery or the birth of a male child. Friendships in the slum, hence, required monetary investment, enough to buy the new mother a sari, the child a small cradle, clothes, ritual offerings to the goddess, home decorations, and enough food (even if just tea and biscuits) for 40 or 50 women from the locality, taking care not to omit or offend anyone.

Another more obvious way of avoiding being excluded from competitive gendered cohorts was for women to choose to live near their relatives in the slum. Though women from the same extended family could personally dislike each other, the transformation of this personal dislike into group enmity against a newcomer was more difficult to achieve. When women criticized their relatives within friends' circles, their friends smiled indulgently, identifying this criticism as personal and not as a marker of 'out-casting' newcomers. Kinship relationships still had enough power to counterbalance friendship circles, and indeed, many core groups became an intermixture of extended clans defined by locality friendships, where entry to mutually helping relationships defined the interiority of kinship relationships between women in the slum. Many families in Taljai thus shifted to other areas inside Taljai itself, to live closer to their kin and village networks, harking back to a common past that transcended their present-day slum realities. At the same time, my respondents knew how to identify single-family domination in their friendship networks and resisted it. The focus of childbirth rituals therefore subtly shifted in the slum, from appeasing goddesses and women within the clan and caste group, to appeasing women organized in friendship circles that formed a socially supportive bulwark of mothers and neighbourly midwives, responsible for ascertaining safe homebirth in Taljai.

The only escape from this group dynamics lay in eliciting and paying for private nurses or trained midwives from nearby areas outside Taljai, or from other distant parts of Taljai during homebirth emergencies. Since Taljai was very large and structurally complex, with intricate and labyrinthine alleyways leading to the central and more squalid areas of the slum, women living closer to the highway, with access to transportation and local markets, were considered comparatively 'free' of the community dynamics that prevailed within its congested interiors. Also, they constituted the 'face' of Taljai, of what could be seen of the slum from its outside, and some of the houses nearer the main road were better-looking. But these areas were also more expensive, and masqueraded as upper-class areas, where the inhabiting family's 'respectability' was identified by its power to maintain privacy from neighbourhood circles. One of my respondents, a trained midwife living on the outer edge of Taljai near the main road, recounted how she had once walked nearly a kilometre towards the slum-interior in the middle of the night, to help a woman who had suddenly gone into labour.

The gendered context of Taljai painted home-birthing in a shade that was quite different from its usual association with 'tradition' and ancestral village practices. Opting for clinical birth was not an independent ideological decision for women concerned with modernity (though younger women in the slum constantly referred to themselves as 'modern'). Instead, the nature of social networks, relationships, and contexts between women played a decisive role in defining childbirth here, wherein ideas that privileged home or the clinic were irrespective of actual practices predicated on emergencies. Home-birthing was thus fluidly located between the ideological extremes of 'tradition' and 'modernity', while this location was simultaneously rendered meaningless when juxtaposed with the exigencies and the precarities of migrant women's lives. This transitory in-between-ness constituted a space wherein childbirth, women's bodies, and social relationships merged to enable safe homebirth. On the other hand, the internally linked powerful and fluid encounter between women and midwives simultaneously excluded others, pushing disliked newcomers to the slum's peripheries, and forcing them to forge childbirth relationships with the outside world that disconnected them from the slum.

Characterizing home-birthing for migrant women at Taljai as transitory led me to introspection about women's relationships and personal powerlessness that were part of their migrant and impermanent existence at the slum. Maintaining friendship circles at Taljai was itself central to the safety of my respondents during an emergency homebirth, mitigating its danger. Women of childbearing age could not afford to be 'out-casted' by friends, because they needed help and support in all kinds of neighbourly ways. Therefore, although women were superficially 'free' to choose between homebirth or clinical birth, they were at the same time bounded by social networks, conventions, and the precarity of a migrant existence that was closely governed by an unpredictable form of sociality. This ungoverned sociality based on personal likes and dislikes was outside any earlier village tradition known by their parental generations, which could have served to mediate between village clans and castes. This unique and rather arbitrary sociality at Taljai, therefore, also had a deep impact on migrant women's reproductive vulnerability, sometimes helping and strengthening them if they were insiders, and sometimes increasing their poverty by introducing the fear of ostracism into their already difficult and precarious lives if they were newcomers.

Though women consumed opinions and experiences of gender-based freedom and choice broadcasted in the media (especially TV serials), they were personally unable to realize this freedom for themselves. They lacked the money that could afford them quality institutional care and health-care practitioners, professional networks, and families that would take over finances and allow them to rest during difficult pregnancies. Many of my respondents led violent personal lives, as male alcohol consumption remained high in Taljai. Most women employed in the unorganized sector were forced to continue working till the very last days of their pregnancy and continued to exist in conditions of systemic violence, if not outright personal or domestic abuse. They enjoyed no reprieve from labour, nor any opportunity to engage with social systems and structures that allowed them to plan clinical birth in advance, especially as they feared being quickly replaced by others within the informal sector, once they dropped out of work. Most Taljai women belonged to nuclear families or had one old parent or parent-in-law living with them. There was hardly ever any extended family to divide up household labour and sometimes there were younger dependents staying over instead, who had come to Pune seeking higher education and job opportunities. While the husbands of many of my respondents at Taljai earned, much of their family savings went into emergencies that involved salvaging homes after demolitions, coping with sudden robberies, destructions caused by fire, or heavy monsoons, or then, spent in extravagances and ostentatious celebrations, and marriages that required a display of their Pune living 'standard'. Above all, systems of quality medical care for pregnant women remained financially out of reach for most families. In comparison to ideas about women's freedom in the media, women's agency in Taljai was limited, their reproductive health decisions being exigent and not the result of their personal choice. Their powerlessness lay in their inability to link their idealized form of childbirth (whether home or clinical) with actual birth practices available to them in the slum, with last-minute solutions due to the unpredictable and sudden onset of their labour during work, what they called the 'compromise'. Linking poverty with migration, social networks, gender, and childbirth practices, this chapter posits Taljai as a world unto itself: marginal to the social mainstream of urban Pune, and yet at the same time, an embodied part of Pune city's migrant labouring force. However, despite being on the margins of Pune, Taljai could also be described as an independent and partially closed system that functioned like a 'hydraulic model' (Skultans 1991), wherein every opening to the outside world was closely predicated on lessening the pressure upon social relationships on the inside.

Skultans used the concept of a 'hydraulic model' for the first time to describe how women, considered socially inferior to men in rural Maharashtra, undertook healing rituals on behalf of men to cure them of spirit possession. Since spirit possession was understood to cause madness, and too stigmatizing a diagnosis for men, women in their families undertook healing rituals for spirit possession (and madness) to not just heal men but also to avert their stigmatization. This idea of a 'hydraulic model' can be extended to social networks among Taljai women that enabled safe homebirth, while also fostering the exclusion of disliked newcomers. The 'hydraulic model' at Taljai functioned by replacing or counterbalancing the precarity of migration and poverty with social relationships among women that absorbed and mitigated the transitory nature of childbirth emergencies. Women within such relational core groups displaced their own precarity to the margins, and to marginal newcomers at the slum. While Skultans's hydraulic model demonstrates patriarchal hierarchies in ritual healing that functions by siphoning off pressure from the more powerful and hierarchically superior interior to is powerless margins, in the Taljai context, this meant that poorer interiors were hierarchically superior social spaces, whereas the non-networked more affluent outskirts became considered socially inferior. Networked women's core groups at Taljai, especially in its interiors, assumed hierarchical superiority by successfully replacing structural precarity and systemic violence with individual-social-gendered bonds. These groups then, siphoned off the pressure of poverty, precarity, and violence on the inside, by displacing it to its margins of excluded women. Excluded women in this case became the poorer margin of this internal core group that bore the burden of precarity displaced from the inside, by paying more for their homes and being more vulnerable to demolitions that always targeted the peripheries first. Not only did they additionally pay for midwives and trained nurses during childbirth emergencies, but women sometimes completely forwent employment during the last trimesters of their pregnancies to plan their clinical birth in advance, in an already precarious informal sector. To be excluded thus, implied expenditure and loneliness for marginalized migrant women, who had somehow been unable to hit it off with the women in the slum interior who had stayed there for a far longer time and were strongly networked.

There is, however, one important difference between Skultans's 'hydraulic model', with hierarchically superior male cores and female peripheries, and the societal web of Taljai, with safe, networked, albeit poorer cores and unsafe peripheries. The difference here lies in the fact that clinical birth is definitely not considered 'marginal' in Pune city. There are many clinical options that are increasingly available to women living in slums, and many women actively choose clinics, while others are taken to clinics in emergency situations, despite the social support they enjoy as members of women's groups. The marginality of clinical birth is, hence, artificially produced in relation to the safety and security of women's social relationships at Taljai. Childbirth in Taljai that takes place on the margins of clinics therefore forms its own group that discursively produces childbirth as social and as central to a gendered and interpersonal arena, reflective of the poverty and precarity of migrant women's individual and family lives. It is within this interrelated space and sociability of shifting core and periphery, explained by extending Skultans's 'hydraulic model' to Taljai, that childbirth in the slum becomes transitory.

Notes

1. Cf. Chakravarty and Negi (2016) for an analysis of interstitial spaces in slums that are utilized as nodal points of negotiation by slum-dwellers to own collective spaces and transform government and state policy on urban planning.
2. For research on labour and birth pollution, see Jeffery et al. (1989), Jeffery and Jeffery (1993), Rozario and Samuel (2002). Also, see Dandekar (2009, 2014, 2016a, 2016b) for a description of her doctoral research on childbirth rituals in rural Maharashtra.
3. For married women as migrants in virilocal marriages, see Palriwala and Uberoi (2008). Also, see Nichter (2001) for the political ecology of health and the interlinkage between belonging and body in rural India.
4. See Goswami (2014) for a review on female reproductive health morbidity and slum-life. Also see Weigl (2010) for the reproductive health of women in a slum in North India.
5. Çaglar and Glick Schiller (2018) have recently written on how migrant displacement and re-settlements lead to their participation in unequal networks of power that connect them in new ways to regional, national, and global institutions.
6. See Van Hollen (2003) for how childbirth practices are mediated by globalization and 'modernity' in India.
7. For an intense ethnography of childbirth and motherhood in a slum, see Scheper-Hughes (1992) on how poverty and high infant mortality rates reconstitute motherhood and child survival.
8. See Sadgopal (2009) for indigenous practices of midwifery that preserve the placenta as a life-giving force for the newborn.
9. See Chawla (2002) for an ethnographic description of *hawa gola*, the equivalent of *vayu-gola* in Hindi.

10. See Duvvury (1991) for a rich ethnographic account of childbirth rituals in Tamil Nadu, which are similar to the ones I encountered in rural Maharashtra and in Taljai, that associate safe childbirth with women's sexual morality.
11. Rairkar (2007) has conducted interesting research analysis on the transformation of midwifery traditions and practices in rural Maharashtra.
12. See Pinto (2008) for how childbirth is a political arena with fluctuating spaces and actors that produce power, authority, and politics within communities.

References

Çaglar, Ayse, and Nina Glick Schiller. 2018. *Migrants and City-Making: Dispossession, Displacement, and Urban Regeneration*. Durham, NC: Duke University Press.

Chakravarty, Surajit, and Rohit Negi, eds. 2016. *Space, Planning and Everyday Contestations in Delhi*. New Delhi: Springer India.

Chavan, Vijay. 2011. 'Stolen Moments for Three Youth on Parvati Hill'. *Pune Mirror*, 6 March. Accessed 12 February 2019. https://punemirror.indiatimes.com/pune/cover-story/stolen-moments-for-three-youth-on-parvati-hill/articleshow/32220340.cms

Chawla, Janet. 2002. '*Hawa, Gola* and Mother-in-Law's Big Toe: On Understanding Dais' Imagery of the Female Body'. In *Daughters of Hariti: Childbirth and Female Healers in South and Southeast Asia*, edited by Santi Rozario and Geoffrey Samuel, 158–73. London & New York: Routledge.

Dandekar, Deepra. 2009. 'Satvai and the Lives of Women in Ghodegaon'. In *Liebe, Sexualitat, Ehe und Partnerschaft: Paradigment im Wandel*, edited by Roswitha Badry, Maria Rohrer, and Karin Steiner, 281–92. Freiburg: Fördergemeinschaft wissenschaftler Publikationen von Frauen.

Dandekar, Deepra. 2014. 'Childlessness and Empathetic Relationships'. *The Oriental Anthropologist* 14 (1): 123–39.

Dandekar, Deepra. 2016a. 'The Baaravi Ritual, Clan and Ancestor Worship'. In *Childbirth and Its Accompanying Rituals: An Anthropological Analysis of Birth and Childhood Rituals in South and South East Asia*, edited by Karin Polit and Gabriele Alex, 128–43. Heidelberg: Neckar Draupadi Verlag.

Dandekar, Deepra. 2016b. *Boundaries and Motherhood: Ritual and Reproduction in Rural Maharashtra*. New Delhi: Zubaan.

Duvvury, Vasumathi K. 1991. *Play, Symbolism, and Ritual: A Study of Tamil Brahmin Women's Rites of Passage*. New York: Peter Lang.

Godsmark, Oliver. 2019. 'Searching for Synergies, Making Majorities: The Demands for Pakistan and Maharashtra'. *South Asia: Journal of South Asian Studies* 42 (1): 115–33.

Goswami, Sribas. 2014. 'A Study on Women's Healthcare Practice in Urban Slums: Indian Scenario'. *Journal of Evidence-Based Women's Health Journal Society* 4(4): 201–7.

Jeffery, Patricia, Roger Jeffery, and Andrew Lyon. 1989. *Labour Pains and Labour Power: Women and Childbearing in India*. London: Zed Books.

Jeffery, Roger, and Patricia Jeffery. 1993. 'Traditional Birth Attendants in Rural North India: The Social Organization of Childbearing'. In *Knowledge, Power and Practice: The Anthropology of Medicine and Everyday Life*, edited by Shirley Lindenbaum and Margaret Lock, 7–31. Berkeley: University of California Press.

Nichter, Mark. 2001. 'The Political Ecology of Health in India: Indigestion as Sign and Symptom of Defective Modernization'. In *Healing Powers and Modernity: Traditional Medicine, Shamanism, and Science in Asian Societies*, edited by Linda Connor and Geoffrey Samuel, 23–62. Westport, Connecticut: Bergin and Garvey.

Palriwala, Rajni, and Patricia Uberoi, eds. 2008. *Marriage, Migration and Gender*. New Delhi: Sage.

Patil, Prathamesh. 2017. '20 homes Encroaching on Taljai Forest Demolished'. *Pune Mirror*, 16 November. Accessed 12 February 2019. https://punemirror. indiatimes.com/pune/civic/20-homes-encroaching-on-taljai-forest-demolished/ articleshow/61664522.cms

Pinto, Sarah. 2008. *Where There Is No Midwife: Birth and Loss in Rural India*. New York & Oxford: Berghahn Books.

Pune Municipal Corporation. 2019a. 'Slum Rehabilitation Work in Pune'. BSUP-JNNURM. Accessed 12 February 2019. https://pmc.gov.in/en/slum-rehabilitation-work-under-bsup-jnnurm

Pune Municipal Corporation. 2019b. 'One Home-One Toilet'. Rapid Household Survey across the slums of Pune, conducted by Shelter Associates and Pune Advitiya & Unique. Accessed 12 February 2019. http://shelter-associates.org/ downloads/Individual%20toilet%20projects/Individual%20toilet%20projects_ 70.pdf

Rairkar, Hema. 2007. 'Midwives: A Tradition on the Move'. In *The Social and the Symbolic*, edited by Bernard Bel, Jan Brouwer, Biswajit Das, Vibodh Parthasarathi, and Guy Poetevin, 413–72. New Delhi: Sage.

Rozario, Santi, and Geoffrey Samuel. 2003. 'Tibetan and Indian Ideas of Birth Pollution: Similarities and Contrasts'. In *Daughters of Hariti: Childbirth and Female Healers in South and Southeast Asia*, edited by Santi Rozario and Geoffrey Samuel, 193–219. London & New York: Routledge.

Sadgopal, Mira. 2009. 'Can Maternity Services Open Up to the Indigenous Traditions of Midwifery?' *Economic and Political Weekly* 44 (16): 52–9.

Scheper-Hughes, Nancy. 1992. *Death Without Weeping: The Violence of Everyday Life in Brazil*. Berkeley: University of California Press.

Skultans, Vieda. 1991. 'Women and Affliction in Maharashtra: A Hydraulic Model of Health and Illness'. *Culture, Medicine and Psychiatry* 15 (3): 321–59.

Van Hollen, Cecilia. 2003. *Birth on the Threshold: Childbirth and Modernity in South India*. Berkeley & Los Angeles: University of California Press.

Weigl, Constanze. 2010. *Reproductive Health Behavior and Decision-Making of Muslim Women: An Ethnographic Study in a Low-Income Community in Urban North India*. Münster: LIT Verlag.

SECTION 4

CONTEMPORARY BIRTH ATTENDANTS

7

Outsiders in the Village

Class, Space, and the Shortage of Women Doctors in Rural Rajasthan, India

Jocelyn Killmer

In their heart, no one wants to go to a village.

Medical student, Jaipur

Introduction

Doctors in Rajasthan—as in much of the world—tend to cluster in cities, where hospitals offer amenities, technology, and prestigious career paths not found in the *dehat*, or countryside. Furthermore, in Rajasthan, as elsewhere in North India, there is a disproportionate lack of women doctors working outside of urban areas. My research addresses this puzzle: what is it about being a woman that makes rural work even less appealing than it might otherwise be? The answers to this question are complex, interweaving issues of class, space, and gender.

Women doctors' discomfort with rural work has repercussions beyond the lives of doctors and their families. In 2013–14, fewer than 10% of rural primary health centres (PHCs) in Rajasthan employed a woman medical officer (Government of India 2014).[1] The larger community health centres (CHCs), tasked with providing specialist obstetric services outside of urban district centres, also faced a shortage: fewer than 20% of CHCs employed an obstetrician, the vast majority of whom in Rajasthan are women (Government of India 2014). Thus, in many areas of the state, women patients seeking to consult a woman doctor for reproductive healthcare find the government sector falling short, requiring them to travel long distances—precisely what the appointment of obstetricians to local CHCs was designed to avoid.

Through ethnographic work on women's reproductive health in India we have been granted access to the perspectives of birthing women (Donner

Jocelyn Killmer, *Outsiders in the Village* In: *Childbirth in South Asia*. Edited by: Clémence Jullien and Roger Jeffery, Oxford University Press. © Oxford University Press 2021. DOI: 10.1093/oso/9780190130718.003.0007

2008; Jeffery et al. 1989; Jeffery and Jeffery 1993, 2010; Jullien 2015; Van Hollen 2003; 2013) and birth workers with varying levels of professionalization and training (Pinto 2008; Price 2014; Rozario 1998, 2003). This chapter is part of an expanding project to include the perspective of allopathic doctors (see also Madhiwalla, this volume; Ruddock 2017). This research is based on 9 months of fieldwork in Jaipur and Dausa districts during 2013–14. I conducted interviews with 29 medical students, mostly from the Mahatma Gandhi Medical College (MGMC) in Jaipur. I also interviewed doctors in the private and government sectors, professors at MGMC, and public health officials. In the countryside I spent time at four CHCs and three PHCs; in the city I observed two government dispensaries, two private in-home clinics, and two large private hospitals. Like so many of the doctors I met in rural Rajasthan, I maintained ties with both city and village, spending much of my time moving back and forth across the countryside.

In the medical college, where students made decisions about whether to accept rural work, I found a clear discursive rift between city and village. While many medical students had experience visiting relatives in villages, the thought of moving to a village for several years was not appealing. Cities were deemed appropriate less by their sheer size and population and more by what they offered in terms of prestigious career opportunities, modern spaces for consumption (malls, multiplex movie theatres), and good schools for one's children. The social support young women doctors find in cities helps to mitigate the many risks to women associated with rural work: living alone in the clinic's quarters, travelling unaccompanied for long distances, and interacting at all hours of the day and night with the 'wrong' kind of people (Killmer 2018). Doctors' narratives produce doctors as perpetual outsiders to the village, forced to step backwards in time and space in order to perform village work. Even if a doctor's 'home place' is in a village, years of schooling in a city, along with the prestige of a medical degree, can make the doctor not quite fit into the rural landscape. In order to understand the shortage of women doctors in rural clinics, it is necessary to consider the interconnections of class, space, and gender as they relate to rural work.

Women Doctors for Women Patients

The shortage of women doctors in rural Rajasthan is particularly troubling because, unlike Europe and North America where obstetrics and gynae-cology remained in the hands of men until recently, women have dominated the field of allopathic women's health in India since its inception. Gender proved to be the motivating factor for a migration of medically trained women from the colonial metropole: according to colonialist discourse, Indian women were secluded from men, therefore women's healthcare must be a women-only enterprise (Burton 1996). In actual practice, full seclusion in the *zenana*, or women's quarters of a home, was available only to those families with the financial capital to pull it off; nevertheless, British ideology framed Indian men as disinclined to allow 'their' women to be examined by a male doctor (Forbes 1994; Lal 2006; Sehrawat 2013). In Rajasthan today, at all levels of professionalization, from the lowest-level community health workers to obstetricians and gynaecologists, women's health continues to be women's work.

The government health sector in India has tried repeatedly to increase the number of births overseen by biomedically-trained attendants—including midwives, medical officers, and obstetricians—rather than untrained dais. Every PHC is responsible for several sub-centres, each employing an auxiliary nurse midwife (ANM) to provide reproductive healthcare to women. The ANM is part of the first line of contact for women and is expected to encourage women to enter the allopathic system for perinatal care, and to refer upwards in the system if necessary. In theory, ANMs should be equipped to attend normal births, thereby expanding the reach of the allopathic system into every village. However, long-term efforts to train women to become ANMs, or to train dais in allopathic methods, have failed to create a large number of midwives who are skilled birth attendants and who consistently use the evidence-based standards promoted by global health organizations (Pinto 2008, Price 2014). Iyengar et al. (2009) found that, despite the training of ANMs to oversee births, it was common practice for doctors to preside at births with nurses assisting. Furthermore, if an ANM detects something amiss and refers the patient onwards in the government system, the patient is likely to experience the lack of women doctors who can attend to gynaecological morbidities and perinatal complications. Yet the number of institutional births has increased dramatically with the adoption of the Janani Suraksha Yojana, a programme implemented in 2005 that pays women to deliver in a government or government-sanctioned clinic (Govil et al. 2016, Paul and Chellan 2013). In Rajasthan, the number of institutional births increased from 30% in 2005–6 to 84% in 2015–16 (Government of India 2017). Without doctors in rural clinics who are positioned to deal with an increase in deliveries, already-overburdened urban district hospitals must somehow accept a greater number of patients.

Addressing the Rural Doctor Shortage

India's public health apparatus is keenly aware that rural healthcare services are less than ideal and that practitioner shortages contribute to the problem, yet, shortages remain. Calls throughout the mid and late twentieth century to reorient medical education towards an emphasis on preventive and social medicine met with little success (Jeffery 1988). Medical education in India continues to steer young graduates towards specialization and away from primary care and rural health (Ruddock 2017). Doctors see rural areas as underdeveloped and non-industrialized spaces where the proper practice of medicine cannot take place. The Hindi film *Ek Doctor ki Maut* ('A Doctor's Death'), released in 1990, illustrates the undesirability of rural medical work. The doctor of the film's title upsets his supervisor at a large urban hospital and, as punishment, is sent away from his research lab to provide primary care in a coastal village. The film's title refers to the doctor's symbolic, rather than literal, death; in the far-off space of the village he is merely treating the minor ailments of the poor, seen here as less important than creating new knowledge in the research lab. The tension between medical work as service to the community and medical work as an avenue for India to claim a place in the international medical research economy remains, with the latter usually dominating doctors' opinions.

Several Indian states offer financial incentives to lure doctors out of the city; in Rajasthan doctors receive an extra Rs. 4,000 per month for working in rural areas and Rs. 7,000 per month for working in 'hard' (mountainous or desert) areas (Sundararaman and Gupta 2011). Various Indian states, as well as the national government, have mandated 1- or 2-year rural postings for all MBBS graduates. For example, the Union Health Ministry announced a mandatory rural posting in 2008 (Sinha 2008). The idea keeps reappearing but has proven difficult to implement in practice (Rao 2019). Students protest any new ruling for mandatory rural postings, and, should their protests fail, they can escape rural work by paying a fine. The fine becomes just another cost of medical education for all but those dedicated to serving rural populations, or for those without the financial resources to pay. Until 2019, Rajasthan had not implemented compulsory rural service for MBBS graduates. The Medical Council of India (MCI) has tried to entice recent graduates to accept short-term rural postings by reserving a proportion of seats in specialist postgraduate programmes for doctors who have worked in a 'remote or difficult area', with an added 10% of entrance exam marks per year for up to 3 years of rural service (Medical Council of India 2018). The desire to specialize is a powerful one for recent medical graduates, and some students are indeed willing to work in a village long enough to boost their chances of a postgraduate residency, making the rural posting a stopping point on the way to specialization and work in an urban tertiary hospital, not an end in itself. A rural posting is also the first step towards a desirable career in the government sector. The majority of medical students in my sample preferred the government sector for its stability and what was perceived as a relatively easy work life. Nearly all medical graduates who enter the government sector are assigned to rural postings; doctors are expected to pay their dues in an undesirable area and then gradually work their way to a more urban space. The exceptions to this rule had political connections that allowed them to jump immediately to a more desirable clinic.

While financial incentives have not proven effective in changing doctors' attitudes towards rural work (Jeffery 1988; Sundararaman and Gupta 2011), the reservation in the postgraduate exam and the requirement that doctors wishing to enter government service 'pay their dues' in a village have the potential to bring doctors to rural areas, at least for short-term postings. In theory, the benefits from a short-term rural posting should be open to everyone. In practice, I found that women had a much harder time accomplishing a short-term rural posting, particularly if they were unmarried or were unable to bring their husbands along. For women, much of the difficulty in rural work comes from the social isolation it entails. Although few were willing to talk forthrightly about it, the spectre of sexual violence hung over my research. The further women travel away from their protective social network, the more risk they accrue (Killmer 2018). The health administration may keep a flow of young medical graduates cycling through rural postings, but they are less likely to solve the shortage of *women* doctors.

Some working in public health have advocated a new medical degree, the Bachelor of Science (BSc) in Community Health, to address the problem of rural doctor retention. Those holding this degree would be eligible to practise only in rural areas. The degree would take 3 years (instead of the 5 years of an MBBS) and cover basic anatomy, normal deliveries, perinatal care, vaccination, and the treatment of diarrheal diseases, pneumonia, tuberculosis, fevers, and skin infections (Dhar 2013). Such a qualification has been rejected by the MCI many times and in many forms over the last few decades. At the time of my research, this degree had finally been approved by the MCI, but it was left to individual states to take it up; it was not available in Rajasthan. Doctors, fiercely protecting their professional niche, were quick to criticize the BSc in Community Health in the press, claiming that it would create 'half-baked' practitioners (Garg et al. 2011) or an 'army of quacks' (Rathee 2013), 'slaves' with a degree that would only allow them to live and work in rural areas (Rathee 2013). Medical officers are justified in worrying about a potential threat to their professional domain, because in practice the two types of practitioners would do very similar work. And yet, MBBS graduates continue to refuse rural work. The BSc degree in some ways represents an admission of defeat: we will never get MBBS doctors to work in villages, so we should try someone else.

The push for a rural medical degree, along with efforts to recruit and train local women to provide frontline reproductive healthcare, pragmatically accept the class-based problems inherent in coaxing urban-educated doctors into village spaces while perpetuating the idea that only *some* kinds of people are suited to live in villages. If Rajasthan implements this programme, it may very well bring more trained medical practitioners into village clinics, but not without reifying the divide between urban and rural and the differences between the kinds of people who inhabit both spaces. The debate over the rural medical degree was focused on the shortage of rural doctors in general, rather than the shortage of 'lady' doctors, but the different experiences of men and women doctors in rural spaces require attention to gender. In the rest of the chapter, I turn to doctors' discourse of 'urban' and 'rural' and its practical effects as it overlaps with gendered norms relating to safety, propriety, and family.

The City and the Village

While researching medical education in urban Jaipur, I met an obstetrician eager to give me advice about how to improve my research. If I really wanted to understand medicine in India, she said, I should visit a village clinic. She gave me the contact information for her husband, who worked at a CHC. The next time I ran into her, she greeted me with mild shock. 'I heard you *actually went!*', she said, surprised that I had ventured several hours out of the city. Her recommendation to visit the village, and her surprise when I followed this recommendation, hint at the contradictory nature of the village in doctors' narratives. In her opinion, the village may be 'real India', but it is not an obvious space for educated urbanites and foreigners to inhabit. As I elicited stories of the village from doctors, tensions emerged about what the village signifies and the doctor's place in it. The village manages to be simultaneously the symbolic heart of India and Indian culture while also embarrassingly in need of transformative development. Because the rural is seen as a space of backwardness and a place yet-to-be-developed, most young doctors had a difficult time imagining their lives there. There was some discrepancy among doctors regarding what exactly counted as a village, especially since so much of India lies somewhere between small villages and large cities, leaving the space between open to interpretation. The state defines rural areas based on data such as population density and the percentage of people working in agriculture.[2] People who lived and worked in villages unsurprisingly had a much more nuanced idea about what constituted the interior, as well as the *real* middle of nowhere. Those in villages along the highway to Jaipur told me that this was not the 'real' interior since it could be reached in a few hours from the city. Yet the same obstetrician who urged me to go out into the 'real India', looking from the perspective of the city, thought that these easy-access villages were indeed the real thing, or at least real enough to induce surprise over my visits there.

After hearing doctors' narratives of the village in Rajasthan, I began to imagine what a biomedical landscape in Rajasthan might look like, envisioning urban hubs of activity surrounded by 'negative space'. Medicine happens in cities, while negative space is created in the interior in large part by the practice of doctors avoiding it—the rural is seen as emptied of all that is important (Munn 1996). The city and the countryside are thus inseparable—each exists only in relation to the other (Massey 1994). Pigg (1992) describes the landscape of Nepal similarly: 'the overall impression is of islands of not-village surrounded by a sea of villageness'. This separation implicitly declares the city to be the important pole in the city–village binary. For doctors too, the village is defined as not-city; the biomedical gaze simply cannot see spaces without technologically equipped hospitals or the trappings of urban middle-class life. And yet, the negative space of the village is constantly haunting the young medical graduate who must cross the hurdle of village work in order to reap the benefits of a government job. In doctors' narratives, the multiplicity of rural spaces overlapped and coalesced into an imagined village, an image that circulated in urban medical colleges and informed young doctors' decisions about where and how they might live. This imagined village did more work for those doctors who had little real-world experience of village life; those who had rural ties were able to offer counterpoints to the standard narrative I encountered in the medical college. Yet even the students with rural backgrounds could not escape the hierarchy of prestige that placed cities above villages, or the timescale that framed villages as backward spaces.

Conversations about 'real India' reminded me of an exchange attributed to Gandhi, who told a group of foreigners that 'if they wanted to "see the heart of India", they should "ignore big cities"', venturing at least 30 miles from the railway line into the interior of the country (Jodhka 2002: 3347). Gandhi contrasted 'authentic' Indian life with foreign, Western influence: the 'village was the site of authenticity, the "real/pure India", a place that, at least in its design, had not yet been corrupted by the western influence. The city was its opposite, totally western' (Jodhka 2002: 3346). The village is a shifting symbol in Indian culture, used to represent authenticity, or underdevelopment, or casteism and oppression, depending on who is invoking its symbolic richness (Jodhka 2002, Mantena 2012). Doctors tended to highlight the 'underdeveloped' qualities they saw in village clinical spaces, which in their narratives lack electricity, plumbing, and basic tools and supplies. Doctors still contrasted city and village, but the poles were now reversed compared to Gandhi's vision: the city was the place of authenticity in medicine, while the village became mainly a place of backwardness. At MGMC, a statue of Gandhi dressed in a homespun dhoti and clutching a walking-stick towers incongruously above a dry fountain in front of the hospital's shining façade. Gandhi's statue is out of place and out of time at the medical college, perhaps imagined as a symbol of India's tradition that could anchor the college in morality (a good public relations move considering the moral suspicion with which the burgeoning private medical colleges are viewed). In her analysis of 1990s-era Bollywood films, Sharpe (2005) argues that villages began to evoke both a different space (not-city) and a different time (an imagined past) as film settings became increasingly urbanized and globalized. When rural spaces appear in these films, they are 'emptied of the culture of everyday life', existing 'not as a geographical location so much as a signifier for a simpler way of life prior to globalization' (Sharpe 2005: 60). Doctors, as a group, did not wish to revert to a time prior to liberalization while they were so well poised to reap its benefits. Doctors invoked a similar conflation of time and space when they spoke of the village as 'backward', placing villages behind cities on an evolutionary continuum between underdeveloped and developed spaces.

Doctors and the Rural Other

Place was important to doctors' project of differentiation between themselves, as subjects who have secured their place in the middle class, and subaltern middle-class aspirants (Bhatt et al. 2010; Fernandes and Heller 2006).

In village narratives, doctors used the village as code for low educational and class status—and by separating themselves from the geographical space of the village, they also put metaphorical distance between themselves and their subaltern Other. The time-scape that frames villages as 'backwards' aids in the production of a village Other in comparison to the urban, modern doctor (Fabian 1983). Following the pattern of speaking about villages in terms of material lack—of supplies, electricity, and technology—there was also a consensus among young doctors that the *people* who lived in villages were somehow lacking: they were uneducated, deficient in social skills, prone to violence. These qualities combined to create an Other deemed 'backward'. Doctors used the discourse of backwardness to account for a wide variety of behaviours they expected in the village, for example, that the rural population did not understand the limits of biomedical treatment and would blame the doctor if a patient died, often retaliating with violence (Kumar 2016, Perappadan 2017).[3] During my year of fieldwork, several accounts of doctors being attacked by patients' relatives turned up in the local media. This does not happen only in rural areas; in fact, the most high-profile case of violence that year happened to several doctors at a tertiary hospital in Bikaner, precipitating strikes at urban hospitals across the state. But, because doctors tended to associate violent retaliation with a lack of formal education, and a lack of education with villagers, they were more suspicious of the rural population.

Dr Divya was working on a postgraduate degree in preventive and social medicine when I met her; [4] she had also cultivated a private practice out of her home in urban Jaipur. When she first graduated from medical college, she was posted to an isolated area of Bharatpur district. She lasted only 8 days at the clinic before returning home to her family in Jaipur. She was one of the first women I interviewed who had rural experience and I was eager to find out the whole story. Dr Divya, on the other hand, had no intention of telling me. She asserted several times that the village was a 'disturbed place' not suitable for women doctors: 'a male can sustain there but a female cannot', but was unwilling to offer any more details. Months later, she told me why villages are dangerous spaces for doctor-outsiders, but only in general terms:

> If some incident happens, no one will step up to help you. This is not be-
> cause they are bad people—there are both good and bad people in the vil-
> lage. But they can't speak out against the *panchayat* [village council], against
> the *neta* [leader], against whoever has done wrong to the doctor. They are
> part of their community; the doctor is the outsider. They have to continue
> living here; the doctor can leave.

Dr Divya's experience highlights the plight of women doctors as outsiders in the village. For her, this village was empty of social support and risky enough that she chose to leave after a week, opting out of the government sector altogether.

Dr Kavita, a medical officer who grew up in Jaipur, had worked in two different village postings before being transferred to a city. She describes her first rural posting, at a PHC in Jhunjhunu district, fondly. In this village, 'the people were very good; they were very simple. Meaning they thought that whoever is the doctor, if she will help us, and if she comes on time, she won't be bothered'. Importantly, Dr Kavita's parents-in-law lived nearby, making her far less of an outsider in this particular village. Things unfolded differently when she was transferred to a CHC in a region of Dausa district, where a caste-based conflict had been stirring for several years. Dr Kavita was from a caste group without political clout in the CHC area, nor did she have any family nearby. The caste politics of the village placed her firmly outside the spheres of political power in the area. As an outsider, she could not count on community support for her work and life in the village. Of seven doctors at the CHC she was the only woman and was required to handle all the women's reproductive health work. She was overworked, attending deliveries day and night as well as covering outpatient duties during the day and general emergencies at night.

One evening a group of people brought in a girl who, according to Dr Kavita, had died before she reached the clinic. Dr Kavita explained that nothing more could be done for her. The girl's family accused Dr Kavita of negligence—they argued that the girl was still alive when they arrived and Dr Kavita had refused to save her. The girl's politically-connected relatives were able to bring Dr Kavita's supervisor onto their side. Dr Kavita was saved from being transferred out of the village by a group of pharmaceutical suppliers whose shops faced the CHC: 'They told the in-charge [head doctor], "this Madam does a lot of work; we have seen that you are causing her problems night and day. And a lady doctor has come to our area after a long time. If you cause her to be transferred from here, we will never leave you alone". Meaning, they took my side'.

Dr Kavita made a distinction between 'political people' who use their power to manipulate the medical system for their benefit, and honourable people who have the community's best interests at heart. But it is difficult to separate these two designations from the caste politics that overlay them. Dr Kavita described the region as a 'quite notorious area' populated by 'rude' people. For her, 'notorious' people belong to a particular caste, and they represent a dangerous Other to her, the doctor outsider. While I never heard a doctor explicitly label a caste group as backward, the implications are clear when villages are simultaneously associated with particular caste groups and deemed less cosmopolitan, or less educated, or prone to violence. Doctors are sometimes posted in a region where they 'fit', either because they have family in that area or come from the right caste community.[5] But, as Dr Kavita's story shows, they can also end up in a place where they feel their outsider status keenly.

Urban Bodily Dispositions

Regardless of one's caste community or the location of one's family, doctors can all experience some degree of outsider status in the village based on the years they spend in urban areas pursuing their MBBS degree. I found that doctors, particularly those who had lived in a city following the blossoming of mall culture since the 1990s, were unable to successfully perform their class position in the space of a village in large part because the leisure spaces they were used to in the city were missing. Urban restructuring, linked to economic liberalization, has changed the class-based desires of doctors (Fernandes 2006). Liechty (2003: 15) argues that aspirants to the middle class in Kathmandu required 'cultural strategies, systems of prestige ("status"), and forms of "capital" that are not, strictly speaking, economic'. The performance of middle-class-ness demands a set of behaviours that are linked not just to wealth but to the appropriate consumption of 'modern' goods such as televisions, refrigerators, and fashion. This performance involves a material economy *and* a moral economy; modern consumption, done within set boundaries, makes one respectable and therefore able to claim middle-class status (Liechty 2003). Moreover, young people are integral to middle-class formation: 'class, consumption, media, and youth must be seen as not merely *interactive* but *mutually constitutive* cultural processes' (Liechty 2003: 6, emphasis in original; see also Lukose 2009). If doctors merely needed access to TVs and fashion, their middle-class life could be transported to the village with minimal difficulty. Wealth exists in villages too, and residents have their fair share of refrigerators, televisions, and smart phones (Jeffery et al. 2011). Instead, many of the new kinds of consumption available in Jaipur were simply not possible in villages, particularly in terms of the process of consumption outside the home rather than the use of consumer goods like TVs within it. When not chatting on each other's beds in the hostel, medical students spent their free time going out to restaurants, malls, multiplex cinemas, and coffee shops.

McGuire (2011) argues that bodily dispositions, created through the process of consumption, help to mark some bodies as middle-class and others as not. McGuire observed people cultivating these dispositions in New Delhi malls, designed for shoppers on different levels to peer up or down at each other: 'it is important that one is *seen* consuming, and that one can *watch* others consume' (2011: 128). Bodies thus gain middle-class status in part through the gaze of other urban middle-class consumers. When I asked medical student Sandhya what she would miss most about the city if she took a village posting, her answer was immediate and emphatic: 'malls!' None of these modern, sanitized public/private spaces occupied by doctors' peers are available in the interior. Post-liberalization urban leisure spaces are especially important for middle-class women as they allow women to spend time with their peers outside the home or hostel. Coffee shops and malls mark the women who occupy them as 'modern' rather than 'loose'—although there remains a considerable amount of slippage between these two categories (De Koning 2009). Phadke (2007: 1514) argues that the presence of women in urban leisure spaces is 'a marker of the modernity of the city and its claim to global status'; modernity requires the visible presence of women in these spaces outside the home. In addition to marking class status, the semi-private interior of malls offers middle-class women a feeling of safety in cities that have been marked as dangerous for them. Malls provide a space for women to congregate away from the watchful eyes of their parents, but also away from the public streets, where danger is represented by the bodies of lower-class men (Phadke 2013). Through the creation of a middle-class space regulated by security guards, the mall symbolically sanitizes the dangers of the public sphere.

Villages, which did not have leisure spaces for women or mixed-gender groups, were thus rendered distinctly *un*modern and unwelcoming for urban professional women. When Prema, my host in Vijaynagar village who taught at a private English-medium school, walked in the streets of the village, she covered her head and face with the free-flowing end of her sari as a *ghunghat*, or veil. She did this with great reluctance; she had been raised in Maharashtra where the rules for women's comportment are less restrictive. When she visited her natal family she saw couples outside socializing in the evenings. In her marital village, married men and women did not socialize together even at home (casual conversation was nearly impossible in the presence of her husband's male relatives, in front of whom she had to cover her face). She chatted with other women next door in the courtyard, or with her sisters-in-law in their house a short (ghunghat-covered) walk across the fields. But there was no non-domestic space in the village where Prema went to meet other women, let alone men, as women are able to do in urban malls. Doctors, especially of the younger generation, feel the absence of malls and multiplexes in the village keenly, especially when these are the only places middle-class women can feel they safely belong.

Dr Nandini commuted daily by bus from her parents' house in Jaipur to her PHC 2 hours away, a practice referred to as the daily 'up-down' available to those working in an 'easy' village close enough to the city. A recent MBBS graduate who was unmarried, she did not feel comfortable living in the village alone. Unlike many women doctors, she did not feel afraid to live in the village; instead, she explained that 'the way of living is mashed up here'.[6] This means, Dr Nandini went on, that doctors need a place to sit in the evening, along with a social circle of their peers with whom they can pass time. She could not find the right social environment in her village, so she straddled the urban/rural divide, spending her free time in Jaipur and her work hours at the clinic. When Dr Nandini spoke of the way of life in villages being 'mashed up', she referenced both the people of the village and the spaces it provided (or failed to provide) for leisure. The lack of peers could also affect women doctors' feeling of safety as they moved through public space. Shilpa, an MBBS student, told me the story of her recent birthday party as we sat in her hostel room one afternoon. Her family, visiting from out of town, returned her to the hostel at 11 p.m. after a celebratory dinner. Then her friends whisked her away to a surprise outdoor party where they stayed until two-thirty in the morning. After listening for months to women tell me about the restrictions on their movements, especially after dark, I was very surprised— how had this happened? The answer lies in Shilpa's social network. She could not have gone alone for dinner until 11 at night. She certainly could not have gone alone to party until the wee hours of the morning. She had friends, both boys and girls, who, through their critical mass, transformed the empty fields where the party took place. The *necessity* of being alone in a rural posting left medical graduates unable to make such a social life possible.

Several doctors described villages as 'desolate' places. Dr Asha, who worked her way up in the government sector from villages to towns to, ultimately, Jaipur, talked about the wildness of some village spaces: 'It is so hard for lady doctors to live in remote areas. If the clinic is one or two kilometres away from a village, how can the doctor live there alone? There is one [PHC] in Kotputli district that is in the forest and a panther lives nearby. One time it was found in the [living] quarters. A panther!' Dr Asha had only heard of this panther, but the story performs work in separating acceptable urban spaces from wild rural ones. Doctors do not have to worry about finding wild animals in urban hospitals (beyond the usual insects, pigeons, and stray monkeys, none of which invoke panther-level fear). Dr Asha felt that spending time in such a wild place had changed her: 'You can't find people who have similar thoughts to you. You spend time with village people and you become *jangli* [wild or uncivilized] within six months!'

Not only were village residents inherently different from Dr Asha, in her estimation, but she feared becoming more like them, losing her urban habitus for something less desirable. She saw the changes when she visited Delhi after living in a village for many years: she was suddenly afraid to take the bus, and surprised herself by feeling shocked at women who wore sleeveless shirts. She lost her ability to move through the city with ease, not because of social restrictions on her movements, but because, against her will, she had begun to inhabit a *jangli* worldview. Her struggle illustrates the dialectic between the durable nature of the habitus and its plasticity (Bourdieu 1977), as she acknowledges the undesirable change in her reactions but is unable to overcome it. Her discourse of 'jangliness' performs boundary-making work, distinguishing between city and village, as it shows how the village can transform a person in undesirable ways. Villages emerge therefore not merely as spaces, but as constellations of thought and behaviour (in this case, undesirable thought and behaviour). Dr Asha implies that travelling freely in a city and gazing without judgement on a woman's bare arms are positive, desirable, actions; and yet, her time in the village has left her unable to perform them.

Thus far, I have made a distinction between 'rural' patient and 'urban' doctor, where doctors may live within village confines but are not seen to be *of* the village. While most of the doctors I met were raised and educated in urban settings, I did meet some who complicated such a sharp separation between urban and rural. Dr Shireen, an intern at MGMC, grew up in a remote area where she was the first woman to have any education beyond ninth grade. A group of doctors from her Muslim caste group raised money to pay for her medical tuition on the understanding that she would return to her home village to practice medicine for the local women:

DR SHIREEN: The people who have helped me to do my studies have made a big sacrifice, so I want to help them. In our society girls don't study. I'll be the first girl doctor in my district, from my community.

JK: If it's possible, do you want to return to your home area?

DR SHIREEN: Yes, if my husband is ready to go there, I want to go back. I want to build a small hospital there. Where poor people, families below the poverty line, can go to get free treatment, wherever possible, or can get treatment for less money. I don't have a desire to earn money. I just want to help people, however many people I can. That's my idea.

Dr Shireen should be an ideal candidate to work in a rural clinic, yet even she was unsure about her long-term plans. She worried a great deal about finding a husband who was willing to live in rural Rajasthan. She had already rejected a potential match suggested by her father because the boy's thinking 'wasn't like mine'. The boy asked her: 'Why do you want to be Mother Teresa? You should live your life, you should take your own enjoyment. Why do you want to trouble yourself with helping others?' Ideally, Dr Shireen wants a husband who is a doctor, is of her caste group, from her area, with similar altruistic career goals. In practice, this is turning out to be a tall order—but necessary in order to allow her to remain in the village long term. To complicate matters further, Dr Shireen took a job at a prestigious hospital in Delhi immediately following graduation. Even though she is from rural Rajasthan, her growing credentials mark her as an outsider in terms of class status. Her very success stands in the way of her original goals.

These stories illustrate the overlapping fields of class and space, where doctors cannot perform a proper middle-class lifestyle from the space of the village. Even if one could import modern conveniences into the village, it is impossible for doctors to be modern, middle-class consumers, as they have envisioned this position, in the space of the village. Doctors may be concerned with the health of the rural population in theory but sacrificing their class position for such an abstract concept does not sit well with most young doctors. If a position in the middle class is something constantly in process, doctors cannot simply reach it and then stop. To move to the village is to take a step back—in space and in time, as well as in class position.

Disrupted Motherhood

Dr Anandi, the in-charge medical officer at Rajgarh CHC, welcomed me into the living quarters of her clinic one afternoon for chai and snacks. I was excited to meet her because she provided a shining example of a rural success story: unlike the countless doctors I encountered who shunned rural work, Dr Anandi enjoyed the challenges of rural medicine and had just voluntarily extended her contract at the village clinic.[7] While we sat together, she described the ambitious plans she had for the health centre. When the conversation turned to her personal life, however, she was less enthusiastic: 'we [doctors] have sacrificed our normal female life. I have a son, but I'm not with him'. Her 4-year-old son lived in Jaipur, with his grandparents, while Dr Anandi stayed during the week in Rajgarh. She explained with heavy emotion how her son dreaded her leaving on Monday morning to return to the village: 'He's scared every time. "I know it mama, when I go to school you will leave!" That time I feel, you know, I feel like crying'. Several months later, Dr Anandi confessed that she was frustrated with her job and ready to leave, in large part because of her separation from her son.

Both men and women experienced emotional distress from this forced separation, but women face the additional burden of being responsible for their children's nurturing and education. Doctors told me they felt the mother was the best person to raise and educate a child. Donner (2008) similarly found that middle-class, stay-at-home mothers in West Bengal spent much of their day structuring their children's studying, and that fathers had become 'less involved in the education of their children than their own fathers had been' (p. 133). It is not easy for working women to compete with stay-at-home mothers' participation in school-related tasks. But women living separately from their children must relinquish control over much of the day-to-day work of educating them, broadly defined (and in India's competitive educational environment this is no small task). Dr Sapna, an obstetrician at Devipura CHC, sent her two children to live with her parents in the city of Alwar. 'I don't like it!', she said. 'I have no time to watch them. My first duty is as a mother, but I have no time for it'. And yet, women doctors working in villages chose (albeit reluctantly) separation from their children again and again: the advantage of an urban education won out over maternal oversight of children's lives.

The requirement that parents send their children off to cities is linked to the new urban, professional bodily dispositions that doctors are themselves practising. McGuire (2011) found that 'personality development and enhancement' (PDE) training, once the province of call centre workers, has spread into other Indian businesses, where new social spaces 'demand something particular of the bodies therein' (p. 118). The next generation must learn these bodily dispositions that can only be performed in spaces from which the village is excluded. Parents, then, need not only the proper educational institutions for their children (schools and coaching centres), but also the social spaces that will train their children in the type of bodily dispositions that will allow them to fit in with the new urban middle class.

Dr Meenakshi, an obstetrician who has spent her entire career in rural clinics alongside her doctor husband, has lived apart from her son since he was 8 months old. At first he went to stay with her parents in a town in Jaipur district. At age 11 he began living in Jaipur city with a maid; this remained his living arrangement at age 16. When I asked if her son was able to visit during school vacations, she told me that he never comes to the village. She first explained that he does coaching during school vacations and could not afford to miss it. But other reasons emerged as well: her son has 'requirements' that cannot be met in the village. He likes eating fast food, he feels uncomfortable in the heat, his computer would not work. Dr Meenakshi's son inhabits a body formed in the city with the comforts of urban space shaping his habitus. His experience is not unlike that of medical students who similarly felt uncomfortable in village spaces after a lifetime of urban education.

Conclusion

Doctors are outsiders in the village in many ways—even if, like Dr Shireen, they can claim a village as home. If the village is 'backward' or jangli (wild), then doctors can position themselves as the opposite: modern, with bodily dispositions that mark them as members of a professional class that can exist only in cities. Indeed, if a doctor were to *truly* fit into a rural setting, it would signal a failure to achieve the status promised by her medical degree. Furthermore, those doctors willing to eschew prestige and status in order to serve the rural population must then contend with the impact their decision has on family members. Children need the educational opportunities and bodily dispositions that only urban areas can provide, while for Dr Shireen, potential husbands of the correct class position have no interest in following her to the village. Women doctors' reluctance to occupy rural space illuminates the ways that class, space, and gender overlap to shape the practice of healthcare. If, as I have argued above, women doctors are necessary for the functioning of women's reproductive healthcare as it is currently organized in Rajasthan, their absence in the rural landscape is troubling. Yet the health administration can only offer those incentives that exist within their domain, such as financial bonuses or reservations for the postgraduate exam. Changing how class is performed, and how it maps onto different types of spaces, lies well beyond the purview of Rajasthan's health administration, and signals just how difficult the shortage of women doctors in rural areas will be to solve.

Notes

1. States with the fewest women medical officers at PHCs were in the North (Bihar, Madhya Pradesh, Chhattisgarh, Rajasthan, Uttar Pradesh), while those states with a woman medical officer in more than 50% of PHCs were in the South (Andhra Pradesh and Kerala). In India, 'medical officer' refers to a general practitioner with a bachelor's degree (MBBS) in medicine and surgery.
2. For more details, see Bhagat (2005: 63).
3. Blaming the doctor for a patient's death is not unique to India; elsewhere the patient's family might respond with litigation rather than physical violence.
4. All names of people and villages are pseudonyms.
5. Doctors can make location requests and also ask to be posted near a spouse. In practice, getting posted to a desirable location comes only with a bribe. The most desirable rural locations were in easy commuting distance of a city. One mid-career doctor I met had family connections in the state health administration and could enter government service in an urban posting straightaway; others had to 'serve their time' in less desirable locations and work their way up into more urban spaces.
6. While other women doctors spoke of their parents' role in decisions about rural work, Dr Nandini foregrounded her own agency in the decision, guided by her desire for a rewarding social life.
7. Dr Anandi's situation was also unusual in that she lived apart from her husband, who worked abroad; most women who stayed in rural clinics long term had doctor-husbands posted nearby, providing the paternalistic support required by Rajasthani social norms. Women doctors working in the larger CHCs, with a community of doctors residing in the quarters, had an easier time arranging social support than those who were the sole doctor assigned to a PHC.

References

Bhagat, Ram B. 2005. 'Rural–Urban Classification and Municipal Governance in India'. *Singapore Journal of Tropical Geography* 26 (1): 61–73.

Bhatt, Amy, Madhavi Murty, and Priti Ramamurthy. 2010. 'Hegemonic Developments: The New Indian Middle Class, Gendered Subalterns, and Diasporic Returnees in the Event of Neoliberalism'. *Signs: Journal of Women in Culture and Society* 36 (1): 127–52.

Bourdieu, Pierre. 1977. *Outline of a Theory of Practice*. vol. 16. Cambridge: Cambridge University Press.

Burton, Antoinette. 1996. 'Contesting the Zenana: The Mission to Make 'Lady Doctors for India', 1874–1885'. *Journal of British Studies* 35 (3): 368–97.

De Koning, Anouk. 2009. 'Gender, Public Space and Social Segregation in Cairo: Of Taxi Drivers, Prostitutes and Professional Women'. *Antipode* 41 (3): 533–56.

Dhar, Aarti. 2013. 'Cabinet Approves B.Sc. Community Health Course in State Universities'. *The Hindu*, 14 November. Accessed 1 February 2016. http://www. thehindu.com/news/national/cabinet-approves-bsc-community-health-course-in-state-universities/article5348436.ece

Donner, Henrike. 2008. *Domestic Goddesses: Maternity, Globalization and Middle-Class Identity in Contemporary India*. London: Routledge.

Fabian, Johannes. 1983. *Time and the Other: How Anthropology Makes Its Object*. New York: Columbia University Press.

Fernandes, Leela. 2006. *India's New Middle Class: Democratic Politics in an Era of Economic Reform*. Minneapolis: University of Minnesota Press.

Fernandes, Leela, and Patrick Heller. 2006. 'Hegemonic Aspirations: New Middle Class Politics and India's Democracy in Comparative Perspective'. *Critical Asian Studies* 38 (4): 495–522.

Forbes, Geraldine. 1994. 'Medical Careers and Health Care for Indian Women: Patterns of Control'. *Women's History Review* 3 (4): 515–30.

Garg, Suneela, Ritesh Singh, and Manoj Grover. 2011. 'Bachelor of Rural Health Care: Do We Need Another Cadre of Health Practitioners for Rural Areas'. *National Medical Journal of India* 24 (1): 35–7.

Government of India. 2014. 'Rural Health Statistics 2013–14'. New Delhi: Ministry of Health and Family Welfare. Accessed 18 January 2015. https://nrhm-mis. nic.in/Pages/RHS2014.aspx?RootFolder=%2FRURAL%20HEALTH%20 STATISTICS%2F%28A%29%20RHS%20-%202014&FolderCTID=&View={1316 16BC-2B52-434A-9CB2-F7B1E4B385B4

Government of India. 2017. 'National Family Health Survey 4 (2015–16): State Fact Sheet, Rajasthan'. New Delhi: Ministry of Health and Family Welfare. Accessed 3 May 2019. http://rchiips.org/nfhs/pdf/NFHS4/RJ_FactSheet.pdf

Govil, Dipti, Neetu Purohit, Shiv Dutt Gupta, and Sanjay Kumar Mohanty. 2016. 'Out-of-Pocket Expenditure on Prenatal and Natal Care Post Janani Suraksha Yojana: A Case From Rajasthan, India'. *Journal of Health, Population and Nutrition* 35 (1): 15.

Iyengar, Sharad D., Kirti Iyengar, and Vikram Gupta. 2009. 'Maternal Health: A Case Study of Rajasthan'. *Journal of Health, Population, And Nutrition* 27 (2): 271.

Jeffery, Patricia, and Roger Jeffery. 2010. 'Only When the Boat Has Started Sinking: A Maternal Death in Rural North India'. *Social Science & Medicine* 71 (10): 1711–18.

Jeffery, Patricia, Roger Jeffery, and Andrew Lyon. 1989. *Labour Pains and Labour Power: Women and Childbearing in India*. London: Zed Books.

Jeffery, Roger. 1988. *The Politics of Health in India*. Berkeley: University of California Press.

Jeffery, Roger, and Patricia Jeffery. 1993. 'Traditional Birth Attendants in Rural North India: The Social Organization of Childbearing'. In *Knowledge, Power and Practice: The Anthropology of Medicine and Everyday Life*, edited by Shirley Lindenbaum and Margaret Lock, 7–31. Berkeley: University of California Press.

Jeffery, Roger, Patricia Jeffery, and Craig Jeffrey. 2011. 'Are Rich Rural Jats Middle-Class?' In *Elite and Everyman: The Cultural Politics of the Indian Middle Classes*, edited by Amita Baviskar and Raka Ray, 140–63. New Delhi: Routledge.

Jodhka, Surinder S. 2002. 'Nation and Village: Images of Rural India in Gandhi, Nehru and Ambedkar'. *Economic and Political Weekly* 37 (32): 3343–53.

Jullien, Clémence. 2015. 'L'accouchement en Inde: Une affaire d'État?' *Journal des anthropologues. Association française des anthropologues* (140–1): 259–80.

Killmer, Jocelyn. 2018. 'Village Doctors and Vulnerable Bodies: Gender, Medicine, and Risk in North India'. PhD, Anthropology, Syracuse.

Kumar, Mukesh, Madhur Verma, Timiresh Das, Geeta Pardeshi, Jugal Kishore, and Arun Padmanandan. 2016. 'A Study of Workplace Violence Experienced by Doctors and Associated Risk Factors in a Tertiary Care Hospital of South Delhi, India'. *Journal of Clinical and Diagnostic Research* 10 (11): LC06–LC10.

Lal, Maneesha. 2006. 'Purdah as Pathology: Gender and the Circulation of Medical Knowledge in Late Colonial India'. In *Reproductive Health in India: History, Politics, Controversies*, edited by Sarah Hodges, 85–114. New Delhi: Orient Longman.

Liechty, Mark. 2003. *Suitably Modern: Making Middle-Class Culture in a New Consumer Society*. Princeton, NJ: Princeton University Press.

Lukose, Ritty A. 2009. *Liberalization's Children: Gender, Youth, and Consumer Citizenship in Globalizing India*. Durham, NC: Duke University Press.

Mantena, Karuna. 2012. 'On Gandhi's Critique of the State: Sources, Contexts, Conjunctures'. *Modern Intellectual History* 9 (3): 535–63.

Massey, Doreen. 1994. *Space, Place and Gender*. Minneapolis: University of Minnesota Press.

McGuire, Meredith Lindsay. 2011. ' "How to Sit, How to Stand": Bodily Practice and the New Urban Middle Class'. In *A Companion to the Anthropology of India*, edited by Isabelle Clark-Decès, 117–36. Malden, MA: Blackwell Publishing.

Medical Council of India. 2018. 'Postgraduate Medical Education Regulations 2000 (Amended up to May 2018)'. Accessed 12 March 2021. https://mcc.nic.in/PGCounselling/home/ShowPdf?Type=E0184ADEDF913B076626646D3F52C3B49C39AD6D&ID=6D363479C97439B921AD2BCBA054992D8EDA9A0C

Munn, Nancy D. 1996. 'Excluded Spaces: The Figure in the Australian Aboriginal Landscape'. *Critical Inquiry* 22 (3): 446–65.

Paul, Lopamudra, and Ramesh Chellan. 2013. 'Impact of Janani Suraksha Yojana on Institutional Delivery in Empowered Action Group States, India'. *South East Asia Journal of Public Health* 3 (2): 4–18.

Perappadan, Bindu Shajan. 2017. 'Majority of Doctors in India Fear Violence, Says IMA Survey'. *The Hindu*, 2 July. Accessed 3 May 2019. https://www.thehindu.com/sci-tech/health/majority-of-doctors-in-india-fear-violence-says-ima-survey/article19198919.ece

Phadke, Shilpa. 2007. 'Dangerous Liaisons: Women and Men: Risk and Reputation in Mumbai'. *Economic and Political Weekly* 42 (17): 1510–18.

Phadke, Shilpa. 2013. 'Unfriendly Bodies, Hostile Cities: Reflections on Loitering and Gendered Public Space'. *Economic and Political Weekly* 48 (39): 50–9.

Pigg, Stacy Leigh. 1992. 'Inventing Social Categories through Place: Social Representations and Development in Nepal'. *Comparative Studies in Society and History* 34 (3): 491–513.

Pinto, Sarah. 2008. *Where There Is No Midwife: Birth and Loss in Rural India*. New York & Oxford: Berghahn Books.

Price, Sara. 2014. 'Professionalizing Midwifery: Exploring Medically Imagined Labor Rooms in Rural Rajasthan'. *Medical Anthropology Quarterly* 28 (4): 519–36.

Rao, Sunita. 2019. 'Compulsory Government Service for Doctors Remains on Paper'. *The Times of India*, 27 January. Accessed 3 May 2019. https://timesofindia.indiatimes.com/city/bengaluru/compulsory-government-service-for-doctors-remains-on-paper/articleshow/67706286.cms

Rathee, Vidhi. 2013. 'Union Cabinet's Decision to Approve BSc (Community Health) Programme Gets Mixed Response'. *India Medical Times*, 18 November. Accessed 4 February 2015. http://www.indiamedicaltimes.com/2013/11/18/union-cabinets-decision-to-approve-bsc-community-health-programme-gets-mixed-response/

Rozario, Santi. 1998. 'The Dai and the Doctor: Discourses on Women's Reproductive Health in Rural Bangladesh'. In *Maternities and Modernities: Colonial and Postcolonial Experiences in Asia and the Pacific*, edited by Kalpana Ram and Margaret Jolly, 144–76. Cambridge & New York: Cambridge University Press.

Rozario, Santi. 2003. 'The Healer on the Margins: The Dai in Rural Bangladesh'. In *Daughters of Hariti*, edited by Santi Rozario and Geoffrey Samuel, 141–57. London & New York: Routledge.

Ruddock, Anna Louise. 2017. 'Special Medicine: Producing Doctors at the All India Institute of Medical Sciences (AIIMS)'. PhD, Anthropology, King's College London.

Sehrawat, Samiksha. 2013. 'Feminising Empire: The Association of Medical Women in India and the Campaign to Found a Women's Medical Service'. *Social Scientist* 41 (5/6): 65–81.

Sharpe, Jenny. 2005. 'Gender, Nation, and Globalization in Monsoon Wedding and Dilwale Dulhania Le Jayenge'. *Meridians: Feminism, Race, Transnationalism* 6 (1): 58–81.

Sinha, Kounteya. 2008. 'From '09, 1-year rural stint a must for MBBS students'. *The Times of India*, 25 July. Accessed 3 May 2019. https://timesofindia.indiatimes.com/india/From-09-1-year-rural-stint-a-must-for-MBBS-students/articleshow/3276540.cms

Sundararaman, Thiagarajan, and Garima Gupta. 2011. 'Indian Approaches to Retaining Skilled Health Workers in Rural Areas'. *Bulletin of the World Health Organization* 89 (1): 73–7.

Van Hollen, Cecilia. 2003. *Birth on the Threshold: Childbirth and Modernity in South India*. Berkeley & Los Angeles: University of California Press.

Van Hollen, Cecilia. 2013. *Birth in the Age of AIDS: Women, Reproduction, and HIV/AIDS in India*. Stanford, CA: Stanford University Press.

8

Care's Profit

Precarity and Professionalization of Health Workers in Private Maternal Clinics in Rajasthan and Uttar Pradesh, India

Isabelle L. Lange, Sunita Bhadauria, Sunita Singh, and Loveday Penn-Kekana

Introduction

It is our sixth week of fieldwork at Dr Aastha's maternity clinic in a rural southern Rajasthani town, and she is telling me how she values her patients' pregnancy and childbirth pathways:[1]

> What I say is that each delivery is a second birth of the mother. It is not just a delivery of the baby, but it is about the mother, and you need to take care of her. Medicine is a holistic branch, and it should be performed by trained people only. People who have got the degree.

I have been coming to sit with Aastha during her morning and afternoon antenatal care appointments, and her statement puzzles me. Surely she must know that I know her clinic is almost entirely staffed with unlicensed health workers who handle delivery care (except for one registered nurse-midwife and herself), even though it is illegal for them to do so. During our fieldwork, Sunita B. and I have mostly been focused on hanging out with her employees, and Aastha and I have been dancing around the reasons why I am really spending time sitting with her in her consultations.

As a friendly distraction from the fact that we are there looking at ideas surrounding legitimacy, medical knowledge, and staffing issues in maternity care in the private sector, she sometimes takes us along on her errands during lunch breaks—going costume jewellery shopping for a wedding, or drinking chai up in her spacious family home on the top floors of her clinic, talking about novels and her children.

Isabelle L. Lange, Sunita Bhadauria, Sunita Singh, and Loveday Penn-Kekana, *Care's Profit* In: *Childbirth in South Asia*. Edited by: Clémence Jullien and Roger Jeffery, Oxford University Press. © Oxford University Press 2021. DOI: 10.1093/oso/9780190130718.003.0008

Today we are both aware that I am nearing the end of this second field-work stint, and all week I have been probing more assertively on a few 'formal' questions about how she runs her hospital before we go. Dodging my questions, she turns her responses into a rant against the government and its lack of support for her while she serves their aims and helps them reach their targets for the good of the health of the Rajasthani population. In order to run her private clinic and receive the government backing she needs, she says, they require her to offer free health camp outreach days in the rural communities and accept as patients beneficiaries of government-subsidized healthcare schemes, who pay far less than she would negotiate from private patients. She works long hours to keep her business afloat and to be able to deliver services that help the population in areas where few doctors want to live, she tells me, and yet the government keeps introducing schemes and policies that make her work more challenging:

> In the IT sector they raise the salaries 30% a year. Things are improving that much for them every year. By contrast, we are not getting any increase. Why is our sector different? . . . Why should we have to reduce fees if we work all the time? They think doctors aren't human, but the doctor is a human being; he has a family. If they say that doctors are here to serve others, then they should make this clear from the beginning.

Escalating her frustration, she continues by saying that maybe doctors should be classified as priests, if working in India means that they must live selfless lives solely in the service of others. From our fieldwork off and on over the course of a year, which included an observation of her family-run clinic and facility record reviews, we believed that, actually, she was doing (financially) alright; however, she was keen on emphasizing to us that decisions—in particular staffing decisions—for her hospital were driven by not being able to find or afford to hire licensed staff.

Through the policies the government has devised in the last 15 years, the private health sector has played an increased role in delivering healthcare to rural populations. It straddles the line of being both state-sanctioned and beyond its boundaries, as many private facilities are barely regulated.[2] Yet, as Aastha demonstrates above, she sees herself as being a part of the system by enacting state demands through her immunization programmes, village outreach activities, and free treatment days, all as part of 'alleviating the burden on the public sector' and 'reducing maternal mortality'. (At the same time, she uses these obligatory outreach days to advertise her clinic and attract clients.)

The links drawn between maternal mortality and the solutions for its reductions frequently focus on women's access to facilities for antenatal and delivery care, and the quality of the care women receive from health workers there (Campbell 2006 et al.; Graham et al. 2016; Thaddeus and Maine 1994). In this chapter, we turn the lens on the clinical staff of four small, non-corporate private maternity hospitals in Rajasthan and Uttar Pradesh to explore what it means to work within a self-regulated system and examine the 'creation' of a cadre of unlicensed healthcare workers. We look at how a space of care and business is generated out of the precarious positions of the health workers who depend on employment there, compromising the care of women who seek its services.

By exploring doctors' and nurses' narratives, this chapter highlights the tensions between the value placed on profit, care, and staff rights in this health sector, and examines how unlicensed private sector health workers are at once marginalized and at the same time in a position of (re)asserting and reimagining the standard biomedical guidelines surrounding maternal health practices of care-seeking.

Research Design

This research is born out of a larger interdisciplinary project that explored social franchising (a method of improving services and quality of care in the private sector involving an external organizing body) for maternal healthcare in India (Uttar Pradesh and Rajasthan) and Uganda. We conducted the same qualitative and quantitative research design in all three locations, centring our research on three different social franchising programmes. Quantitative methods included an economic analysis of the programmes for the donors, implementing agencies, clinic owners, and women clients. For the qualitative study, researchers visited six private clinics for one week each and carried out participant observation and interviews with women, owners, and community health workers. Clinically, a team of two nurse-midwives carried out observations of routine antenatal care, delivery, and post-partum care, knowledge and skill vignettes with health workers, and an inventory of equipment and drugs. We also carried out interviews with clinics that chose not to join the franchise or were asked to leave, and conducted repeat interviews with implementing agency staff. Following this, in India, we had dedicated funding and time to address further topics that had caught our attention, one of which was probing the phenomenon of the high number of unlicensed health workers propping up the activities of the private clinics we visited, and it is out of this line of inquiry that this chapter emerges. This phenomenon seemed to be an open secret—with official documentation ignoring its prevalence but observations and personal exchanges acknowledging its widespread nature.

In April and May 2017, I returned to two of the clinics from the larger study in southern Rajasthan for six weeks of ethnographic fieldwork working closely with Sunita B., a translator who acted as a research assistant, facilitating my relationships with staff in addition to building up her own. Over the course of our fieldwork we spent time with staff in and out of the clinic, eating together and getting to know their families. After we had spent some weeks or months together (factoring in our time from the social franchise study), we also carried out repeat recorded interviews with a total of 12 staff, three directors, and four members of the community. After a preliminary analysis of the Rajasthan fieldwork, in September and October we travelled to Uttar Pradesh to carry out similar fieldwork in maternity clinics. We selected two clinics that were part of another social franchise and that were previously unknown to us. Here, in addition to five weeks participant observation at the clinics, we interviewed 10 staff and three directors. A newly graduated nurse-midwife accompanied us for 10 days of our fieldwork, observed quality of care at both clinics and reported back to us. We also returned to Rajasthan to follow up with health workers and respond to some emerging questions.

Throughout 2016–18, we disseminated our work on the private sector in Indian and international fora and interviewed 10 actors at the policy and administrative level in New Delhi, Jaipur, Lucknow, and Agra to better understand approaches to the private sector, in particular issues of staffing in maternal health.

Setting

Maternal Health in India

Geographically, Rajasthan is India's largest state while Uttar Pradesh is, with 204 million people, the country's most populous. Despite a significant reduction in maternal mortality in the last few years, Rajasthan and Uttar Pradesh remain among India's so-called priority states, as they fare poorly on maternal and child health indicators. The maternal mortality ratios (MMRs) in Rajasthan and Uttar Pradesh have been dropping since the turn of the century, from 375 and 440 respectively to about 200 deaths per 100,000 live births in 2016 (largely occurring in rural areas), compared to a national average of 130 the same year (NITI Aayog 2017). Both states also have higher fertility rates than the nationwide average (2.7–3.1 compared to the nationwide 2.3). Presenting these statistics point blank can be problematic. Politics surround the collection and dissemination of maternal health indicators that frequently only reveal a skewed or surface-level glimpse of the situation (Adams 2016), but these statistics have been used to drive changes in policy in the region, prompted by internal advocacy and global pressure to reach the Millennium Development Goals (MDGs) and, since 2015, the Sustainable Development Goals (SDGs).

For those working on maternal health in sub-Saharan Africa, India's policies and practices are frequently considered a model, for examples of how to improve health outcomes and statistics. The Indian government has generated several incentives to reduce maternal mortality, many of which are centred on encouraging women and families to attend facilities for childbirth (Jullien and Jeffery, this volume). For example, antenatal and delivery care are now free in government facilities; the National Rural Health Mission created a cadre of community health workers—accredited social health activists (ASHAs)—to support women and families navigating the system; the government distributes payments for the births of girl babies, provided the mother delivers in a health facility; and, particularly in Rajasthan, insurance and pregnancy care schemes have been developed that apply to those below the poverty line, and are accepted in some private facilities. Under Rajasthan's Free Medicine Scheme, medications from registered facilities are also free for all.

Although the public health infrastructure in India has grown substantially in recent years, it remains inadequate to meet the health requirements of the population. In Rajasthan in particular, the bulk of resources have been focused on health provision in towns, leaving rural areas underserved. Health facilities struggle to retain skilled providers. Over 75% of Rajasthan's human resources and advanced medical technology are found in the poorly-regulated private sector—a testament to the sizeable role it plays in healthcare provision. That said, in 2012 just under one in five women delivered in private facilities, 56% delivered in public facilities, and 26% at home, a decrease over the last decade, indicating that some of the policies to promote facility delivery may be achieving their aims (NHSRC 2013). Health facilities are meant to register with the government, but in Uttar Pradesh, for example, in a survey of maternal health clinics, only 47% had registered (Goodman et al. 2017).

The Four Focal Clinics in This Study

Our four focal clinics were all equipped to carry out C-sections and were currently or had been members of social franchising programmes but received few if any other external monitoring visits from regulatory staff not affiliated with the programmes. None of them reported regular monitoring visits from government staff, bar isolated exceptional circumstances (as had arisen publicly in three of the four clinics).

The two clinics we studied in Rajasthan—referred to here as Sunrise and Cascade—were 30 km apart, both in settings that were locally considered rural (with circa 300,000 people in the area) and served largely rural communities with approximately 40 deliveries per month and 20–40 beds each. Husband and wife doctor teams ran both clinics, with one of each pair in the lead in terms of patient care. Sunrise was a maternity hospital, headed by an MBBS doctor (with a certificate in obstetrics and gynaecology) in her forties, with ten clinical staff members. Cascade was a general hospital, run by an MD about the same age, who hired approximately 15 clinical staff to his team.

In Uttar Pradesh, we selected a large city as a base for our research, and the two focal clinics provided care for urban women. Both were owned by husband and wife teams, with the MBBS wives in charge of the medical care in the clinics. Ravine was a neighbourhood maternity clinic catering to a largely Muslim population, with approximately 30 deliveries per month and 20 beds. Three women attended to deliveries and general care of patients. A technician with 40 years of experience assisted the doctor in the operating theatre and performed other patient-care duties. Clifftop was a continuously expanding general hospital; we focused on its popular maternity services, seeing 80 deliveries a month and having over 80 hospital beds.

These were not the fancy private clinics that some people might imagine when thinking of private care in India. Uncomplicated vaginal deliveries cost between 4,000 and 20,000 rupees (up to 300 USD), which is the starting point to pay at a simple but smart clinic in a small city. Prices are negotiable. In general, the private sector is extremely diverse. A recent study in Uttar Pradesh found that small and mid-level clinics had 54% of the market share (Goodman et al. 2017), and these were typically headed up by MBBS and Ayush doctors.

The assessment carried out by the nurse-midwives as part of our larger research showed that the quality of care was generally poor at all four hospitals. Deliveries were commonly conducted in poor hygiene conditions, and staff showed little knowledge of best practices, let alone demonstrated following them (Penn-Kekana et al. 2018).

Even though pregnancy care is free in the public sector, some families with limited means will still choose to attend private facilities for childbirth. Our evaluation research on why women choose to attend our focal private facilities for delivery and childcare (Haemmerli et al. 2018) is in sync with other literature on the topic in India (Raman 2014; Unnithan-Kumar 2001; Van Hollen 2003). Hospitals in the public sector are known for having long waits, being crowded, and often not being clean or having good hygiene standards. One of the mothers-in-law we spoke to said that during her daughter-in-law's high-risk pregnancy, neighbours would suggest different places for delivery:

> Four different people gave four different suggestions. A few women in the community said, 'Why are you taking her there (to the government facility), go here to the private instead! Your daughter-in-law is feeling restless, her problems will increase with time. What is value of money? You can earn money but if she dies how will you get her back?'
>
> Mother-in-law, Rajasthan

Women choose private facilities for maternal care because of proximity, past attendance, status concerns, and, significantly, the belief that they will receive more individualized attention. Some ASHAs made agreements with facilities to bring pregnant clients to them and received a commission, which could influence decision-making. Particularly when women experienced complicated pregnancies, they turned to the private sector with the expectation of being treated by the doctor him or herself—not by nursing staff.

With facilities drawing women to them in part thanks to target-setting policies, questions arise: what sort of care are they receiving at private facilities? Is it better than the care they could be getting at home? Who is attending to them—trained health workers or those with little experience? And, with the primary attention on women's place of birth, and secondly the quality of care they receive, where does that leave the working circumstances and conditions for the health workers providing the care?

Care and Social Organization

Desires surrounding maternal care practices can shape health-seeking in different ways to other areas of health. After all, pregnancy is not a disease, and the moves to save lives through medicalizing, controlling, and shaping how and where pregnancy and childbirth take place are imposed on women in many settings (as the policies mentioned above illustrate). As a way of thinking about the medical services in these clinics, the following section briefly unpacks conceptualizations of 'care' to help illuminate an understanding of the staffing and social organization we observed in our field sites.

Within the vast anthropological literature on care, scholars have turned their theoretical gaze to understanding the meanings, symbolism, and societal structures that patterns of (health)care work into our daily lives and interactions. Tatjana Thelen urges us to move beyond the typical dichotomy of seeing care practices as being either warm from relatives or cold from institutions, and to look at the practices themselves and through the lens that 'care connects a giving and receiving side in practices aimed to satisfy socially recognised needs' (Thelen 2015: 509). Care has the potential to shape the 'ever-shifting forms of social organization'.

She urges a reconceptualization of care to address some of the pitfalls and limitations that she sees in historical depictions. Thelen suggests a) to look at all parties as equal contributors in the construction of need and responsibility; b) to see care as embedded in larger institutional frameworks as well as within different temporalities; c) to disentangle care from the private sphere of family and kin; and d) to recognize that care does not always have positive outcomes and can have an impact on social relations.

With the individual and the body as a starting point, this notion of care allows for an examination of the social relations and social structures that both influence care and are shaped by it. Private health clinics are meant, in a sense, to merge the 'warm' with the 'institution'—by offering tailored, individual care to women during pregnancy and labour. Thelen writes about rendering visible the boundary work in the relations enacted by care, in order to expose what happens in the spaces in between and to gain insight into practices and relations—between people, practices, emotions, and institutions. This reference is pertinent to this study, because some of the literature looking at informal health workers theorizes the differences between legitimacy and illegitimacy by articulating them as boundaries and analyses that professional space through the lens of the social and historical situatedness of healthcare roles and competency (see, for example, Cross and MacGregor 2010; Pinto 2004). By drawing attention to these acts of care we can also shed light on the symbolic and social boundaries and their 'effect on individual and collective mobility strategy' (Lamont and Molnár 2002) with the idea that they affect actors' agency in creating and bringing about change for themselves. Bringing these together can provide fruitful insight into what we see happening in our private clinics in Rajasthan and Uttar Pradesh.

As the nature of care is contextual and specific to the politics of where and who is performing it, it also bears reflecting on the intentional or unintentional harm care can bring about through its enactment. Martin et al. (2015), in introducing a special issue on care in technoscience, lay out the shadows of care and its possible shortcomings in attempts to 'unsettle' assumptions about care: 'Care is a selective mode of attention: it circumscribes and cherishes some things, lives, or phenomena as its objects. In the process, it excludes others. Practices of care are always shot through with asymmetrical power relations: who has the power to care? Who has the power to define what counts as care and how it should be administered?' (Martin et al. 2015: 627).

These notions about the double-edged nature of care—that its meanings can occupy multiple conceptions and spaces at the same time—are useful in thinking about the care environments that the health workers in our focal clinics operate within, and that they may be acting out contradictory versions of their roles at once.

The next two subsections describe aspects of private sector maternal services using the lens of care, through which the internal structures of these clinics are revealed—structures and practices that in turn are a reflection of their place in greater society. I have chosen two phenomena to explore different aspects: the first concerns the issue of clinical training and qualifications of health workers; the second, the performance of care and ritualized acts of overmedicalization. These examples situate health workers within their tenuous roles in healthcare and in these community-focused maternity clinics.

The Value of Formal Training: What Does a Qualification Really Accomplish?

Our four focal clinics were largely staffed by unlicensed health workers who had been working in the profession between three and 30 years at the time of fieldwork. The majority of those we spoke to and who feature in this chapter had been practising for four to eight years. In terms of maternal care, both licensed and unlicensed health workers delivered babies. Studies show that private unlicensed healthcare workers earn lower salaries and have limited room for job advancement compared to public sector health workers, as social and economic considerations limit their professional lives (Sharma 2015).

After spending several weeks at Cascade, I asked the owner Mahesh to explain his stance on hiring unlicensed staff and putting them to work in his operating theatre and delivery room. Expecting him to inform me that I misunderstood their roles at his clinic and that they actually only performed peripheral tasks, as I had previously heard at other clinics, I was surprised when he paused for a moment and smiled as he said, 'Even if they come here already trained (licensed), everything they learn they learn here on the job'.

Mahesh said that, for him, his hiring decisions were all about personality and workability—he had had enough staff arrive freshly with degrees from nursing, midwifery, or even medical schools, who couldn't function in his clinic. If he could train them himself, they would work the way he wanted. Similarly, his staff said that they didn't really think that those staff who did have formal training knew how to give injections or perform clinical tasks better than they did. So, we asked them, what were the benefits of a qualification? 'Being able to get out'; to get a public sector job that would secure higher salaries, stability, and a pension, was what we commonly heard. Not having a license also served hospital directors in that it was harder for these staff to market themselves and to find other hospital work at the same level.

However, we were also repeatedly told that being officially qualified served as 'a license to make mistakes'. In essence, if you make a mistake and harm a patient and you are not licensed, you can get in trouble with the community, possibly with the director, and with the avenues of recourse that might be taken. But if you are licensed, it is not your fault if something goes wrong—something else will usually be at fault. 'A qualification [degree or diploma] is a pass to make mistakes, it covers you if you mess up', Ina, a 23-year-old unlicensed nurse told us. Ina was the doctor's preferred staff member for patient care and surgical assistance, and while this was her first job and she had only been working at the clinic for four years, she had quickly risen up through the ranks to earn more than even a licensed nurse. More than Rickie, for example, a 25-year-old with a BSc in nursing, who was Dr Mahesh's second choice, even though he had been working with the doctor for three years. Rickie himself said that Ina was a better nurse than he was, and that he learned a lot from her.

Ina engaged in a power struggle with the 'guys upstairs'—the providers who took care of patients in the wards. In particular, Akarsh, who had recently completed his MBBS, was hired by the director as his first job after the exams. Akarsh had asked Mahesh if he could carry out his internship at the hospital, and Mahesh agreed—not paying him a salary, his typical approach for taking on new staff. Throughout our weeks with Ina, she recounted numerous stories of how she tested and discredited Akarsh and that he 'didn't know how to do anything'. Even though Ina told us stories of how she herself had messed up on the job—forgetting to sterilize key instruments for surgery, or how the doctors had, with one leaving a whole load of cotton wool inside a patient during surgery such that they had to open the patient up again the next day—she had a particular lack of faith in Akarsh, who was above her in qualification but below her in skill. This tension between nurses and fresh doctors is known the world over, but Ina didn't speak this way about her fellow staff without formal nursing education.

Local in-clinic training resets the codes and rules from outside to be inside and particular to the clinic. In the outside world, formal training was valid, but on the inside, experience on the job and other skills were given priority. As Sarah Pinto writes, 'education does not necessarily confer legitimacy or transform subjects into legitimate modern ones. Rather it provides a site for enacting authority; the performance of education accomplishes a transformation of subjects. [They are] rehearsed acts with immediate recognisability regardless of the knowledge they convey or contest' (Pinto 2004: 350).

Formal qualifications did not legitimize staff inside the clinic—indeed we got a sense of the power struggles between licensed and unlicensed staff, especially when unlicensed were given more privileges and responsibilities—but it legitimized them in the clinical world outside, the one that health workers wanted to reach. Unable to find work in the public sector, unlicensed staff at our focal clinics sometimes employed their skills in the community for extra income. Capitalizing on their clinic identities, those acting as pharmacists, nurses, and surgical assistants prescribed medications and tended to patients on house calls within their neighbourhoods. This also served as publicity for the clinics, an extension of the reach of their services, embedding them into the community, and further reinforcing acts of unregulated skills and the wishy-washy space of what healthcare entails.

The absence of qualifications made no real difference in terms of clinical responsibilities even though certain roles were engrained, as the following example from Sunrise clinic shows. There, among the nursing staff, Vanya had the reputation of being one of the best providers to deliver babies. Skilful, calm, and successful with women during labour, she was regularly the only staff on duty responsible for childbirth. However, her situation was complicated. Hired as a sweeper eight years previously, over the years she had been trained on the job to deliver babies. Officially, she was still recognized as a sweeper tasked with cleaning the clinic and handling patients' bodily fluids, as well as giving personal massages to the doctor, picking her children up from school, and carrying out similar non-professional duties. In the hierarchy of clinical duties, sweepers generally perform the lowest-ranked—even if they are incredibly important—ward chores, in a structure where dealing with blood, urine, and the by-products of pregnancy is considered a role for someone of lower status or caste and beneath nurses and other medical professionals (Jullien 2017). Opportunistically, Vanya was used for her skills and capacities in midwifery, but these strengths did not release her from the identity of someone who would take the sweeper role.

Our research in Uttar Pradesh further underlined the values, tensions, and obfuscation surrounding degrees. As we scouted out locations for our fieldwork there, Sunita and I paid introductory visits to a few urban facilities to see which could be a good match for our fieldwork. One was Ravine, a small clinic staffed by three providers—all with BSc nursing degrees, we were told by the doctor who owned and ran the clinic.

Because of its other characteristics, Ravine was a good match for our fieldwork, except that it appeared only to employ licensed healthcare workers. 'Oh well', I thought. 'Then we won't focus on unlicensed staff during this fieldwork but at least we'll see how another private clinic functions'. In our initial chats with the staff they confirmed the accounts about their own degrees, but little by little we noted inconsistencies in their stories about each other. Ultimately, to keep track of the different versions we heard, we created a table to detail what we heard from each individual about their own professional background and what they had to say about those of their colleagues. Over the weeks, the scaffolding surrounding qualifications fell away.

Ultimately, it turned out that none of them had nursing degrees. Maya, the most senior nurse—a 28-year-old woman living on the clinic grounds—had started working at a different neighbourhood clinic when she was 12. There, she told us, the owner abused and took advantage of her, while her father insisted that she kept working for the small salary she brought home. Ten years ago, the doctor-owner of our focal clinic hired Maya. She earned a base salary of 6,000 rupees a month, a salary that even the proprietor said was 'impossible' to survive on, and was expected to supplement her income from 'happiness payments' from satisfied patients' families and money for supplementary clinical services she offered at the clinic.[3]

The staging around staff qualifications was elaborated about two years previously. On one occasion, while the doctor was out of town, a woman treated at Ravine later died after giving birth. The case received considerable attention in the neighbourhood and city press, placing the clinic in a negative light. Soon afterwards, the owner arranged for all four of her staff to obtain degrees.

For example, the director of a local private college sold Maya a BSc nursing certificate, retained in the doctor's possession, though Maya had to cover the costs for it herself and borrowed money to do so. The owner employed similar strategies to obtain degrees on paper to meet the official minimum staff qualification requirements for the clinic—none of which were earned through actual formal education or training. The owner secured illegitimate degrees to meet the official minimum staff qualification requirements for the clinic as safety against external rules, while the staff were legitimized internally by their positions of caregiving.

This is a solution of conjuring up qualifications instead of valuing the knowledge and skill that formal training would ideally impart. Throwing money and favours at the issue shows ingenuity on the part of the owner, who thereby solves their problems, but does it actually help the staff or the patients they care for? In recent years the concept of *jugaad,* a type of solution-finding in India that goes outside of officially sanctioned rules, often gaining success through measures that involve false pretences or corrupt practices, has received increased attention from scholars of both entrepreneurship and regulation. Beatrice Jauregui writes about the contronymic character of jugaad, describing its application to actions that have distinctly moral qualities, in that it is justified for those with a lower status but unwarranted for those in positions of power. In addition, those who employ it often do so in opposition to the state. She writes that: 'corruption as immoral practice is somehow fundamentally tied to positional and institutional power—whether it flows through "public" or "private" channels—and that it is tied especially to state power to dominate and regulate' (Jauregui 2014: 78).

The clinic owners in our study, like Aastha at the beginning of this chapter, tell a narrative in which they are the victims of the system, justifying creative resolutions akin to jugaad to their business models. However, is it really the case that they cannot find or afford to hire trained staff? Are they in positions of power or in positions of vulnerability, and is it simply a corrupt strategy? In critiquing a book that praised jugaad as 'the Indian way of innovation that management gurus advised the West to emulate' (Joseph 2018), the author underlines how counterproductive jugaad actually is, an opinion that could be mapped onto the health sector: why would jugaad need to be employed if qualifications on the systemic scale were not actually an integral part of patient care?

Qualifications have currency in the outside world that these health workers don't have access to legitimately because they lack the social capital or funding to pay for them and the bribes for government jobs were they to obtain degrees. In turn, internally, licensing becomes an act for the structure and image of care, not for the actual quality or content of care. Perhaps qualifications aren't actually valuable, if staff can do their jobs without them.

Performance of Care: Unnecessary Practices and Absent Doctors

The second part of this chapter discusses the performance of care, starting with the experience of one individual—Joshi, who worked at Aastha's clinic Sunrise. Though he was a licensed nurse, the argument laid out here extends beyond those who are unlicensed and speaks to the dynamics of the self-contained bubbles of caregiving that these private clinics create.

I had known Joshi for a year when Sunita and I finally sat down to carry out a formal interview with him. He lived just a few buildings down from the clinic in order to be quickly reachable when needed (Aastha paid for his accommodation). Since he was often too busy at work, Sunita and I had taken to visiting his stay-at-home wife and school-age daughter during visits to the clinic; they had a lot more time for us and his wife loved to chat, filling us in on her view of the behind-the-scenes of day-to-day clinic operations. A semi-trained nurse herself, she had work experience at some of the private clinics familiar to us in the area—the world of private clinics in our district was small.

Joshi claimed that he was 'trapped' at Sunrise because of money he owed the owners after lending them his bank account to complete underhand dealings during Prime Minister Modi's demonetization initiative in 2016, and because he had by accident signed a contract that he hadn't read which Aastha and her husband kept it in their safe and denied him access to it. Joshi's experiences highlighted the blurred boundaries between professional and personal relationships we saw at work in the clinics, laced with hierarchy, power, and manipulation. These themes are present in many workplaces, not all necessarily uniformly negative, but focusing on care allows us to understand the nature of their articulation here.

Joshi was in his thirties with a BSc in nursing and had moved back to this district after training and marriage to be closer to his extended family. Widely regarded as being very good at his job, we repeatedly heard from his colleagues that he was capable and respectful with women, unlike some of the other staff. He regularly worked long hours, sometimes triple shifts, as only one other staff member was semi-licensed and at least one health worker on duty should be licensed (though ultimately sometimes only unlicensed workers were on duty).

Already two minutes into this interview, Joshi lifted a load from his chest, setting about telling us the many ways in which the staff at Sunrise carried out unnecessary care practices, and how he colluded with the doctor to create either a need or a perceived need for these services. Their aims were twofold: the main goal was to drive up instances of care that needed to be paid for, thereby increasing profits, but the other was to give attention and to perform care in the eyes of the patient, to encourage the sentiment that they were attended to and looked out for at this clinic. Simple ways of doing this were the frequent prescription of unnecessary blood tests, ultrasounds, and physical exams. However, their actions also led to the prescription of IVs, medications, prolonged hospital stays, and non-medically required C-sections. The strategies for overtreatment that he revealed are not unique to this setting; indeed, well documented are these profit-generating tricks (see, for example, Das and Hammer 2014; Seeberg 2012) and coercion (Jeffery and Jeffery 2010), sometimes considered predatory (Nundy et al. 2018).

We observe here the role that health workers assumed their performance of extra medical tasks would take for patients. These tasks were expected to have a non-negotiable quality that would be accepted, valued, and paid for by patients and their families. We also see how, referencing Thelen (2015), care is embedded in the social institution and responds to alternative needs—those of the health workers to gain more money, and the patients to seek care from a service that will attend to them on a more personal level than the public sector is perceived to—for better or worse.

What struck us during the encounters where he recounted—practically confessed—these methods for driving up profits was Joshi's simultaneous complicity in these acts alongside his assessment that it was completely wrong for him to participate in them and carry them out. He blamed the head doctor for his actions and indicated that a requirement for working at the clinic was to subsume one's own morals to the overarching morals of the clinic in order to keep a job.

Both the owner and Maya at Ravine described care practices prescribed to assure patients that they were obtaining specialized attention. While this was sometimes clearly to the financial benefit of the clinic, some tasks could also be seen as providing special treatment that patients wouldn't find at a public health centre. The owner admitted to taking in pregnant women who pretended to faint in her consultation room in efforts to secure the rest they needed from their 'meddling' families. She played along, giving them a quiet bed for an afternoon and validation in the eyes of family members that she needed care. 'Private sector practitioners do more or less what is expected of them by the patient', Das and Hammer (2005: 2) have written. 'For poorer patients, the quality of advice is low and such patients spend a fair amount of money for nothing—low-value advice and unnecessary drugs'.

In these instances of unnecessary treatment or overtreatment, we see how they can satisfy patient expectations while they are executed carefully, without medical, psychological, or social repercussions. However, the idea that profits or patients' non-medically-indicated service desires dominate care decisions, illuminates the earlier reference to the double-edged nature of care (Martin et al. 2015): that its acts can be positive and risky at the same time. Where are the boundaries between harmful practices and care practices that support women's wishes? Ultimately, what is harmful is allowing unlicensed health workers to attend to childbirth within state-sanctioned spaces, embodying the misleading, hidden, underbelly of care services.

Policy Approaches

The staff described in these vignettes, in their tenuous positions, are beyond the reach of government policies meant to standardize practices surrounding childbirth in facilities and staff working conditions: few clinics in our sample received any monitoring visits from governmental bodies. Instead, they were involved in programmes belonging to a wave of global actors reaching out to the private sector to implement initiatives that aim to improve, regulate, and support quality of care and service provision standards. This wave was comparatively small—only reaching a few scattered private clinics among the vast sea of providers. We observed how the arms of these programmes, intended to monitor and impose change, were met with resistance from clinic owners. Some Indian organizations, such as doctors' alliances and the COPASAH network (Community of Practitioners on Accountability and Social Protection in Health), also worked on the topics of citizen involvement and accountability regarding private and public healthcare, but hospital owners made no mention of such initiatives as playing a role in their operations.

Speaking with the head of a doctors' obstetrics alliance, when I raised the topic of unqualified health workers and their rights, my informant placed the focus of concern back on the vulnerability of doctors running private clinics and the benefits they bring to society:

I want to say: what will make a difference in women's lives is that we need to de-stress my own fraternity first because we, we will be getting bashed up . . . We become the punching bags of the whole society and the government also. For, you know, not providing! Now where do you think we are not providing? We're providing with all the constraints we have.

Head of professional organization for obstetricians

This echoes Dr Aastha's viewpoint at the opening of this chapter: if the private clinics these doctors run are so problematic and shouldn't exist, would that really improve the healthcare circumstances for the population, and by extension, the government? When we spoke to actors at the programmatic and government level about the way forward, we were met with either the denial that unlicensed health workers were operating in hospitals, or an admission of knowledge, but frustration at how to proceed given deep-rooted practices and strong doctors' lobbies that held off regulation of private clinics. Some actors acknowledged that forward movement on this front was challenging and that someone should find a way to work within the system:

All these things we've been doing in the government sector . . . but all these things make no dent in the private sector. For the doctors, it's like if you train a person to work in your house, you are satisfied with that. They want a person who follows directions, not who follows their own prescription. Enforcing this through regulations won't work. Anything that is enforced has less sustainability. You have to get buy in.

Maternal health adviser in the Indian Ministry
of Health and Social Welfare

Others, confirming the frustration of this government adviser, claimed that the government wasn't doing enough, and wasn't committed to changing the situation; the mountain was huge and held sway by the powerful population of doctors. Change needs to come from outside; there is no incentive from the inside, we were told. Gadre and Shukla (2016) argue that introducing regulations can also foster opportunities for corruption to flourish if done inadequately.

Still, this presents a conflicting picture. By encouraging women to attend facilities for childbirth through incentives, and encouraging private clinics to attend to more and more women whose care is paid for by public funds (also through incentives), the government supports these clinics in delivering substandard care and creating a cadre of health workers that are not officially sanctioned, nor do they receive social protection. The values presented here put in opposition the purported values for the importance of healthcare, or, perhaps, demonstrate the contradictory steps that exist at the intersections between the realities of clinic owners, professional associations, and central policy debates as change is brought about.

Conclusion: Structural Vulnerability and the Precarity of Unlicensed Health Staff

Structural violence has become a popular framework for exploring and describing engrained circumstances of neglect and disadvantage due to hierarchical inequalities in societies (Farmer 2004). The concept's origins have been attributed to Johann Galtung, who explained it as 'the indirect violence built into repressive social orders creating enormous differences between potential and actual human self-realization' (Galtung 1975: 173). Expanding on structural violence, scholars have introduced the concept of *structural vulnerability* to refer to citizens who are at a disadvantage of receiving the resources, care, policies, and attention available to the larger population, or those more privileged. As Bourgois et al. write, specifically in reference to the USA where this term has been most deployed: 'These subtle symbolic demarcations of hierarchies may influence perceptions by clinical and social service providers as well as by the larger society about the type of care considered appropriate for an individual or a social group, creating a potential stigma of differential "health-related deservingness"' (Bourgois 2017). They refer to Willen's (2012) idea of deservingness in health—that certain populations are deemed by the larger system as being worthy of getting more expert, considered, and competent care, and that these decisions are cemented by policies, zoning, stigma, and other factors—a perpetuation of engrained inequalities.

We could consider the population of patients who attend these private bubble clinics as being 'better-off'—after all, they have chosen to spend their money on healthcare in the private sector instead of or in addition to the free governmental clinics. (The schemes mentioned at the start of this chapter cover some of these patients, however, reducing their costs.) Nevertheless, the choices they make will result in their regularly receiving substandard care from health professionals acting in the interests of a business, instead of the well-being of their clients. Through the ethnographic details laid out in this chapter, we consider that structural vulnerability applies also to the health workers, themselves placed in a precarious position due to a lack of options, rights, and recourse to alternatives for themselves.

The opportunities that exist for them at these borders of healthcare are diminished, with challenging circumstances for individual or collective possibilities to improve their working conditions (Lamont and Molnár 2002). Just as for patients facing structural vulnerabilities for whom 'health adversities tend to cluster' and whose 'epidemiological patterning of disease, illness and injury is profoundly influenced by upstream determinants' (Willen et al. 2017), those working as auxiliaries in these private maternal healthcare clinics are also in patterns of disadvantage, responding to the influences of the systemic and individual circumstances of the healthcare system in India that fosters an environment for these clinics to flourish.

The bubble worlds of these clinics—owner operated, with few, if any, outside checks and balances; and fluid interpretations of care and quality— lend a particular precarity to both those who are treated there and those who work there. Staff guard the secrets of their bosses, invest in the profit-making enterprise, and in their subordination find ways to survive their situations and find their niche. Unlicensed health workers are marginalized in society, with limited choices to move out of their employment situations to the sanctioned mainstream services. The government, aware of these bubble systems but driven by target-setting policies and a complex terrain of stakeholder interests, allow them to thrive in the aims of reaching national and global targets that will legitimize the status of the country on the international stage.

Through prolonged engagement with a field site in Uttar Pradesh, Jeffery and Jeffery (2008) have suggested that the government has lost its 'moral authority' in managing its state healthcare and failing to meet quality and service standards that its public deserves. In the case of the independent private clinics we visited, the evidence of just how weak this moral authority is becomes clear. While India has received recognition in recent years for the progress it has made—an achievement in a populous land where small changes can entail huge endeavours at the population level—we also see the space that the private sector has come to occupy in the new maternity situation. Invulnerable to outside forces, private clinic health workers—both licensed and unlicensed—in their precarious positions end up unwittingly supporting these untouchable bubbles that serve so many of the country's population.

In public and global health, the focus on private sector maternity care has generally been on health outcomes and oriented through the lens of quality of care, leaving what happens in these ubiquitous non-corporate maternity clinics in a fog. In this chapter, we have looked at pregnancy and delivery care as a link between health targets and those on the frontline who are involved in reaching them. Unlicensed health workers are used within the healthcare system (ultimately made up of both private and public sector realities) and, through their enactment of care practices, professionalized into legitimate healthcare workers, in a sense working on behalf of the state and their employer. By throwing light on the different players at work—from the government policies, to the clinic owners, to women and families' expectations as paying customers, to health workers' constraints—how engrained health workers' precarious positions are becomes clear.

Notes

1. In this chapter the first person refers to the lead author to be true to the narrative characteristic of fieldwork, though the work is the result of all four authors' contributions.
2. During our fieldwork, prenatal ultrasound was the only activity cited by research participants as being regulated, in order to minimise sex selection.
3. Happiness payments are socially obligatory payments given by women and their families upon receipt of healthcare services to employed staff. They are something between a tip and *bakchich*—an expression of gratitude but not consistently paid happily.

References

Adams, Vincanne. 2016. *Metrics: What Counts in Global Health*. Durham, NC: Duke University Press.

Bourgois, Philippe, Seth M. Holmes, Kim Sue, and James Quesada. 2017. 'Structural Vulnerability: Operationalizing the Concept to Address Health Disparities in Clinical Care'. *Academic Medicine: Journal of the Association of American Medical Colleges* 92 (3): 299. doi: 10.1097/ACM.0000000000001294.

Campbell, Oona M.R., Wendy J. Graham, and Lancet Maternal Survival Series steering group. 2006. 'Strategies for Reducing Maternal Mortality: Getting On with What Works'. *The Lancet* 368 (9543): 1284–99. doi: 10.1016/S0140-6736(06)69381-1.

Cross, Jamie, and Hayley Nan MacGregor. 2010. 'Knowledge, Legitimacy and Economic Practice in Informal Markets for Medicine: A Critical Review of Research'. *Social Science & Medicine* 71 (9): 1593–600. doi: 10.1016/j.socscimed.2010.07.040.

Das, Jishnu, and Jeffrey Hammer. 2005. 'Money for Nothing: The Dire Straits of Medical Practice in Delhi, India'. *Journal of Development Economics* 83 (1): 1–36. doi: 10.1016/j.jdeveco.2006.05.004.

Das, Jishnu, and Jeffrey Hammer. 2014. 'Quality of Primary Care in Low-Income Countries: Facts and Economics'. *Annual Review of Economics* 6 (1): 525–53. doi: 10.1146/annurev-economics-080213-041350.

Farmer, Paul. 2004. 'An Anthropology of Structural Violence'. *Current Anthropology* 45 (3): 305–17. doi: 10.1086/382250.

Gadre, Arun, and Abhay Shukla. 2016. *Dissenting Diagnosis*. Gurgaon: Random House India.

Galtung, Johan. 1975. *Peace: Research, Education, Action: Essays in Peace Research.* Copenhagen: Christian Ejlers.

Goodman, Catherine, Meenakshi Gautham, Richard Iles, Katia Bruxvoort, Manish Subharwal, Sanjay Gupta, and Manish Jain. 2017. *The Nature of Competition faced by Private Providers of Maternal Health Services in Uttar Pradesh*. London: LSHTM Impact Partners for Social Development.

Graham, Wendy, Susannah Woodd, Peter Byass, Veronique Filippi, Giorgia Gon, Sandra Virgo, Doris Chou, Sennen Hounton, Rafael Lozano, and Robert Pattinson. 2016. 'Diversity and Divergence: The Dynamic Burden of Poor Maternal Health'. *The Lancet* 388 (10056): 2164–75. doi: 10.1016/S0140-6736(16)31533-1.

Haemmerli, Manon, Andreia Santos, Loveday Penn-Kekana, Isabelle Lange, Fred Matovu, Lenka Benova, Kerry L.M. Wong, and Catherine Goodman. 2018. 'How Equitable Is Social Franchising? Case Studies of Three Maternal Healthcare Franchises in Uganda and India'. *Health Policy and Planning* 33 (3): 411–19. doi: 10.1093/heapol/czx192.

Jauregui, Beatrice. 2014. 'Provisional Agency in India: Jugaad and Legitimation of Corruption'. *American Ethnologist* 41 (1): 76–91.

Jeffery, Patricia, and Roger Jeffery. 2008. ' "Money Itself Discriminates": Obstetric Emergencies in the Time of Liberalisation'. *Contributions to Indian Sociology* 42 (1): 59–91.

Jeffery, Patricia, and Roger Jeffery. 2010. 'Costly Absences, Coercive Presences: Health Care in Rural North India'. In *Diversity and Change in Modern India: Economic, Social and Political Approaches*, edited by Anthony F. Heath and Roger Jeffery, 47–71. Oxford: Oxford University Press.

Joseph, Manu. 2018. ' "Jugaad", India's Most Overrated Idea'. *Livemint Online*, 18 August 2018. Accessed 25 May 2019. https://www.livemint.com/Leisure/2c3sntdHfJ8Py2tWxEqgcN/Jugaad-Indias-most-overrated-idea.html

Jullien, Clémence. 2017. 'Dealing with Impurities of Childbirth: Contemporary Reconfigurations of Disgust in India'. *Skepsi* 8: 39–51.

Lamont, Michèle, and Virág Molnár. 2002. 'The Study of Boundaries in the Social Sciences'. *Annual Review of Sociology* 28 (1): 167–95.

Martin, Aryn, Natasha Myers, and Ana Viseu. 2015. 'The Politics of Care in Technoscience'. *Social Studies of Science* 45 (5): 625–41. doi: 10.1177/0306312715602073.

NHSRC. 2013. 'HMIS Data Analysis'. National Health Systems Resource Centre. Accessed 16 March 2020. http://nhsrcindia.org/hmis-data-analysis

NITI Aayog. 2017. 'Maternal Mortality Ratios for India'. National Institution for Transforming India. Accessed 21 March 2020. https://niti.gov.in/content/maternal-mortality-ratio-mmr-100000-live-births

Nundy, Samiran, Keshav Desiraju, and Sanjay Nagral, eds. 2018. *Healers or Predators? Healthcare Corruption in India*. New Delhi: Oxford University Press.

Penn-Kekana, Loveday, Timothy Powell-Jackson, Manon Haemmerli, Varun Dutt, Isabelle L. Lange, Aniva Mahapatra, Gaurav Sharma, Kultar Singh, Sunita Singh, and Vasudha Shukla. 2018. 'Process Evaluation of a Social Franchising Model to Improve Maternal Health: Evidence from a Multi-Methods Study in Uttar Pradesh, India'. *Implementation Science* 13 (1): 124–38. doi: 10.1186/s13012-018-0813-y.

Pinto, Sarah. 2004. 'Development Without Institutions: Ersatz Medicine and the Politics of Everyday Life in Rural North India'. *Cultural Anthropology* 19 (3): 337–64.

Raman, Shanti. 2014. 'Faith, Trust and the Perinatal Healthcare Maze in Urban India'. *Health, Culture and Society* 6 (1): 73–84. doi: 10.5195/hcs.2014.123.

Seeberg, Jens. 2012. 'Connecting Pills and People: An Ethnography of the Pharmaceutical Nexus in Odisha, India'. *Medical Anthropology Quarterly* 26 (2): 182–200. doi: 10.1111/j.1548-1387.2012.01200.x.

Sharma, Dinesh C. 2015. 'India Still Struggles with Rural Doctor Shortages'. *The Lancet* 386 (10011): 2381–2. doi: 10.1016/S0140-6736(15)01231-3.

Thaddeus, Sereen, and Deborah Maine. 1994. 'Too Far to Walk: Maternal Mortality in Context'. *Social Science & Medicine* 38 (8): 1091–110.

Thelen, Tatjana. 2015. 'Care as Social Organization: Creating, Maintaining and Dissolving Significant Relations'. *Anthropological Theory* 15 (4): 497–515. doi: 10.1177/1463499615600893.

Unnithan-Kumar, Maya. 2001. 'Emotion, Agency and Access to Healthcare: Women's Experiences of Reproduction in Jaipur'. In *Managing Reproductive Life: Cross-Cultural Themes in Sexuality and Fertility*, edited by Soraya Tremayne, 27–51. Oxford: Berghahn Books.

Van Hollen, Cecilia. 2003. *Birth on the Threshold: Childbirth and Modernity in South India*. Berkeley & Los Angeles: University of California Press.

Willen, Sarah S. 2012. 'How is Health-Related "Deservingness" Reckoned? Perspectives from Unauthorized Im/migrants in Tel Aviv'. *Social Science & Medicine* 74 (6): 812–21. doi: 10.1016/j.socscimed.2011.06.033.

Willen, Sarah S., Michael Knipper, César E. Abadía-Barrero, and Nadav Davidovitch. 2017. 'Syndemic Vulnerability and the Right to Health'. *The Lancet* 389 (10072): 964–77. doi: 10.1016/S0140-6736(17)30261-1.

9

Protocols and Set-Ups

Producing Professional Obstetrical Knowledge in the Periphery of Mumbai, India

Neha Madhiwalla

Introduction: The Locus of Medical Knowledge

The universalization of institutional delivery necessarily needs the consolidation of a comprehensive system of emergency obstetric care to meet the goal of reducing maternal mortality and disability (Paxton et al. 2005). In India, there remains a significant gap in the availability of emergency obstetric services in rural areas (Bailey et al. 2006). Moreover, guidelines emanating from the Global North or from India's metropolitan centres do not resonate with the reality of practising obstetrics in rural settings. For example, the prohibition on the use of unbanked blood makes the provision of comprehensive emergency obstetric care difficult (Sood et al. 2018). The lack of clarity in the demarcation of tasks that can be performed by various cadres of medical personnel also poses barriers to the delivery of emergency care (Mavalankar and Rosenfield 2005).

Metropolitan experts overwhelm India's health policymaking and professional leadership. Research output of Indian medical colleges, which is meagre overall, also largely emanates from elite, metropolitan institutions (Reddy et al. 1991). Consequently, the evidence base is skewed in favour of developed countries in general and urban centres within India. Subsequently, norms of treatment are based on developed country contexts (Jacob et al. 2011). Global clinical practice guidelines are also not systematically adapted to local contexts (Mehndiratta et al. 2017). Individual practitioners make ad hoc decisions leading to immense idiosyncrasies in practice (Das et al. 2012; Nagpal et al. 2015). Typically, informal trends play an important role in influencing the nature of medical practice beyond official guidelines and protocols. Global advances in technology and pharmacology are assimilated into metropolitan medical practice, with no particular scientific basis, but

Neha Madhiwalla, *Protocols and Set-Ups* In: *Childbirth in South Asia*. Edited by: Clémence Jullien and Roger Jeffery, Oxford University Press. © Oxford University Press 2021. DOI: 10.1093/oso/9780190130718.003.0009 intertwined with the logic of fee-for-service private practice (Ecks 2010). Although similar market conditions are not obtained in peripheral areas, professionals across geographies mimic these trends, transplanting often unnecessary and unviable technologies and specialist domains (Zachariah et al. 2010).

Embedded in this larger milieu of poorly regulated, non-standardized, and marketized medicine are premier government colleges, which retain the reputation of practising 'scientific' medicine. Insulated by state sponsorship from the pressure of the market and relatively better resourced, thanks to their political importance, they represent the best available context for practising and teaching scientific medicine to new recruits. As the social and political imperative to democratize higher education makes its effect felt on these institutions, they are increasingly admitting more diverse students. Caste-based reservation and centralized admissions based on common entrance tests are being more effectively implemented. These entrants, who are often both socially disadvantaged and have rural or semi-urban origins, are popularly referred to as students from the 'periphery'. Arguably, these professionals, with their superior training and professional experience are well placed to improve the standards of practice and contributing evidence to make medicine more relevant to rural populations. In this chapter, I explore the role of non-metropolitan obstetrics and gynaecology graduates of two premier government medical colleges in Mumbai as agents in knowledge production in the periphery.

Conceptualizing Democratization of Professional Knowledge Production

Historically, socially disadvantaged groups have been greatly underrepresented in the medical profession. Among the enumerated practising allopathic doctors across India in the 2001 census, only 7.5% belonged to the scheduled castes and 1.5% belonged to the scheduled tribes. This was significantly lower than their representation in the total population (16.2% and 8.2% respectively).[1] These professionals were largely practising in the rural areas. While, overall, 39% of allopathic practitioners were located in rural areas, this figure was 59.4% for scheduled caste doctors and 55.2% for scheduled tribe doctors. Relatively little change was noted in the All India Survey of Higher Education conducted in 2017–18. Among the students enrolled for MBBS, the basic degree for allopathic medicine, 9.3% of the students belonged the scheduled caste and 3.7% to the scheduled tribes. However, once admitted there was relatively little difference in the likelihood of their progressing to a postgraduate degree as compared to others.[2] These overall statistics obscure regional and sectoral differences: the representation of so-cially disadvantaged students in the socially developed states and in government institutions is higher.

Current admission data submitted by the largest government medical college in Mumbai to the Medical Council of India reveal how far diversity among the student body has increased. Standardized data are available on course of admission, category as per the caste-based reservation policy, and the state or central quota under which admitted. As Indian first names tend to be gender-specific and last names religion-specific, it was possible to clas-sify the students by sex and religion with almost 100% certainty.

Between 2011 and 2017, this college admitted a total of 256 students (on average 37 per year) in the postgraduate diploma and degree courses for ob-stetrics and gynaecology. Of these 37 students, on average, 14 students were admitted in a reserved category. Although the relative proportion varied year by year, of the total reserved category students, 34 belonged to other back-ward castes, 35 were scheduled caste students, and 30 belonged to scheduled and nomadic tribes. The presence of religious minorities was very small. In the tabulated data for 256 students, there were 4 Christian names and 12 Muslim names.

On average, 14 students were admitted in the national quota and the re-maining 23 in the state quota each year (excluding 2017 for which data is not available). In-state students were more likely to belong to a reserved category (48%) as compared to out-of-state students (24%). Given obstetrics' reputa-tion as a female speciality, not surprisingly, women outnumbered men sig-nificantly: 223 women and 33 men were admitted during the whole period. However, the male students were more likely to belong to a reserved category (64%) than the female students (35%).

This premier medical college presents an interesting picture of the extent to which high-quality medical education has become accessible for disad-vantaged students. More disadvantaged male in-state students, usually from smaller towns and cities, appear to be gaining entry. However, student admissions through the national quota, intended to benefit students from underdeveloped regions, appeared to be favouring students who were not so-cially disadvantaged.

It must also be noted that the inferences drawn here are constrained by the use of statutory reservation categories, which capture only certain dimensions of disadvantage. These categories obscure the personal histories of students, which could have revealed a more complex social reality. Also, the non-metropolitan origin of the students is not apparent from this data.

Medicine is a discipline that is unique in its reliance on unstructured individualized training. Both during the process of training and in active practice, peer learning, mentoring, and apprenticeship play an important part in professional development, these interactions often shaping the 'hidden curriculum' of medical training (Haidet and Stein 2006; Wear 1998). In contravention of stated rules or routinized decision-making, students clamour to be placed under particular unit heads for clinical training or vie for the attention of specific faculty by offering gratis services. It is not unusual for professionals to describe themselves in terms of the mentors that they 'trained under' or 'worked with', rather than citing their qualifications. Obituaries of renowned doctors are replete with names of mentors and protegés and reminiscences of personal encounters (Pandya 2017, Singh 2012). Outside academic institutions, while some of these processes have been formalized into certified courses, fellowship or observer-ship programmes, an informal exchange still has high legitimacy. The concept of 'communities of practice' (Egan and Jaye 2009), widely used in healthcare settings gives evidence of the strong sense of cohesion and affiliation among team members. Relationships built during training and at work play an important part in the professional development of doctors (Supe 2008). As informal exchanges that transcend or are transacted beyond the reach of organizational norms, these rest on the cultural apparatus of the profession built on 'trust', kinship or prior acquaintance, common training institutions, references from other 'trusted' acquaintances, and collaborations among socially familiar professionals. These knowledge transfer processes achieve a certain stable, self-perpetuating character, coalescing into distinctive subcultures of practice. Inevitably, cultural affinities based on similarity in caste and/or class origin play an important part in the shaping of these subcultures.

Commentaries dating from the post-independence pre-globalization period, when allopathic medicine was establishing itself in India, highlight the role of the socially privileged backgrounds of its members in its ability to retain its influence through the capture of metropolitan medical institutions, despite its alienation from rural realities and contestation by other systems of medicine that the state also appeared ready to patronize (Jeffery 1977) It was also argued that allopathic medicine was tacitly the favoured system of medicine and was destined to rise in dominance because of its wider social base and a relationship of complementary dependence and complicity with the state (Frankenberg 1981). With India's integration into the global market, the state has diminished in importance as an employer or patron of western medicine practitioners and their institutions. The key concern has shifted to the inadequacies and distortions in medical practice introduced by unregulated marketization (Zachariah et al. 2010). The relationship between the profession and the state remains ambivalent, with a contest between the demand for self-regulation and the state's inclination to impose external control (Mazumdar 2015). With the disengagement between the state and medical profession, government medical colleges face complex problems. On the one hand, they are losing resources such as faculty to private medical colleges (Narayana 2003). On the other hand, they are no longer politically influential enough to resist attempts to curb their autonomy. The establishment of health sciences universities and the compulsory affiliation of government medical colleges to them is a case in point. Underlying this institutional struggle is a social conflict between the upper-caste dominated professional institutions and the middle- or backward-caste dominated bodies of elected representatives. An article documenting the establishment of the Maharashtra University of Health Sciences (MUHS) cites the bypassing of Pune and Mumbai in favour of Nashik as the location of the MUHS as a deliberate move to prevent 'upper-caste academics' from exerting their influence on it. Power is vested with the middle- and backward-caste dominated political parties (Ashtekar 2001).

The changed student profile in premier government medical colleges is a consequence of the explicit policy to centralize admissions to all medical colleges via a common entrance test and more rigorous implementation of reservation policy, both being driven by the interests of the political elite. However, while democratization has visibly been achieved in admission of greater numbers of socially disadvantaged students, the challenge of facilitating their assimilation into the historically upper-caste, metropolitan subculture of professional education remains. While not studied specifically in medical colleges, insights can be gained from research in similarly placed elite institutions, the Indian Institutes of Technology (IITs). While the traditional entrants of these institutions achieve a certain 'castelessness', with their specific caste identities subsumed under a new neutral identity of meritorious students, exemplified by the rank in the entrance examination, socially disadvantaged students are more deeply marked by their caste status, overwhelming all their other identities (Subramanian 2015). Abjuring pointed inquiries about their caste identity, socially disadvantaged students continued to be marked out by oblique inquiries about the parents' occupational background or simply family size (Deshpande and Newman 2007). As participants in knowledge production, the challenge for new entrants, on the other hand, is navigating through gendered and caste-determined workplaces and learning spaces that are reified as sanctums of merit. They must acquire and deploy cultural resources that would enable them to make a credible claim to professional identity, beyond the acquisition of formal educational qualifications.

Thus, in this chapter, I explore the cultural resources that non-metropolitan students of obstetrics are invested with, their efforts to acquire such capital, and the influence of the training experience in shaping their professional identity. As trained professionals, location and positions in institutional and disciplinary hierarchies have a particular importance for knowledge production. Predictably, involvement in teaching, training, and research establishes a more direct and agential role. Given the empirical nature of medical knowledge, being located in sites that offer greater volumes and diversity in medical practice, as also those that offer greater opportunity to use complex skills within teams, consolidates one's role in knowledge production. Thus, I also explore the organizational arrangements within which they practise their role in teaching, training, and research, and the implications of their practice for public health.

The Study: Participants, Methods, and Contexts

This chapter has emerged from a doctoral study on the context, process, and outcomes of democratization of postgraduate medical education in two premier government medical colleges in Mumbai. This qualitative study focused on two clinical specialties: obstetrics and gynaecology, and general surgery. It primarily used interviews with faculty, key informants, and alumni of these colleges who had taught or trained between 1985 and 2015, supplemented by ethnographic observation. This period just precedes and spans across the implementation of successive policies aimed at democratizing medical education.

I use the term 'non-metropolitan' students to connote these students who belonged to social groups that did not have a history of higher education and/or a visible presence in the medical profession. This did not coincide with official reservation categories, though there was a considerable overlap. While reservation covers those groups whose disadvantages have deep structural origins, the definition of 'non-metropolitan' students includes many categories who were disadvantaged in the *particular* context of specialist education, which is a highly exclusive field.

Participants were identified and contacted using a snowball method. To capture the experience of democratization, my purposive sample selection was skewed towards alumni who were considered less advantaged by their faculty or peers in that particular batch or period. Each interviewed participant was asked to share contact details of batchmates, seniors, and juniors. After obtaining as exhaustive a list as possible, I identified regions with a concentration of participants for fieldwork. During fieldwork, I obtained more names and contact details of alumni practising in that geographical area. In smaller centres, practitioners knew almost all the alumni from their alma mater across generations. This enabled me to achieve a more representative sample.

Fieldwork was conducted in four regions; metropolitan Mumbai; Thane, on its periphery, which is emerging as a metropolitan centre; Nasik/Dhule, a relatively underdeveloped, tribal predominant region; and Kolhapur/Karad, a highly developed, largely agricultural region. Fifty participants were interviewed, which included 36 alumni who graduated between 1985 and 2015, 6 alumni who were also presently faculty members, 5 retired and senior faculty members and 3 key informants. Of these, 33 alumni and 4 faculty members were obstetricians.

Semi-structured interviews with the participants explored their perceptions and experiences of interacting with their peers, clinical training, teacher–student relationships, the organizational environment and ethos, and the effect of policies and rules regarding admission and assessment. Their interviews also explored the milieu surrounding their decision and success in gaining admission and their professional life after graduation.

Participants were asked questions about their family background, the context in which they made the decision to pursue medicine and, later, their particular specialization, their experience of training, the outcomes of that training, their professional history, their career plans, and their perspective of the trends in the practice within their specialization. This information was supplemented by ethnographic observation in their clinics/hospitals/institutes as well as the local context of healthcare.

In conformity with general professional etiquette, the initial conversation took place in English. However, a sizeable number of participants could not express themselves freely in English. If I found this to be the case, I switched to Marathi, offering the participant an opportunity to do so as well. As a result, several interviews were conducted in Marathi and some in both English and Marathi. All the participants readily agreed to audio-taping of the interview.

Cultural Preparation for a Career in Medicine

While the official data reveals the caste diversity of contemporary students, during the interviews there was a great deal of sensitivity around mentioning one's own or other students' caste. The more acceptable and widely articulated distinction was between metropolitan and 'peripheral' students. The term 'periphery' was used repeatedly by the participants to denote their origin in district or sub-district towns, as opposed to the metropolitan city of Mumbai.

The overwhelming presence of students from non-metropolitan locations was acknowledged and described in great detail. Most participants could enumerate the hometowns of all their batchmates. While stating that their peers were drawn from all over the state and beyond, younger alumni did not find this situation remarkable.

The sudden cultural break from the homogenously metropolitan composition of the college was more palpable in the interviews of the faculty, who had emphatic, if differing, views on the common entrance test and the consequent entry of non-Mumbai students into the colleges. They drew a contrast between an era when 'Mumbai students', implicitly middle-class, had dominated the college, and the present era where mostly 'outside' students populated the college.

Participants estimated that only about one-quarter of the students had origins in Mumbai. There were two distinct groups among the non-metropolitan students. There was a relatively elite group, which had the material and cultural resources to transition to a metropolitan medical education. These students had parents who had made a similar journey from small towns or rural locations to a regional centre for professional education. Their biographies revealed the strategic allocation of family resources to enable the aspirant to fulfil their career goals. The first step was invariably movement to a regional centre, which provided an urban ethos and, complementarily, quality schooling facilities: 'Originally, we are from a farmer caste. But my family has a "doctor background". Both my parents are MBBS doctors and, earlier, they were practicing in (a small sub-district town in Western Maharashtra). After school, my mother and I moved to Nashik for my studies. My father moved after his retirement' (Pratham, Ob/Gyn specialist, male, 30–35 years, practising in Nashik).

Central to their journey was enrolment in coaching classes that offered specific tutoring to enable them to 'crack' the competitive exam. Even for those whose parents were themselves doctors, coaching classes were seen as a necessity to succeed in the competitive exams, which required a different kind of preparation as compared to the school-leaving examination. Success in the latter did not necessarily predict success in the former. Rather than approaching basic sciences as a knowledge system, coaching classes specifically prepared students to answer discrete multiple-choice questions through endless mock tests based on a repository of questions and answers that they had compiled from previous examinations. More than mastery of the subject, the successful candidate was one who could predict the right answers and could make judicious decisions about what to attempt and leave out. Coaching classes helped to prepare the mindset of students who 'lived for the test' (Ørberg 2018). In this context, where students did not necessarily have medical professionals in their social circles, coaching classes also inducted them into a subculture of 'toppers', who became their role models: 'So, whenever all the toppers return home during the holidays, they (coaching classes) generally have some felicitation programmes or something like that. So, they gather all the toppers and then they organise interviews with them for the students. And then the entire year, it's like "you should be like him, you should be like him!"' (Varun, ENT specialist, male, 25–30 years, practising in Kolhapur).

The motivations and strategies of this group were stated in relatively more pragmatic and dispassionate terms, emphasizing the need to secure the best option available within a highly competitive system. The relative valuation of institutions was based on internet searches, reviews, and so on, combined with their understanding of the utility of training in their future professional life. This group also evinced a confidence to navigate through the cultural chasms that the selection of desirable institutions outside their region would entail. Although their English did not necessarily conform to standard grammar rules, this group, which had access to private schooling, spoke with confidence in that language:

According, to my search, the Pondicherry place had a lot of cases to do, lots of hands-on work. So, inspite [of living] in Maharashtra, I preferred to go to Pondicherry and stay there for two years, rather than option of a private hospital in Pune. According to me, [obstetrics and gynaecology] is a very practical field and you should have good practical knowledge.

Atul, Ob/Gyn specialist, male, 30–35 years,

practising in Nashik

For the other group of non-metropolitan students, aspirations were not matched by family resources, either financial or cultural. Although this group consisted predominantly of students admitted under the reservation policy, it also included a few students admitted in the 'open' category. For these students, there was an uncertainty even about the wisdom of pursuing a medical career and a continuous preoccupation with finding resources to meet their needs. Although they, too, described themselves as 'middle-class', this referred more to a certain cultural orientation, rather than actual material conditions. They described themselves as simply 'clever' (*hushar*), reflecting the muted appreciation that their academic achievements received at home: 'In my Pune college, there were a lot of us like this. We had very 'middle class' backgrounds—things are difficult at home (*gharchyanchi saglaynchi bombabomb*), but because the boy is clever, send him for medicine' (Sujit, Ob/gyn specialist, 25–30 years, practising in sub-district town near Dhule; translated from Marathi).

Despite having entry to the most elite institutions, through reservation, at the undergraduate stage, none of them had chosen a Mumbai college. They were both financially unequipped and socially unprepared to face life in a metropolitan college. In their social network, they could not rely on relatives or acquaintances who had established themselves in Mumbai. They either had no such contacts or, if existing, they were unable to provide support: 'After the MBBS entrance test, I was getting [admission in] Mumbai. I was also getting admission in Pune and in my hometown. I felt that I have spent enough years in my hometown and Mumbai felt very "high-funda" [too alien and modern], so I chose Pune' (Dayanand, Ob/gyn specialist, 25–30 years, practising in suburban periphery of Pune; translated from Marathi).

Unlike their predecessors, for recent alumni, their ability and success in obtaining a good rank in the entrance examination was the key determining factor for choosing a career in medicine. Their preoccupation with navigating through the admission process overwhelmed all other concerns. Objective entrance tests do not evaluate the higher-level cognitive skills required for disciplinary study but reward the ability to memorize facts. One study found that marks obtained in the school-leaving examinations for science subjects, which required more subjective responses and a holistic understanding of interrelated topics, was a better predictor of success in the first year MBBS than the rank obtained in the entrance test (Parate et al. 2016). On the other hand, as the entrance tests did not require writing skills and evaluated only the fragmented knowledge of facts, these were easier to 'crack' for socially disadvantaged students who had had an indifferent school education, where

English language teaching and science teaching may not have been adequate. However, multiple-choice question tests, the format of the entrance test, and all successive examinations during medical training inherently undervalue other learning skills such as reading ability, concept-building, and 'soft skills' such as communication skills, motivation, and empathy (Huda 2001). These are also skills that are integral to research. Thus, the students from the periphery entered training with the perception of medicine as a body of discrete facts, rather than a knowledge system. Not much change took place in their understanding of the nature of medical knowledge through their training. As there was relatively little effort to enhance their higher-level cognitive and non-cognitive skills, it is understandable that they did not develop an affinity for research or a curiosity about medicine beyond the requirements of the examinations.

The Development of a Professional Identity

The description of medical training by contemporary non-metropolitan students, ranging across the undergraduate and postgraduate phases was notably impersonal. Participants talked at length about the structure of the courses, the various exams that they had appeared for, and the procedures involved in admission and assessment. However, they made virtually no mention of significant relationships with faculty or moments in training experiences that had a lasting impact on their understanding or approach to their discipline. Instead, they described an experience wherein there was an almost bureaucratic adherence to norms and rules unmodified by informality. This was in distinct contrast to older metropolitan participants, who described a very similar formal training process, but a very different 'hidden curriculum' built on an informal exchange with teachers wherein the latter communicated values, instilled a certain work ethic, and inducted students into an approach to acquiring medical knowledge. The importance of student–teacher relationships in shaping professional values and identity has been studied extensively (Hafferty and Franks 1994; Haidet and Stein 2006), shaping future physicians' perspectives on patient care, and by extension, their approach to medical knowledge. Arguably, the homogeneity in class and caste background of the faculty and students had facilitated this exchange prior to the democratization phase. However, these exchanges were not sustained, and the colleges had not evolved peer mentoring and support systems to address distress among medical students, as exist in many other countries (Dyrbye et al. 2005). It is not that the faculty did not perceive or informally address these problems. However, even the concerned faculty members could not identify measures beyond being personally accessible. As a result, these students often felt that their personal/social problems, which could also include experiences of discrimination, had no legitimacy and that the institution had no responsibility for their well-being:

> We don't really ask them questions in depth about their background and all that. [Their] family background is revealed only if they have some issue or we are required to contact their parents for something. Sometimes, actually parents have come to us because student is finding it very stressful. At least we should know what they do. I may not be able to take them [residents] home every week for a dinner. But, at least once in a while I should take them out, and somehow that is missing.
>
> Meenakshi, Ob/gyn specialist, 50–55 years,
> faculty in Mumbai medical college

More in evidence was the formation of peer relationships among similarly located students. The convergence of similarly disadvantaged students in the medical college provided them a peer group that helped them to nuance their plans and goals, even while it emphasized the unsuitability of their home and family environments for nurturing their professional ambitions. Consistently, disadvantaged students described a certain solidarity and collaboration among students who shared similar life-contexts, despite the fact that they were competing for the same seats. This 'homophilic' behaviour has also been observed in culturally diverse medical schools (Vaughan et al. 2015). Although they were not required to, they chose to locate themselves in the metropolis during preparation for the entrance examination at great financial cost and physical hardship:

> But it is important to stay in the city with friends while preparing for the entrance tests. There is discussion . . . You tell them what you have read, they tell you what they have read. And then you compare what you have written in the mock tests, check where you have gone wrong. When there is discussion, you remember better than if you have just read.
>
> Parag, Ob/gyn specialist, 25–30 years,
> practising in Dhule; translated from Marathi.

The blurring of medical residents' identity as trainees under the burden of the human resource needs of the hospital—a known educational dilemma— was also in evidence here (McDougall 2008; Sadeghi et al. 2014). Given their high dependence on inexperienced trainees, and challenged by inadequate institutional support, the senior staff of the hospital, including the unit heads, were preoccupied with organizing the medical work so as to prevent lapses, focused on safeguarding women's safety (Madhiwalla et al. 2018). This translated into a certain 'regulatory' approach to their interactions with the residents:

> The professors' role is, actually . . . the only things that helped the students in [premier medical college] is their strictness and discipline. That you did one LSCS, the paper has to be very relevant with that indication, you cannot say that there was only foetal distress, no it is not. So, whenever I say there is a foetal distress, we have to justify it. Our paper [case notes] will go according to that, there is no manipulation in that. So, I have never done manipulation, so that their strictness or just their presence will help us to be a protocolic [*sic*] and honest doctor in practice.
>
> Surekha, Ob/gyn specialist, 30–35 years,
> practising in Karad

Although the participants recalled the hardships associated with residency, they accorded great value to that experience in the formation of their professional selves. They appreciated postgraduate training for being focused on 'practical things' as opposed to their largely theoretical undergraduate training. For those who had earlier trained in peripheral and less organized district-level institutions, the contrast in work culture was also very apparent. They often contrasted the more structured and disciplined working environment at the metropolitan medical college to the lackadaisical approach to work in their previous training institutions:

> I was a rough gynaecologist through my earlier training. But whatever the protocols, whatever the operative skills, whatever the patient behaviour skills and approach and management of each and every patient in gynaec and obstetrics, and new operative techniques, laparoscopy, then rare operations, like Sling surgeries, non-descent vaginal, everything I got in college A. So, I became much more refined, my skills became more refined.
>
> Parag, Ob/gyn specialist, 25–30 years,
> practising in Dhule; translated from Marathi

With very long working hours and provision of very basic facilities for accommodation and food, existence in this phase had a certain spare quality. As there was neither time nor opportunity to socialize or even leave the hospital or college premises, descriptions of life offered by different participants had a certain homogeneity that effaced social differences. The emphasis on 'work', which required cooperation and efficiency, created a different conceptualization of 'merit' than one based on academic performance and rank in examinations. The corporeal nature of medical work upturned caste-based hierarchies, and foregrounded characteristics like manual skills, stamina, and physical labour, which are not the preserve of the upper castes:

> I was not appreciated for being from some particular community, I was not appreciated because I come from open category, I was appreciated because I was working hard, I was . . . (I would be admonished when I had made a mistake) and my boss used to pamper me when he used to see (how hard he has worked all night. That's the good thing about Mumbai. The one who stands up, who does work), he is accepted in Mumbai.
>
> Sujit, Ob/gyn specialist, 25–30 years, practising in
sub-district town near Dhule; phrases in
parentheses translated from Marathi.

While Dalit or tribal participants were not as unequivocal in their affirmation of this work culture, they too agreed that discriminatory attitudes among senior faculty, which they had encountered in regional colleges, were not in evidence in Mumbai. Among these participants, too, there was an acknowledgement that 'good workers' were generally appreciated.

Interestingly, although they focused so consistently on protocols, none of the participants made any reference to national or international guidelines as a part of their training process. The key training document was an internally produced manual, which each resident was given at the time of induction. If there was a process of translating evidence-based treatment guidelines into hospital-specific protocols, this was not apparent to the residents. They credited the ownership of the protocols to the hospital or medical college. It did not appear unusual to the participants that there was no reference point external to the college or the hospital for the material and methods used for their training. This also implied that there was no focus on training students to evaluate evidence scientifically. Although a research project is a mandatory component of the training, none of the interviewed participants attached any particular importance to it. Specifically, for non-metropolitan students who had difficulty with written English, the dissertation posed a challenge. However, one participant mentioned the presence of an organized system whereby dissertations could be completed with external help from typists who produced the dissertation on the basis of the material and data provided by the client. An older metropolitan participant, who had received training at a London-based institution after her residency, remarked on the priority given to research and evaluation there, which was in stark contrast to her previous experience:

> [With our registrar and senior registrar, we had] a purely academic discussion on how to analyze a published study in terms of credibility; looking at the kind of data that it was using . . . In 3 years [of obstetric residency training in Mumbai], nobody spoke to us about the value of the randomized double blind study over something else. In fact, clinical audit is something I learnt about for the first time [in London]. Although we used to have the mortality review here [in Mumbai] but you know in spite of them saying it's more about the patient and not about the clinician . . . they ended up just being about blaming.
>
> Malini, Ob/gyn specialist, 45–50 years,
> practising in Mumbai

The participants' framing of the outcomes of postgraduate training as a portable resource of operative skills and protocols is significant. They did not evince recognition of the fact that the practice that they had been immersed in was very context-specific, located in a metropolitan tertiary care government centre. In fact, when specifically asked about the relevance of their protocols in non-metropolitan contexts, they reaffirmed their universality. Given the mode in which these protocols had been transmitted—didactically, through a regulatory process—it is not surprising that the participants also described these as immutable.

The Organizational Arrangements for Practice

To complement their use of the term 'protocol' to signify the core of their approach to medical practice, they used the term 'set-up' to describe the organizational arrangements within which they practised. While 'protocols' were endowed with immutable value and a universal character, 'set-ups', as the word suggests, had a transient, neutral nature. They were fluid and dynamic, accommodating local imperatives, sheathing the specialist's practice, not fundamentally determining it. Participants spoke variously of private, government, corporate set-ups as well as 'own' versus 'other' set-ups, without according any intrinsic value to any or assuming any intrinsic hierarchy among them.

Younger non-metropolitan participants had made notably many more transitions in set-ups than older participants. Given that they were still in the initial phase of their careers, it was certain that they would make many more changes. Many participants expressly stated that their plans were yet to materialize.

Only two of the non-metropolitan participants had parents who were medical practitioners. Of these, one had parents who had been family physicians in a sub-district town. The other had a mother who was herself an established obstetrician in a sub-district town. The remaining participants had had to evolve their specific plans to establish practice.

There was a clear gender-specific trend in the choice of set-ups and their locations. Significantly more young women participants with non-metropolitan origins had relocated to Mumbai and Thane. They did not describe any premeditated plan to remain in the city, but had come to do so to align their plans with their spouses. Interestingly, among the older participants who had made the reverse journey, from their original metropolitan location to the 'periphery', all were women who had moved to the present location after marriage.

The primacy of women's reproductive goals was very apparent in their narratives as well as those of their male counterparts. In comparison to the men, more women were in government service. However, they did not explain this choice in terms of the desirability of the work or setting, but rather its compatibility with their personal lives and parental responsibilities. Fixed working hours and the possibility of availing paid leave made managing childcare easier and, therefore, government jobs more desirable. For the same reasons, women were considered ineligible for establishing their own practice. The inability of women doctors to contest patriarchal expectations of reproductive work has been documented in Pakistan, where some women were forced out of practice altogether (Arif 2011; Masood 2017). This, by default, would entail long working hours and attending to emergencies during the night. One participant described how women obstetricians need male support to 'rescue' them in case of night-time emergencies. While not abandoning practice, it was evident that women participants' labour had been co-opted for the fulfilment of the family's entrepreneurial plans in a modified form of a patriarchal division of labour. Only one female participant articulated a clear independent plan for establishing her practice, while another mentioned that the couple had jointly taken a decision to relocate.

The absence of overt professional ambition among the women participants also mirrored the perception of obstetrics as a rather static sub-speciality, less permeable to technologization and surgical innovation. The women participants more distinctly viewed themselves as obstetricians, unlike their male counterparts, who perceived themselves as primarily gynaecologists. This is ironic in view of the fact that for all the participants, excepting one who was employed in an infertility centre, obstetrics formed the bulk of their workload.

While the male participants were not constrained by reproductive work and had clearly more ambition and distinct plans for career development, among them too, a re-engagement with family affairs was in evidence. Two of the participants cited the reluctance of parents to relocate as their reason for their return to their hometowns. For the most disadvantaged, there was immense pressure to earn incomes in keeping with their qualifications, which was not easily accomplished:

> Family members do not understand the struggle we go through. They are in a fantasy that their son is going to be a doctor. It was financially a little difficult, but now I am stable. But still, my family regrets, 'why did we make him a doctor? If we had made him an engineer, he would have earned so much by now'.
>
> Dayanand, Ob/gyn specialist, 25–30 years,
> practising in suburban periphery of Pune;
> translated from Marathi

Interestingly, as the participants exited the sequestered domain of the government medical college, there was a re-emergence of a consciousness and articulation of social identities that had appeared to be erased during the training experience. The option of remaining at the medical college after graduation offered the easiest survival strategy for the students with the least resources. Many of the interviewed students had spent 6 months to 2 years working as ad hoc assistants after residency. However, for their long-term plans, outside the college, they were conscious of a certain cultural incompatibility—a lack of fluency in English and a discomfort with the 'suit and tie' culture, which were associated with metropolitan private practice. While not impossible, there was a consciousness that there was an additional process of acculturation associated with settling in practice in Mumbai:

> I was Convent educated so I didn't feel that thing, but most (non-metropolitan students) have Marathi schooling background and all that so they feel a bit awkward while getting into it [Mumbai-based practice]. But there are many even from the Marathawada belt, many of the guys are settled in Bombay. Gradually they develop the confidence, gradually they get mixed up with the people of Bombay, so it depends how you mould in the group or how you want to get moulded in the group.
>
> Atul, Ob/Gyn specialist, male, 30–35 years,
practising in Nashik

For the majority of the male participants, the long-term plan was to return to their hometowns or similar locations to practice. The most predominant long-term goal was the establishment of their independent hospital. However, without the support of parents and an existing family practice, the journey to establishing their own institution was complex. Formal credit in terms of bank loans was readily available, enabling them to procure the capital required for purchasing land, building, and equipment. However, availing a large loan in the initial phase of their career determined the course of their work-life for a significantly long period: 'For a doctor who comes from a "middle-class" family, there is a certain "life cycle". He comes back [to his hometown], starts work [in a larger set-up], settles down, buys land, constructs a hospital and by the time he repays his loans, half his life is over' (Sujit, Ob/gyn specialist, 25–30 years, practising in sub-district town near Dhule; translated from Marathi).

Apart from the challenges of arranging the resources required, they felt challenged by a rural medical market that was, at once, both underdeveloped and highly competitive. Firstly, they are pushed into a small enclave by the fact that most rural patients prefer free government services. Apart from their unwillingness to pay for services, rural patients were seen as undesirable because of their medical illiteracy and their demands for illegal services, such as sex determination and late abortions. There is a strong pressure to succumb to malpractice and illegal activities. They relied on the solidarity among batchmates—often settled in different towns to resist the pressure.

Interestingly, in one of the sites where I conducted my fieldwork, an obstetrician who was also an alumnus of one of the two selected colleges had been indicted for conducting sex determination tests. While many peers shared contact details, uncharacteristically, none of them offered to introduce me and pointedly avoided any discussion about that alumnus. My independent attempts to reach this potential participant were also fruitless:

> Latur, Beed, Osmanabad, Chandrapur, people generally avoid settling there. Very difficult to survive over there. Out there, people don't value what you are doing. They conduct deliveries at home. Sex determination is . . . When I came here, it was so much, meaning so much! In the interim, the rules have become a little stricter. Before that, 3–4 years ago, I used to get patients from Aurangabad even [asking for sex determination]. I have never done it. Our 'motto' was clear. All our batchmates were so good that nobody practiced SD, second trimester MTPs. There are a couple of people . . . you will find those anywhere.
>
> Akshay, Ob/gyn specialist, 30–35 years,
> practising in Dhule

Their struggle to maintain a modicum of professional practice in the face of these problems posed by patients is further aggravated by the presence of existing practitioners from both modern medicine and the indigenous systems of medicine (called 'established brands' by one participant) who provide intense competition. In this undifferentiated market, their credentials as alumni of a premier medical college were not perceived as offering any value-addition. Although they were actively acquiring affiliations, they were not completely certain about the degree to which these would benefit their practice.

The participants with the least social advantage and constrained family resources affiliated themselves to different set-ups simultaneously in order to build their professional network and client-base. Surekha was simultaneously attached to a government community health centre (secondary-level hospital) as an empanelled consultant, a private medical college as a lecturer, and in a family-run nursing home that she co-owned with her husband. A male obstetrician was engaged as a full-time lecturer in a government hospital, handled complex obstetric cases in a family-run nursing home managed by his wife, and conducted laparoscopic surgery on patients admitted at other private hospitals as a freelance consultant:

> I know that the patient class that is coming here [to the government hospital] is actually coming because it is free. They are not too much 'affording'

and, basically, they are not worried about their problem. They are not conscious about their pregnancy so this patient will not turn up in my private
[hospital], that much I know. But the only thing [reason] I come [is] that
people will start knowing me.

Surekha, Ob/gyn specialist, 30–35 years,
practising in Karad

The female participants did not express any discomfort with their current
profile of practice, which was usually a combination of obstetric care, clinic-
based gynaecology, and open surgery. In contrast, male participants em-
phatically mentioned a long-term plan to exit obstetric practice. They made
investments in expensive laparoscopy equipment and underwent training
in in vitro fertilization. This was an attempt to differentiate themselves from
female specialists, who were the preferred providers for delivery care, and
from other non-specialist providers who competed for 'medical cases'. 'For
delivery per se, they will choose a female doctor, like here in Nasik, I don't
know about Bombay but the trend here is like for surgeries if she has to undergo hysterectomy or any major surgeries, she will prefer a male gynaecologist' (Pratham, Ob/Gyn specialist, male, 30–35 years, practising in Nashik).
However, when viewed against the volume of their practice and the profile
of their clientele, it was not clear how these strategies could be financially
viable. Complementarily, these arrangements created an inbuilt incentive to
overuse these facilities.

Involvement in Teaching, Training, and Research

The conceptualization of their workplaces as 'set-ups' was complemented
by a marked disinterest and lack of involvement in activities beyond clinical practice, which require a more stable organizational framework. While
two of the participants were formally employed as lecturers in one government and private medical college each, the other participants did not report
any involvement in teaching. Even for these two participants, affiliation to
the medical college was not their primary identity or focus. They found the
teaching environments, which they specifically described as belonging to the
'periphery', highly unsatisfactory. With significant involvement in private
clinical practice, they also did not visualize themselves as primarily teachers,
as their own teachers did. Unlike the latter, who had exerted considerable

oversight, the imperative on the participants to direct their students' practice was markedly lax:

> Teaching private students are . . . actually they know since the beginning that anyways they have paid so they are going to pass and again because of management pressure you cannot fail them, so actually they are not too much study oriented or they are not too much enthusiastic in learning but still if you guide them, they also want some guidance, if you guide them they are happy.
>
> Surekha, Ob/gyn specialist, 30–35 years,
> practising in Karad

They were also deterred by the inability to recreate the training environment that they had experienced during their residency. Being at relatively low levels in the hierarchy, they could only undertake individual actions to improve the learning environment:

> In [metropolitan medical college during his undergraduate training], there was a fixed schedule, and everybody used to come and stay and every teacher actively participates during each presentation and all. During lectures also students used to ask questions, but here the students are not interested in lectures and all. But I would keep doing, I used to read the topics through the books and I used to take clinics of the UG students, whether they are interested or not, I used to call them and tell whatever I learned. I used to teach my junior residents whenever I was on call during labour and [in] OPDs.
>
> Parag, Ob/gyn specialist, 25–30 years,
> practising in Dhule; translated from Marathi

Given the preponderance of participants in private solo practice, the opportunity for them to transfer skills was also limited by the absence of other professional providers in their set-ups. Typically, there would be just them and a team of unqualified staff, such as orderlies and nursing assistants. Some of the participants had spouses who practised alongside them. Only one participant worked in a multidisciplinary team in a government hospital with qualified nurses, who, however, were not supervised by medical staff in her absence. She described a scenario in which she was able to transfer skills on the job to nurses to establish best practices:

> [I have taught them] don't call every primie CPD [cephalopelvic disproportion]. Unless and until the head is up, don't call them CPD because primie is

the only thing where head is the best perimeter. So try to give them full trial with all safety measures. Even for meconium, I have started here amnio infusion. So now they are happy, that if you do amnio infusion the patient will deliver fast and LSCS [caesarean section] is avoided. So those who are interested, they will do that procedure. Those who are afraid, they will say, 'You come and you do, I cannot do this!'

Surekha, Ob/gyn specialist, 30–35 years,
practising in Karad

Notably, the only references to engagement in research and publication were made by those participants who had remained at the teaching hospital after their training. Typically, these referred to presentations made at a conference or joint publication of a paper with a senior faculty. However, these participants also noted that movement out of the teaching college had effectively ended such involvement. The non-metropolitan environment as well as the mental make-up of its practitioners were seen as being incompatible with research:

> It's not that you cannot do it. It's not even a matter of getting the time. But you need to have it inside you, that attitude [for research]. It's true that that environment [to nurture research] does not gets created here. But it's also that the 'boys' from here [non-metropolitan] don't have it inside them. The few who do, they do not stick around here, they run off to the cities. They are not made for this life.

Sujit, Ob/gyn specialist, 25–30 years,
practising in sub-district town near Dhule

Apart from formal research projects, none of the participants reported involvement in analysis of their patient data or writing case studies, which are widely accepted forms of evidence in medicine. Outside of the institutional context, where there is a strong emphasis on documentation and internal processes of audits, the participants admitted to deviations from the protocols that they had imbibed during the training. Given the immutability that they accorded to these, they were more prone to consider these as violations, rather than legitimate local adaptations:

> When there are multiple risk-factors, had I been at college A, my boss would have told me on the phone to try induction, not take her up for C-Section directly. In my private practice in a small town, I would not try it.

Even in Mumbai, in private sector, nobody tries induction. So, yes, in that sense, that is a violation of protocol.

Sujit, Ob/gyn specialist, 25–30 years,
practising in sub-district town near Dhule

Predictably, given their own negative view of the scientific validity of their practice, they were less likely to be motivated to share their experiences in the professional domain, where they would be subject to the scrutiny of peers. A metropolitan participant who was deeply involved in public health research and evidence-based medicine elaborated the process by which rural practitioners' knowledge is actually marginalized. He described the scenario in which some non-metropolitan centres gained renown informally as centres of excellence. However, these centres remained marginal to the formal process of the reproduction of knowledge through research and the development of national guidelines or protocols:

So, if I were to evaluate a rural practitioner, it would be, of course, by their work. Usually they are pretty well-known in their places and you know the volume that they do. While I acknowledge the volume, they are not able to convert that normally to a document or a publication or a presentation, and that is where they fall short. Even if they are doing great amount of work, we are not able to evaluate them objectively at the scientific level. And that is the missing skill in their work, so good work does not always translate into a protocol or something at the national level.

Paranjoy, public health expert, 45–50 years,
practising in Mumbai

Implications for Public Health Goals

Within the larger framework of maternal healthcare, obstetricians are expected to play an important role in providing comprehensive emergency obstetric care at tertiary and secondary care institutions. A study mapping obstetricians and their practice in Maharashtra has estimated that there were eight times as many professionals practising in the private sector as in the public sector. It is unclear how those engaged in dual practice were classified. Moreover, this study also documented that schemes to contract them to make their services available for providing emergency obstetric care in government hospitals or to poor beneficiaries had not been very successful due to institutional constraints and their focus on private practice (Randive et al. 2012). The alignment of their individual practice with public health goals was not a matter of reflection among these participants.

Within the for-profit, fee-for-service framework in which they were predominantly practising, there was an inbuilt imperative to steer away from women who were poor (described as non-affording) and, consequently, unsuitable as paying patients. Other studies have also documented that attempts to make privately employed obstetricians' services available for emergency obstetric care have not been fruitful. Commenting on the recent policy measures that incentivized women to deliver at government hospitals with conditional cash transfers, many providers noted that they had seen a decline in their practice. This also, in turn, increased the competition for 'affording' patients who patronized private hospitals. The emergence of corporate hospitals and corporatization of the private medical college hospitals had created additional competition for solo practitioners. In particular, in the more developed areas, such as Thane, Karad, and Kolhapur, there was frequent mention of saturation as a problem. In Thane, adjacent to Mumbai, particularly, all the providers could foresee the demise of independent practice alongside the ascendance of corporate hospitals.

Ironically, even though these were the most skilled providers of obstetric care, they also steered clear of women facing obstetric emergencies. Women with complex medical needs who could require resource-intensive care and have unpredictable outcomes posed a threat to their practice. Those who were affiliated with tertiary care facilities were able to attend to such women, albeit as remotely engaged consultants, rather than attending physicians:

> The type of practice and the priority of the investigation and, you know, everything has changed. Probably what patient I would operate [on] in college A, now I don't even keep in my nursing home . . . They [corporate hospital] admit her, they wake her up and they call me at the time of C-Section. They pay my operative charges.
>
> Aparna, Ob/gyn specialist, 40–45 years,
> practising in Kolhapur

For those participants whose set-ups precluded the possibility of treating such women, there was little choice but to refer them to distant referral centres, out of their ambit of influence, despite having the operative skills and experience. Without exception, all the participants had described in great detail their experiences of treating poor women with complex medical conditions during their residency training. Both the opportunity to acquire rare skills and their involvement in treating poor women had been described as a source of great satisfaction. However, their narratives of their present practice were overwhelmed by financial and legal considerations. Their attitude towards such women had changed as well, viewing them as threats, whereas they had earlier regarded them as 'exciting cases': 'Every 3–4 months, we have to refer one or two patients. Then we have to organise for an ambulance. One of our people has to accompany the woman and get her admitted [to a higher facility]. There is no monetary gain from such patients. Its pure social service [*samaj seva*]. But you have to do it' (Sujit, Ob/gyn specialist, 25–30 years, practising in sub-district town near Dhule).

As stated earlier, several participants had expressed a desire to exit obstetric practice altogether for elective, hi-tech sub-specialities, such as infertility treatment and laparoscopy. These were viewed as being less 'risky' and more profitable. Arguably, these strategies were likely to accentuate the disconnect between their individual practice and public health.

Discussion

The increasing diversity within elite metropolitan educational institutions, although mandated by public policy, has been actualized by the process of social change, particularly in rural and semi-urban India. Complementing expanding market opportunities were persisting disadvantages. The absence of social and economic networks and the imperative to sustain their families pushed the most socially disadvantaged participants into a corner. They could enter the government system and have to confront the hyper-consciousness of their caste status. Alternatively, they could enter the private sector, where within the market economy they would confront modernized forms of untouchability. Without social networks and family resources, they would be condemned to subordination within the professional sphere.

For participants belonging to the emerging rural elites, which had ready access to surplus capital, acquiring a specialist degree clearly was linked to consolidating their social status, 'updating' it to assimilate into a global professional culture, allowing them, so to speak, to 'dress up for the part' (Kaur and Sundar 2016).

For both groups, it was evident that they had acquired a cultural capital that enabled them to take financial and professional risks that would have been unimaginable to them earlier. Within the social contexts that they had emerged from, their qualifications, skills, and professional status, set them apart. Within the domain of market medicine, the ready availability of formal credit and their ability to navigate through local professional networks had driven them towards entrepreneurship, making it possible for them to visualize long-term futures.

However, the vestiges of the caste/gender frameworks were clearly visible. Women subordinated their careers to their spouse's plans, settling for roles that allowed them to accommodate their reproductive responsibilities, but which simultaneously also characterized them as inferior professionals. The most socially disadvantaged professionals struggled harder to establish themselves and survived through a longer period of subordinate, transient positions.

When decentred from their origins, the specificities of the social identity and history was lost in their non-metropolitanism. They confronted a new social hierarchy in which they were all relatively subordinated by their absence of a cultural history of higher education. A reluctant institution engaged with them enough to transform them into skilled and disciplined technicians, but not acculturating them to approach medicine as a knowledge system. Their conceptualization of their professional role remained limited and constrained, precluding any participation in research and academia.

Consequently, they also had no tools to analyse and engage with the challenges they faced in their practice in the periphery, beyond condemning it as substandard. Their diffidence about participation in research and a disdain for academics, as it existed in the periphery, further distanced them from meaningfully engaging with knowledge production. Their economic strategies, embedded in the logic of market medicine, inexorably draw them away from the very women who needed their attention. The dyad of 'protocols' and 'set-ups' consolidated their identity as skilled technicians, rather than professionals who could exercise autonomous control over empirical conditions.

The primary goal of these professionals was the establishment of a private solo practice, associated with the entrepreneur-professional model of bourgeois capitalism. But already, in the areas where corporate capital had made inroads, such as Thane, it was evident that this model was becoming unviable. Professionals there are acceding to co-option by corporate capital in various forms. Some are seeking attachment as consultants to corporate hospitals, marginalizing their own sole practice. Others are employed as faculty in private medical colleges, where they form the base for launching elective services such as infertility centres as a part of corporate chains. Without an ideological position on the various 'set-ups' that they did and could occupy, it is predictable that this co-option will be not resisted too strongly.

Conclusion

This chapter lies at the intersection of two discrete discourses: first, the application of science/medicine for the betterment of society, and second, the expansion of opportunity through the democratization of higher education. Implicit in the former is the production of locally relevant knowledge. Implicit in the latter is the promise of collective upliftment through the success of individual students/professionals. The metropolitan government medical college is the institutional embodiment of both these discourses. It is also the site where the fault lines emerge. The hesitation of medicine to interrogate its caste/class-specific ideological moorings disables its engagement with newer entrants, who do not fit into its particular subculture. Thus, even as it expounds an ethic that conflates its pursuit of knowledge with the fulfilment of social good, it stands revealed as sectarian and insular, unable to assimilate social change in its institutional processes.

On the other hand, the democratization of higher education, propelled as much by the imperatives of the market as by welfare politics, does not translate easily into its ultimate goal of social transformation. The individual strategies of these professionals, when viewed against the background of post-capitalist economy, foretells a certain kind of future. Excluded from engagement with medicine as a knowledge system and also its ideological goals, they lack the skills to engage with their local practice environments as professionals. They remain narrowly contained in the professional practice, adapting a hegemonic metropolitan framework to meet the exigencies of their individual contexts. In reproducing themselves as lesser professionals, they also reproduce their subordinate social status, exemplified by their description of their location as the 'periphery'.

Notes

1. Data compiled from Economic Tables, which reports persons by occupational categories by sex, scheduled castes, and scheduled tribes. Data on population representation drawn from Primary Census Abstract (Census of India 2001).

2. The ratio of postgraduate to graduate students for general, scheduled castes, and scheduled tribes categories were 0.2:1, 0.18:1, and 020:1 (Department of Higher Education 2018).

References

Arif, Seema. 2011. 'Broken Wings: Issues Faced by Female Doctors in Pakistan Regarding Career Development'. *International Journal of Academic Research in Business and Social Sciences* 1 (Special): 79–101.

Ashtekar, Shyam. 2001. 'Medical University: Failure and Opportunity'. *Economic and Political Weekly* 36 (22): 1951–2.

Bailey, Patsy, Anne Paxton, Samantha Lobis, and Deborah Fry. 2006. 'The Availability of Life-Saving Obstetric Services in Developing Countries: An In-Depth Look at the Signal Functions for Emergency Obstetric Care'. *International Journal of Gynecology & Obstetrics* 93 (3): 285–91.

Das, Jishnu, Alaka Holla, Veena Das, Manoj Mohanan, Diana Tabak, and Brian Chan. 2012. 'In Urban and Rural India, A Standardized Patient Study Showed Low Levels of Provider Training and Huge Quality Gaps'. *Health Affairs* 31 (12): 2774–84. doi: 10.1377/hlthaff.2011.1356.

Department of Higher Education, Ministry of Human Resource Development, Government of India. 2018. *8th Report on the All India Survey on Higher Education, 2017–18*. Ministry of Human Resource Development, New Delhi. Accessed 13 March 2021. http://aishe.nic.in/aishe/viewDocument.action;jsessionid=E823478 F3ECC0BCAD46B12A1C0FFF568.n1?documentId=245.

Deshpande, Ashwini, and Katherine Newman. 2007. 'Where the Path Leads: The Role of Caste in Post-university Employment Expectations'. *Economic and Political Weekly* 42 (41): 4133–40.

Dyrbye, Liselotte N., Matthew R. Thomas, and Tait D. Shanafelt. 2005. 'Medical Student Distress: Causes, Consequences, and Proposed Solutions'. *Mayo Clinic Proceedings* 80 (12): 1613–22. doi: 10.4065/80.12.1613.

Ecks, Stefan. 2010. 'Spectacles of Reason: An Ethnography of Calcutta Gastroenterologists'. In *Technologized Images, Technologized Bodies: Anthropological Approaches to a New Politics of Vision*, edited by Jeanette Edwards, Penelope Harvey, and Peter Wade, 117–36. Oxford: Berghahn.

Egan, Tony, and Chrystal Jaye. 2009. 'Communities of Clinical Practice: The Social Organization of Clinical Learning'. *Health* 13 (1): 107–25.

Frankenberg, Ronald. 1981. 'Allopathic Medicine, Profession, and Capitalist Ideology in India'. *Social Science & Medicine* 15 (2): 115–25.

Hafferty, Frederic W., and Ronald Franks. 1994. 'The Hidden Curriculum, Ethics Teaching, and the Structure of Medical Education'. *Academic Medicine* 69 (11): 861–71.

Haidet, Paul, and Howard F. Stein. 2006. 'The Role of the Student–Teacher Relationship in the Formation of Physicians'. *Journal of General Internal Medicine* 21 (1): 16–20. doi: 10.1111/j.1525-1497.2006.00304.x.

Huda, Nighat. 2001. 'Admission Procedure as Predictor of Performance in Medical Colleges'. *Journal of the Pakistan Medical Association* 51 (11): 380–381.

Jacob, Shevin T., Eoin West, T., and Patrick Banura. 2011. 'Fitting a Square Peg into a Round Hole: Are the Current Surviving Sepsis Campaign Guidelines Feasible for Africa?' *Critical Care* 15 (1): 117.

Jeffery, Roger. 1977. 'Allopathic Medicine in India: A Case of Deprofessionalization?' *Social Science & Medicine (1967)* 11 (10): 561–73.

Kaur, Ravinder, and Nandini Sundar. 2016. 'Snakes and Ladders: Rethinking Social Mobility in Post-reform India'. *Contemporary South Asia* 24 (3): 229–41. doi: 10.1080/09584935.2016.1203864.

Madhiwalla, Neha, Rakhi Ghoshal, Padmaja Mavani, and Nobhojit Roy. 2018. 'Identifying Disrespect and Abuse in Organisational Culture: A Study of Two Hospitals in Mumbai, India'. *Reproductive Health Matters* 26 (53): 36–47. doi: 10.1080/09688080.2018.1502021.

Masood, Ayesha. 2017. 'A Doctor in the House: Balancing Work and Care in the Life of Women Doctors in Pakistan', PhD, School of Human Evolution and Social Change, Arizona State University.

Mavalankar, Dileep V., and Allan Rosenfield. 2005. 'Maternal Mortality in Resource-Poor Settings: Policy Barriers to Care'. *American Journal of Public Health* 95 (2): 200–3. doi: 10.2105/AJPH.2003.036715.

Mazumdar, Sumit. 2015. 'The Murky Waters of Medical Practice in India: Ethics, Economics and Politics of Healthcare'. *Economic and Political Weekly* 50 (29): 40–5.

McDougall, Rosalind. 2008. 'The Junior Doctor as Ethically Unique'. *Journal of Medical Ethics* 34 (4): 268–70. doi: 10.1136/jme.2007.020636.

Mehndiratta, Abha, Sangeeta Sharma, Nikhil Prakash Gupta, Mari Jeeva Sankar, and Françoise Cluzeau. 2017. 'Adapting Clinical Guidelines in India: A Pragmatic Approach'. *British Medical Journal* 359: j5147.

Nagpal, Jitender, Aman Sachdeva, Rinku Sengupta Dhar, V.L. Bhargava, and A. Bhartia. 2014. 'Widespread Non-adherence to Evidence-Based Maternity Care Guidelines: A Population-Based Cluster Randomised Household Survey'. *BJOG: An International Journal of Obstetrics & Gynaecology* 122 (2): 238–47. doi: 10.1111/1471-0528.13054.

Narayana, K.V. 2003. 'Changing Health Care System'. *Economic and Political Weekly* 38 (12/13): 1230–41.

Ørberg, Jakob Williams. 2018. 'Uncomfortable Encounters between Elite and "Shadow Education" In India: Indian Institutes of Technology and the Joint Entrance Examination Coaching Industry'. *Higher Education* 76 (1): 129–44.

Pandya, Sunil. 2017. 'Two Founders of Bombay Neurosciences: Professor Gajendra Sinh and Professor Noshir Hormusjee Wadia'. *Neurology India* 65 (2): 240.

Parate, Vrushali R., Sushma S. Pande, and Pushpa O. Lokare. 2016. 'Admission to Medical Colleges: Predictive Validity of Selection Criteria'. *National Journal of Integrated Research in Medicine* 7 (4): 98–105.

Paxton, Anne, Deborah Maine, Lynn Freedman, Deborah Fry, and Samantha Lobis. 2005. 'The Evidence for Emergency Obstetric Care'. *International Journal of Gynecology & Obstetrics* 88 (2): 181–93. doi: 10.1016/j.ijgo.2004.11.026.

Randive, Bharat, Sarika Chaturvedi, and Nerges Mistry. 2012. 'Contracting in Specialists for Emergency Obstetric Care: Does It Work in Rural India?' *BMC Health Services Research* 12 (1): 485–94.

Reddy, K. Sudhakar, Peush Sahni, Girish K. Pande, and Samiran Nundy. 1991. 'Research in Indian Medical Institutes'. *The National Medical Journal of India* 4 (2): 90–2.

Sadeghi, Anahita, Asgari Ali Ali, Alireza Bagheri, Alireza Zamzam, Ahmadreza Soroush, and Zhamak Khorgami. 2014. 'Medical Resident Workload at a Multidisciplinary Hospital in Iran'. *Research and Development in Medical Education* 3 (2): 73–7. doi: 10.5681/rdme.2014.015.

Singh, Virendra. 2012. 'Professor U.S. Mathur'. *Lung India: Official Organ of Indian Chest Society* 29 (2): 200.

Sood, Rachita, Nakul Raykar, Brian Till, Hemant Shah, and Nobhojit Roy. 2018. 'Walking Blood Banks: An Immediate Solution to Rural India's Blood Drought'. *Indian Journal of Medical Ethics* 3 (2): 134–7. doi: 10.20529/IJME.2017.098.

Subramanian, Ajantha. 2015. 'Making merit: The Indian Institutes of Technology and the social life of caste'. *Comparative Studies in Society and History* 57 (2): 291–322.

Supe, Avinash N. 2008. 'Networking in Medical Education: Creating and Connecting'. *Indian Journal of Medical Sciences* 62 (3): 118–23. doi: 10.4103/0019-5359.39616.

Vaughan, Suzanne, Tom Sanders, Nick Crossley, Paul O'Neill, and Val Wass. 2015. 'Bridging the Gap: The Roles of Social Capital and Ethnicity in Medical Student Achievement'. *Medical Education* 49 (1): 114–23. doi: 10.1111/medu.12597.

Wear, Delese. 1998. 'On White Coats and Professional Development: The Formal and the Hidden Curricula'. *Annals of Internal Medicine* 129 (9): 734–7.

Zachariah, Anand, R. Srivatsan, and Susie J. Tharu, eds. 2010. *Towards a Critical Medical Practice: Reflections on the Dilemmas of Medical Culture Today*. New Delhi: Orient BlackSwan.

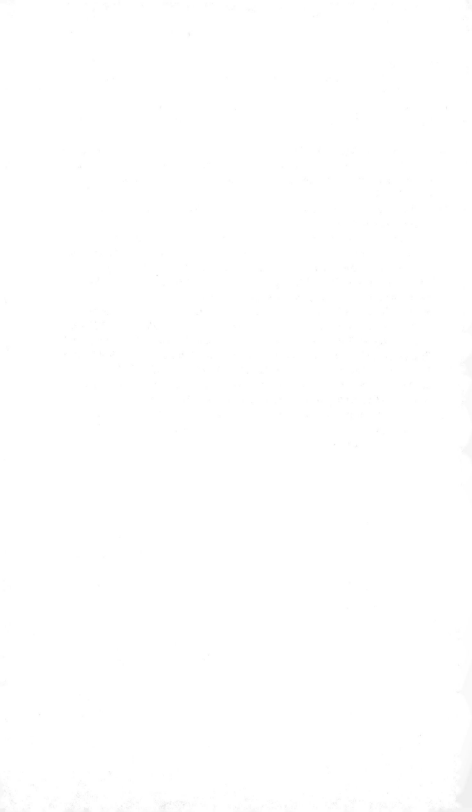

SECTION 5

INSTITUTIONALIZATION
OF CHILDBIRTH

10

Son Preference in India

Stigmatization and Surveillance in Maternity Wards in Jaipur, Rajasthan

Clémence Jullien

Introduction: (Dis)continuities?

According to a recent Indian report produced by the Ministry of Finance, there are currently 63 million women 'missing' in India (Government of India 2018). While early studies of unbalanced sex ratios in the colonial and immediate post-Independence period dealt mainly with female infanticide and the neglect of daughters (Miller 1987, 1997; Bhatnagar et al. 2005; Vishwanath 2004), after the introduction of ultrasound technologies in the 1970s, a growing number of social scientists studied the practices of sex detection and the selective abortion of female foetuses (Croll 2000; Manier 2006; Jeffery and Jeffery 1983; Patel 2007). With some exceptions (Jeffery 2014; John et al. 2009; Vishwanath 1983), current practices of female abortions are often presented as a continuity (by substitution or by intensification) of neglect or female infanticide: while postnatal discrimination existed for centuries, the rise of modern medical technologies has led to increasing prenatal discrimination.

Despite abundant literature on the topic, conflicting accounts of the reasons for the shortfall in girls has led researchers to describe the phenomenon as a 'Bermuda Triangle' (Oldenburg 1992; Guilmoto 2008; Hudson and den Boer 2004; Rao 2004). Although it is insufficient to explain the sex ratio imbalances between the north (west) and south (east) of the country on its own, Dyson and Moore's argument (1983) that regional variations in women's social status (age at marriage, degree of autonomy, maintenance of ties with the family of origin) are determined by cultural differences related to the kinship system has marked the research. Using data from Uttar Pradesh (UP), political scientist Oldenburg (1992) refers to a less commonly cited factor: that of structural violence. Supported by statistics, he correlates

Clémence Jullien, *Son Preference in India* In: *Childbirth in South Asia*. Edited by: Clémence Jullien and Roger Jeffery, Oxford University Press. © Oxford University Press 2021. DOI: 10.1093/oso/9780190130718.003.0010 high gender imbalances with high crime rates, district by district. According to him, the desire for sons constitutes a defence strategy in the regions concerned: sons are seen as providers of physical protection and as better suited to the necessary exercise of political power. From a post-colonial and feminist perspective, Bhatnagar et al. (2005) analyse female infanticide by situating the practice of female infanticide in India in the broader context of violence against women (rape, dowry deaths, cases of female neglect, women 'accidentally' burned, etc.). Their research pays attention to the impact of reproductive technologies, government programmes and family planning policies, and—more broadly—to what they view as coercive state policies that have caused people to have no more than two or three children. Although researchers do not agree on the main underlying causes of son preference, a common emphasis is put on the fact that it results from specific ritual duties, practices of patrilocal residence (with financial and emotional support of parents in old age preferentially provided by sons), patriarchal property rights, and a binding dowry system.

By pointing out social, economic, and religious structural elements relatively well anchored in India, the state of research related to son preference in India often gives an impression of immutability. This perception is reinforced by academic and media accounts that have also drawn attention to the persistent poor implementation of the law against sex detection in utero. In 1996, the Indian government began to implement the 1994 Pre-Natal Diagnostic Techniques Act (amended in 2003 to become the Pre-Conception and Pre-Natal Diagnostic Techniques Act, PC-PNDT Act) in order to ban disclosure of the sex and to counter practices of female foeticide. Persons who contravene the provisions of this Act—either by practising sex determination or by not maintaining clinic records—are punishable with imprisonment and fine. Yet, so far there have been very few arrests.[1] Doctors in the private sector are frequently accused of disclosing the sex of the foetus when patients ask (and sometimes bribe) them for it. The 2001 and 2011 Censuses attest that female selective abortion and/or infant neglect persist, despite the implementation of the PC-PNDT Act, since the child sex ratio (0–6 years) has become even more masculine. According to the census, the sex ratio for the 0–6 years group went from 927 girls per 1,000 boys (2001) to 919 girls per 1,000 boys (2011).[2] Regional disparities in child sex ratios also show uniform trends across decades, 'with the northern and western states displaying a much lower child sex ratio [that is, more masculine] relative to the southern and eastern states in India' (Mitra 2014: 1022). In sum, by underlining the straightforward continuity between female infanticide and female foeticide—by highlighting the fact that son preference is caused by structural motivations and by pointing out that implementation of laws does not lead to counter practices against selective abortion—researchers often give an erroneous impression of immutability.

Based on research conducted at a pivotal time (2011–12) and in an under-researched setting (a government hospital), this chapter sheds significant light on new issues at stake. It shows how government awareness campaigns, together with a sharp rise in institutional deliveries in the 2000s and increased surveillance in hospitals, have had negative unintended consequences on health and gender. This example of changing biopower has, in turn, deeply changed how son preference is currently discussed and experienced.

To do so, this chapter draws on how son preference has been debated in the media and the Indian political arena since the 2000s.[3] Using anthropological fieldwork conducted in Jaipur (Rajasthan) over 18 months in 2011–12, as part of my doctoral research on the politics of health reproduction, it focuses more particularly on 3 months of ethnographic fieldwork carried out in one of the three government hospitals in obstetrics (that I will call Janm) in the city.[4] While the issue of son preference in India is often raised through village fieldwork, analysis of Ayurvedic texts (cf. Charaka or Sushruta), or studies of quantitative data (Census of India, National Family Health Survey), it is (as far as I know) never addressed through hospital ethnographies. Yet, it is mainly in government hospitals that public health policies and new resolutions are displayed (through advertisements) and transmitted (by civil servants who act as street-level bureaucrats) to the country's population. Furthermore, by conducting research in both the common labour room and the operation theatre, as well as the antenatal check-up rooms and the post-natal wards—that is, by taking into consideration doctor–patient interactions as well as more private consultations—particular attention can be paid to people's adjustments in a variety of settings (Goffman 1959) as well as on how space is conceived, lived, and perceived (Lefebvre 1991). In doing so, it also portrays the broader norms, values, and concerns of the outside world (Van der Geest and Finkler 2004).

I argue that preventing daughter aversion has ironically reinforced the pressure and the stigma that underprivileged women face in hospitals while giving birth. More largely, based on the example of son preference, I explore the paradoxical correlations between increasingly institutionalized moral and medical surveillance and the emergence of new forms of risk. To this end, I draw on theories of surveillance, mainly through the Foucauldian notions of discipline and biopower (Foucault 1963, 1995) inherent in the so-cial relationships between patients and caregivers.

The first part of the chapter explains how the institutionalization of child-birth delivery plays a pivotal role in awareness-raising against son prefer-ence. The second part explores the diversity of procedures and techniques women adopt in order to have a son, and how they deal with the risk of being duped. While underlining the mechanism of visibility in the hospital, the third part analyses how surveillance and discipline operate within the wards. Based on multifocal perspectives, the chapter then shows how doctors, nurses, patients, and their relatives condemn son preference by constantly finding scapegoats and pointing at social classes, state differences, and gen-erational differences. As I argue in the conclusion, condemning son prefer-ence constitutes a new opportunity for social distinction while exacerbating tensions between patients, mothers-in-law, and hospital staff.

The Impact of the Institutionalization of Childbirth on Son Preference

As the introduction to this volume has demonstrated, the maternal care programmes introduced in the 2000s—Jananī Surakṣā Yojnā (JSY) and Jananī Śiśu Surakṣā Kāryakram (JSSK)—have led to rapid increases in institutional deliveries in Rajasthan as in the rest of India. Due to these schemes, the rate of institutionalized deliveries in government hospitals in Rajasthan has almost tripled in a decade, going from 29.6% in 2005–6 to 84% in 2015–16. Janm is representative of such evolution: while there were 7,544 deliveries in 2002, the number of deliveries reached 12,708 in 2011. The hospital serves some urban middle-class women (who often happened to be doctors' or nurses' friends, neighbours, relatives, or former patients) but, given its location, it attracts first and foremost low-caste villagers living a few kilometres away from Jaipur, and poor Muslim women living in the adjacent neighbourhood.

Through these national programmes that promote the institutionalization of childbirth, the Indian government expected to fight against maternal and infant mortality in India.[5] But the impact of such schemes goes beyond com-mitment to safe motherhood. As Foucault (2004: 108) has explained with his concept of governmentality, the family has emerged 'as a segment' to regu-late population, that is to say as an instrument of biopolitics. By attracting a growing number of women into maternity wards, health and other gov-ernment authorities can disseminate and promote their messages on a larger scale. Beyond health-related recommendations (for example, vaccination, HIV testing, balanced diet), the interior and exterior walls of Janm are covered with awareness-raising messages on what leads to a good family, such as family planning and gender equality. Some posters (for example, 'let girls be born') focus mainly on the fact that sex determination is illegal and condemned by the law. While reminding the reader of the law, such posters come with drawings of blood, handcuffs, and a judge's gavel to reinforce the point that foeticide is illegal. The government's advertising campaigns to defend the cause of little girls are not only propagated on hospital walls, but also on television and in the press. Moreover, cases of foetuses and baby girls found in garbage cans, in forests, on the edge of motorways or buried alive are scattered in local press articles. The question of son preference is also addressed through short stories, novels, and films, such as *Atamaja* and *God's Left Hand* (Visaria 2008). The first episode (May 2012) of the famous and popular TV programme *Satyamev Jayate*, hosted by the Bollywood superstar Aamir Khan, was dedicated to female foeticide, with a special focus on Rajasthan. And, last but not least, in 2015, Narendra Mondi launched a movement '#Selfie with Daughter' that soon became a top trend on both Facebook and Twitter in India. While such schemes and awareness campaigns have been launched all over India, it is worth highlighting that son preference was particularly a concern in Rajasthan. With a child sex ratio especially imbalanced (888 girls per 1,000 boys in 2011) and well below the national average (919 girls per 1,000 boys), Rajasthan was considered by the central government among the five lowest-performing states of the country.[6]

In other words, the condemnation of son preference and girl discrimination is becoming increasingly evident in the Indian public sphere, and patients (whether they be from Jaipur or from rural villages located on its outskirts) are all aware that sex determination is now prohibited. In fact, few patients ask the doctor about the sex of the foetus during one of the two mandatory ultrasounds. 'The doctor would yell at us if we would dare to ask!', they explained to me. In view of these changes, it remains to be seen how these official and guilt-ridden discourses are appropriated by the women, their families, and the caregivers in hospitals.

Getting a Boy: Predictions and Operating Instructions

Despite the fact that sex disclosure is strictly forbidden, trying to figure out whether the foetus is a boy or a girl remains common for the families in my study. Many women I met at Janm had made predictions (that interestingly were systematically in favour of boys) depending on the source of the pain, the form of craving, the shape of the belly, or the speed of the delivery. They usually did not rely solely on intuition. Many women believed that the sex of the foetus would only be determined from the fourth month. In the meantime, and as the Vedic texts stipulate, it would be possible to promote the development of a boy, or even to influence the sex of the child, by taking medicinal herbs or making certain offerings. The existence and plurality of methods for predicting a child's sex are neither specific to Rajasthani society (or India), nor are they new. Predictions and practices attempting to change the sex of a foetus were widespread in India well before the implementation of the PC-PNDT Act (Jeffery and Jeffery 1983).

The ban of gender detection tests and sex-selective abortion has probably enhanced the appeal of alternative methods. Although some social groups cannot access sex determination as it is illegal, and as they might not have the financial means to travel to a foreign country or bribe a doctor in private clinic who will agree to disclose the sex of the baby, the desire to have a son in India is still dominant. In order to have a son, I met many pregnant women who had followed the advice of priests and/or used medicines they had seen in newspaper advertisements or that a family member (or neighbours) gave them. Krishna Sharma is a 27-year-old Rajasthani woman who completed her college education. I met her in the delivery room of Janm while she was giving birth to a boy. Once the birth and the counselling phase of family planning was completed, Krishna described her previous pregnancies, that is to say her 3-year-old daughter as well as two miscarriages. She talked at length about the person (*Mātājī*) that her sister-in-law recommended to protect her from evil spirits throughout the pregnancy. When I asked if she received some recommendations in order to have a boy, Krishna acknowledged that this same woman gave her medication (*deśī davāyiān*) for this purpose at the cost of 1,500 INR (around 20 USD). She had been taking these tablets from her husband's hands, in three doses during the second month of pregnancy. Then, somewhat embarrassed by this confession, she asked me not to repeat this information within the hospital as only the person who sold her the drugs, her husband, and one of her sisters were aware of it.

The recommended remedy can be more cumbersome and expensive than the one Krishna followed. In one of the private cottages of the hospital, Khushbu—a young educated woman—mentioned that she got injections every week during the 9 months of her pregnancy in order to have a son. Her husband, a pharmacist, administered them to her and each injection cost them 200 INR (around 3 USD). While pointing to her new granddaughter, Khushbu's mother concluded with a smile: 'And here she is. If my destiny is to have a boy then I will have one . . . We only get what was planned for us [jo likhā huā hotī hai, vahī hotā hai, literally, "what happens is what is written"]'.

Interestingly, women and their families frequently spoke of these practices as superstitions for uneducated people. Only when trust was established and no caregiver was around did some women acknowledge that they had observed these practices themselves. Even though patients usually did not mention such treatments to the doctors as they were afraid of being mocked, most of the caregivers were aware of such practices. They were often irritated when they learned that some of their patients had recourse to 'non-scientific' practices, and that they would give the credit to the priests they consulted if the delivery went well. As an intern once said: 'Then they think it's all because of them!' The tone of Dr Sneha was both amused and upset:

They are happy to believe that the remedy given by a priest has worked. These priests give incense residues (bhabhūtī) to pregnant women so they can have a boy. These false beliefs are there. They are only superstitions. India is full of superstitions! There's nothing we can do. Yesterday I met a woman who was educated. She came to see me and told me that she had recited Sundarkān kā Path and that today she had farted! The priest had told her that if she farted, it was because her prayer (mantra) had worked out. She said to me: 'I followed the path of the Hanuman God and everything seems to be fine. [She's laughing]. What can I do with that?!'

When I mention that some patients get injections in order to get a son, Dr Mukherjee replied, outraged:

People are ignorant. They do not have the knowledge and some people want to take advantage of it . . . Some give incense residues (bhabhūtī), others give medicines or injections made of distilled water and glucose. And if the patient has a son, she'll think it's because of these injections and she'll send more people to this man who makes money from nothing.

Many physicians, such as Professor Shreya Rao, mentioned that such women are 'idiots' (bevkūf), that there is 'no medical evidence' and, as such, that they refuse to talk more about this subject.

In short, political correctness on son preference seems harmful in two ways. Not only is inquiring about the child's sex strictly prohibited but it seems that, more broadly, son preference has become an illegitimate topic that is not to be addressed within the hospital (as women do not want to risk facing mockery from the staff). Yet, despite being a taboo, pregnant women— whether educated or not, economically privileged or not—are often asked by their mothers-in-law to wear talismans, to make offerings, or to undergo drug treatment in order to have a son.[7]

In addition to this, it is well known that some 'ersatz' doctors (and priests) 'fill the gaps left by legitimate institutions' (Pinto 2004) and that they take advantage of this taboo by financially benefiting from these beliefs held by pregnant women with full impunity.[8] Thus, not only are alternative methods of gender prediction more numerous and more debated (see, for example, blogs on the internet), but also a growing number of actors (priests, gurus, etc.) benefit financially from it. To take just one example, the Indian media recently covered a controversy about a product named *Putrajeevak Beej* that allegedly promotes the birth of a son.[9] Commercialized through the Ayurvedic brand Patanjali and its worldwide-known guru Baba Ramdev, the product was strongly condemned by different Indian ministers in 2015–18 as it violates both the Drug and Cosmetic Rules 1945 and also the PC-PNDT Act, which aim to prevent practices of son preference.

Visibility and Surveillance

Interestingly, while patients tended not to mention a possible son preference, the configuration and the functioning of the hospital enabled constant monitoring that easily allowed caregivers to detect signs of son preference.

In the antenatal check-up rooms, the interns in charge would see the patient only once she had registered at the desk office and presented her document that traced her health history. Women sometimes left out some details from these documents that would reflect badly on them. This document, systematically updated after the third month of pregnancy was completed, includes the number of children and abortions the woman had, the type of delivery she went through, the date of her last menstruation, the expected date of delivery, as well as the age and the sex of her children. Thus, when Smiti, an intern, received a 25-year-old pregnant woman who had previously had two daughters and was waiting for her third child, she chuckled: 'And after this one, you will make a fourth one?!' Similarly, another intern who had just learned that the pregnant woman sitting in front of her already had five girls and a boy, called me aloud to quickly come and 'photograph this woman'. The intern then asked the patient whether she wanted a second son. By asking this rhetorical question, the young intern seemed willing both to shame the patient (as she suddenly became the focus of attention in the room of antenatal check-up) and to show me the ease with which caregivers can spot the women who multiply pregnancies in order to have a son. In general, in such situations, doctors were not expecting women to answer the question. They were also not taking the time to explain the medical risks involved in repeated or too close pregnancies. Yet, through simple rhetorical questions that point out and morally condemn those who are suspected to be looking for a son, caregivers not only reaffirm their authority but they also reveal how programmes of safe motherhood and biopolitical mechanisms are closely intertwined.

The insidious forms of social surveillance—well-known for operating in hospitals (Gibson 2004; Foucault 1963)—also operated in the delivery room, but with a different mechanism and other aspects at stake. While patients who were delivering were lying on beds placed next to each other and separated by metallic screens, the caregivers' desk was located in the middle, enabling them to easily scan the six beds. If this physical layout allowed the team quickly to track the progress of the delivery of their patients, it also allowed them to observe the reactions of the women once they had found out about the sex of the baby they had just delivered. Some women who would have liked to have had a boy expressed their regrets through sore expressions or lost gazes, but also more openly through crying or verbal complaints. This was the case with Simran, a 25-year-old patient who exclaimed (after finding out that she had a daughter for the third time): 'Oh God! Now I won't do it again. All these issues and yet it is a girl'. In such situations, the nurse or the intern who took care of the delivery used to assert authoritatively that 'girl or boy, it is just the same' (larkī ya larkā ek hī hai). To strengthen their points, women caregivers sometimes took their professional success as an example: 'Look at us, we contribute to our parents' good reputation [rośan karnā or illumine the names of our parents], why could not you do it?' (Dr Malhotra); 'Look at this hospital, it is managed by women doctors, women nurses, women auxiliaries, all are women' (Dr Kumar).

While scrutinizing patients' reactions, caregivers were also attentive to the clothes for the newborn that mothers-in-law were responsible for bringing into the delivery room shortly after birth. If a woman's in-laws brought old and dirty clothes or if she claimed she had nothing, the doctor sometimes admonished her for gender discrimination. Such a situation happened with Nisha's mother-in-law when she found out she had a second granddaughter although she wanted to have a second grandson. When the mother-in-law explained she had no clothes for the baby, the doctor replied: 'For the first one [a 5-year-old boy], there were some and this time you didn't bring any? Go to the *Lifestyle* [a shop in the hospital] to buy some'. It goes without saying that this doctor did not remember personally Nisha's first delivery (ironically it was a home delivery), but the insinuation of gender neglect was effective and the mother-in-law left without saying a word, in the direction of the shop.

In sum, and as Foucault has underlined, disciplinary institutions (like hospitals) have secreted a 'machinery of control' that functions 'like a microscope of conduct' (Foucault 1995: 173). In this specific example, encouraging women to deliver in hospital settings afforded new opportunities for mechanisms of real (or perceived) surveillance and castigation that were simultaneously medical as well as moral. Against this backdrop, I will explore how caregivers and patients explain away, or rationalize, the deviances at stake. More precisely, I intend to explain how an old and still largely generalized attitude is debated when it is simultaneously firmly condemned. As Taylor rightly points out, 'there is a consistent scepticism displayed about the value of actors' statements' within the area of deviancy (Taylor 1972: 24). Yet, 'the imputation and avowal of motives by actors are social phenomena to be explained' (Mills 1940: 904). In line with C.W. Mills's work on the 'situated actions and vocabularies of motive', the next section will show that the different reasons people give to each other's attitudes are not themselves without reasons.

The Education Paradox

With a few exceptions, the physicians of Janm took for granted that uneducated families from underprivileged backgrounds were the most eager to have sons and that women from such backgrounds cannot oppose them as they have low decision-making power. Dr Pankaj Rao explicitly related son preference to a lack of education: 'It's a matter of social reasons. They are not educated and think that girls are burdens and that they must spend money to raise them, marry them and even after marriage to continue to give gifts to the in-laws'. According to this doctor, to fight son preference, school education must come first. He referred to a girls' education assistance programme in UP and then continued: 'When a girl is educated, she becomes independent, so she can see this evil. And when she becomes a mother, she may be more mature about it'. In other words, based on their personal professional success, women doctors presented the professionalization of current women as a remedy to (re)valorize girls. These statements echoed the rhetoric used by the government of Narendra Modi in its awareness programme for girls launched in 2015, 'Save girl child, educate girl child' (*Betī bacāo, betī parhāo*). Through the representation of smiling schoolgirls and fulfilled women who pursued a career (often as a doctor), iconography discredits the idea that girls would be of lesser value than boys. With the iconic image of a smiling girl with braids reading a book, this vast campaign depicts girls' education as a tool to fight against gender-based discrimination.

In the narrative of many doctors, the lack of education was intrinsically entangled with women's lack of autonomy within their in-laws' home. Shiv, an intern, had obviously overheard the conversation I was having with Mobina, a patient who had just delivered her first child. When I asked her how many children she would like to have, Shiv replied aloud without giving her time to answer: 'She doesn't know this kind of thing, her family knows how many children she will have, they want a son in the prize for ten girls!' Given his ir-ritated tone and attitude, these were not words of empathy. Rather, Shiv was implying that poor Muslims wanting to have a son multiplied pregnancies without any limit.

Many researchers (for example, Arokiasamy 2007; Bhat and Sharma 2006; Mitra 2014) agree that illiteracy and the absence of female labour-force ac-tivity are not—as people assumed for a long time—the main cause of the imbalance of child sex ratio. On the contrary, the development of education could have adverse effects. As early as the late 1980s, Das Gupta (1987: 95) revealed that a girl born in Punjab among young educated women who al-ready had at least one girl had 2.36 times the likelihood of dying than her siblings. From the various socio-economic classes and sex ratio data for the 0–6 age group from 1981, 1991, and 2001 censuses, Sudha and Irudaya Rajan (2003: 4366) showed that at the national level, socio-economic 'development in India is not accompanied by a decrease in gender bias'.

Similarly, drawing on the analysis of census data, economists Bhat and Sharma (2006: 368) concluded that 'economic prosperity and education of women, which were traditionally thought to be the variables helpful in making improvements in the sex ratio (a connection that is true of many de-veloped countries), have actually resulted in the decline of the sex ratio, par-ticularly at the 0 to 6 age level, in many parts of north India'.

In addition, Arokiasamy (2007: 70–1) pointed out that decreased fer-tility has led to increased discrimination against girls among educated and economically well-off individuals from urban areas, as they can access prenatal sex-determination more easily. Some affluent couples even fly to neighbouring Thailand to take a pre-implantation genetic diagnostic to ensure that only male embryos are placed in the womb (Mitra 2014). In sum, many demographers, economists, and anthropologists have invalidated a common assumption by showing that the improvement of the level of family education and the better quality of life of individuals reinforce son preference rather than reducing it. If educated wealthy urban families usually discriminate less (than poorer rural residents) against girls they allow to be born, they are more likely to practise sex-selective abortions (Jeffery 2014: 173).

Not only is the practice of selective female abortion mainly the preserve of the Indian urban middle and upper middle class, but also families are particularly likely to use such practices when one of the partners is a doctor. This was revealed by a study conducted in the Vidarbha region of Maharashtra (Patel et al. 2013). It is no coincidence that the TV programme *Satyamev Jayate* (which many patients referred to during my fieldwork in Janm) staged the case of Dr Mitu Khurana, a woman doctor from a wealthy district of Delhi, who had been impelled to practise prenatal sex detection and to abort her daughter due to the pressure of her in-laws. Lastly, whether the rumour is false or true, it was also significant for me to hear in the corridors that a senior professor of Janm—a Punjabi woman with three children, married to a doctor—once practised female abortion. In other words, though doctors systematically mention son preference as a shameful attitude of the lower social classes, the medical community is more involved in the phenomenon of son preference and the practices of sex-selective abortion than they appear.

Reproducing Indictment on Generational Differences

Interestingly, though the doctors' rhetoric is erroneous, patients at Janm attempt to solicit solidarities by mimicking or internalizing providers' oft-used tropes, namely that son preference indexes 'illiteracy' and 'backwardness' and that the drive for sons is more a matter of affinal kin than of the woman herself. In fact, and although researchers and the media commonly use the expression 'son preference', few patients speak about it in these terms. In most of the cases, expecting to have a son was expressed more as a necessity (*zarūrat*), than as a personal 'preference'. It is important to draw this clarification as some women might recognize that they 'need a son', even though some of them would personally prefer daughters.

This was the case of Suma, an 18-year-old pregnant Hindu slum-dweller who already had a boy and hoped to get a daughter. While people usually put the emphasis on the departure of girls when they marry (patrivirilocality), Suma praised the proximity of mother–daughter relationships: 'If it is a girl, she will stay with me, she will play with me while the boys are right over there. They spend the day playing outside and then they stay with their wives. I always wanted to have a daughter because she would stay with me'. The idea according to which only sons take care of their parents was also sometimes questioned. As Kalpana's mother mentioned: 'It is said that one day the girl will leave and the boy will stay, that he will take care of you. But, actually, tell me, when are the boys available for their parents? The girls are there, even when they are married, they come back to their parents' place [māykā] if necessary'.

Though son preference is widespread, many women challenged this common assumption and said they would not personally make any difference between a boy or a girl. With spite or condescension, they tended to attribute such behaviour to the retrograde mind of their husband or mother-in-law. While talking to me, they often highlighted the illiteracy or the lack of education of their husband by mentioning, grinning: 'He is illiterate', 'he is not very intelligent', or 'he has no brain' (dimāg nahī hai).

When it comes to mothers-in-law, the focus was on the generational gap: 'These are words from older women' or 'The previous generations never celebrated the birth of girls'. Educated patients tended particularly to accentuate generational differences and to be more eager to distinguish themselves from their mother-in-law's allegedly retrograde thoughts. This was the case of Puja, a 25-year-old student in the third year of a business degree (BComm), who had married three years previously. After two challenging years of not being able to be pregnant, she received medical treatment. When I met her, Puja was 9 months pregnant and was about to enter the operating theatre to have a C-section delivery. Although she first stated that decisions related to the number of children a family has were the responsibility of 'husband and wife and no one else', she nuanced her statement as we continued to talk. When I asked her how many children she aimed to have, she recognized the influence of her mother-in-law:

If it's a boy, then I'll be sterilized. If it's a girl, I'll have to try one more time. I don't want to, but my mother-in-law and the others want that I have a boy. Today, boys and girls are the same. Nowadays, boys are not even able to do what girls can do . . . She says we need a boy. I don't understand, only old women talk like that.

For Puja, as for many women I met, the pressure in-laws exert regarding the child's sex had concrete effects on them. In fact, 'Indian mothers-in-law have a strong influence on the decisions taken by their daughters-in-law on important personal questions, such as the number of sons they will have' (Robitaille and Chatterjee 2017: 48). Even when their in-laws' preference for a son was criticized or mocked, it could still determine the number of pregnancies and deliveries the woman will undergo. In this sense, patients who attributed the 'need to have a boy' with the retrograde spirit of their husband or in-laws were, despite their statements and regardless of their personal opinions, directly concerned by son preference.

As the hospital staff liked to point out, young women were often compelled— sometimes in spite of themselves—to receive treatment, to undergo abortions, or to multiply pregnancies in order to have a boy. Although doctors believed that women from underprivileged classes and low castes were particularly under pressure from their in-laws, they attributed responsibility to them in medical consultations. Ironically, the women most heavily targeted are those least able to engender change in their circumstances, or mitigate the pressures placed on them.

An Unfortunate but Profitable Rajasthani Practice

Though, so far, it is difficult to state that the awareness campaigns have succeeded in empowering girls and more generally women, the stigmatization of son preference has—ironically—undoubtedly become a tool of self-empowerment in obstetric wards. If this is especially true for the medical staff, it was particularly salient for the nurses whose ambivalent attitude enabled them to enhance their social power or economic gain depending on the moment.

As it is often the case in India, a significant percentage of the nurses at Janm are catholic nurses from Kerala.[10] When we were discussing son preference in the delivery room, the phenomenon was mainly formulated in terms of regional differences: 'Here [in Rajasthan], they want a son, no matter if he is black, yellow or whatever! They need a boy, full stop'; 'Here, in Rajasthan, they all want boys. In my state, in Kerala, this is absolutely not like that. Girl or boy, it's the same thing'; and 'People want boys [with round eyes] and in

Rajasthan, even more so! . . . In my state in Kerala, it's not like that. Over there, women can be equal to men'. In a few cases, the same nurses would imply that gender bias is also partly related to education. Yet, in doing so, they would still—as a head nurse did—reinforce the idea that Rajasthan is a backward state: 'There's also the fact that people used to not be educated and that now they are. Well, in Rajasthan, it does not reach 70%! [Laughs]'.[11]

According to the 2011 census, Kerala is indeed the only Indian state (with the Union Territory of Pondicherry) where the overall sex ratio is not unfavourable to women. As for the child sex ratio, it is 964 girls per 1,000 boys, close to the global average sex ratio at birth (estimated at 950 girls per 1,000 boys). More generally, while opposing Kerala to Rajasthan, the hospital staff—and particularly nurses—underlined the conservative and patriarchal nature of Rajasthan.[12]

And yet, despite their discourse on gender equality in front of the patients (or the ethnographer), many nurses insist on the fact that the birth of a boy is a happier event. Indeed, when a baby is delivered, both aux-iliaries (*bāī*) and nurses (including these nurses from Kerala) openly ask for a few more rupees if it is a boy. After a baby is born and cleaned, either a nurse goes to the waiting room to deliver the newborn child to a family member, or she calls a relative of the patient (often the mother-in-law) to the entrance of the delivery room. If a boy was born, the procedure was often the same: in a cheerful voice, as if she was personally rejoiced, the nurse hastened to inform that 'it is a boy' (*larkā hai!*). While sharing the news, she usually spread one of the newborn's legs to reveal his sex. She did not hand over the baby yet. Rather, she patted the child's body and cradled it in her arms at the same time, or she looked at the little boy with tender-ness and pinched his cheek while laughing. During these few seconds, one of the family members had time to look for a few rupees and hand them to the nurse. At times, when the person finally thought she/he would be handed the newly born child, the nurse made a face, obviously unsatisfied by the amount she saw. While keeping the newborn in her arms, she then claimed more money or simply and explicitly added: 'Come on, he's a boy, right!' (*Are larkā hai, na!*).

The idea that the family should 'by happiness' (*khuśī se*) be more generous for the birth of a boy is well established in India: not only do families give more to traditional midwives (in case of a home delivery) when they have a boy, but they also spend more money to celebrate this birth (*hijrā* remunera-tion, ceremonies with guests and musicians such as *kuā ka pūjā*) than if it was a girl (Jullien 2019a).

In short, while looking down at patients who complained about giving birth to a girl and by repeating the credo 'boys or girls, it's the same' (*larkā ya larkī, ek hī hai*), these same nurses showed clear enthusiasm when a boy child was born as they could economically benefit from this. In behaving in this way, they corroborated the idea that families should rejoice and spend more money for the birth of boys than for the birth of girls. By overlooking the diverse advertisements and messages posted in the different wards of the hospital that firmly condemn *bakchich*, both nurses and auxiliaries simultaneously engaged in illegal acts. Not only did they claim or take money from the in-laws but some nurses on duty in the labour room or the operating theatre would also not announce to the mother the sex of her baby, despite repeated requests. The aim was usually twofold: it was a way of retrospectively punishing the women who were considered 'not cooperative' (or too noisy) during labour and it was a means of pressure to get a small financial incentive (as Neelam mentioned above). Against this backdrop, one may wonder whether these contradictions are not likely to undermine the credibility of nurses' messages and to further erode the trust placed in hospital staff.

Conclusion

Through the case of son preference, I argue that safe motherhood policies and increased surveillance in hospital wards are, despite rhetoric of development, concomitant to the rise of new forms of risk. Insofar as the trust placed on caregivers is sometimes jeopardized and women risk being reprimanded or mocked when coming to the hospital, one can assume that the backdrop of son preference's stigmatization and sex-selection's criminalization might have an impact on future trajectories of care-seeking in public hospitals. Thanks to the JSY and JSSK programmes, the rate of institutional births in public facilities in Rajasthan has increased from 19% to 63.5% over the last 10 years (Government of India 2016: 3). Yet, as I have shown elsewhere based on the data I collected in 2011–12, many slum-dwellers located on the outskirts of Jaipur went for antenatal check-ups but refused to deliver in public hospitals as they either had previous bad experiences with the hospital staff (such as insults, humiliation, or unconcern) or heard through relatives or neighbours that caregivers would abuse them (Jullien 2019a). Given the 'widespread and long-term mistrust of state services' (Jeffery and Jeffery 2010), which is particularly prominent in the field of reproductive healthcare in India, it is fair to consider that the growing moralizing attitude of the hospital staff is likely to undermine the efforts of the state in promoting childbirth deliveries in public hospitals.

It is worth noting that the different narratives of the patients and the hospital staff are revealing of deeper forms of social resentments (often based on religious communalism or feelings of biased political favouritisms). On the pretext that uneducated and poor women are careless and have no hygiene, patients of Janm were often held responsible for threatening the life of their own child (Jullien 2017). On the pretext that the policies of the Congress prompt the Muslim community and the low castes to have large families, these patients were blamed for contributing to India's population growth and its corollary issues (Jullien 2019b). Similarly, on the pretext that people from underprivileged background are mostly responsible for son preference (a practice that is increasingly portrayed as both illegitimate and shameful), some members of the hospital staff tend to further discriminate against such patients at Janm, as well as mocking them and blackmailing them.

As mentioned earlier, son preference is closely associated with backwardness or retrograde mentalities in both social media and official speeches.[13] Significantly, over the last decade, different government schemes launched—to fight girl discrimination—are addressed solely to couples with daughters who have the below poverty line (BPL) card.[14] By focusing exclusively on the supposedly poorest families, these programmes are based on the premise that the most vulnerable groups would be the main perpetrators of this discrimination and that a financial incentive could remedy this. In fact, when doctors, nurses and patients condemn son preference, it seems it is sometimes less on the grounds of strong personal ideological views than the willingness to place themselves in the 'modern' and 'educated' spheres conveyed in public awareness campaigns 'as the possessors of legitimate culture' (Bourdieu 2003). While strengthening forms of stigmatization, the cross-accusations also help doctors, nurses, and patients to distinguish themselves socially, by presenting themselves in opposition to 'backward' views and behaviour. To draw on Bourdieu's (2003) well-known thesis, tastes and preferences exhibited by certain social groups or categories signify social difference and distance. On the one hand, they unify as they mark status: 'taste is the basis of all that one has—people and things—and all that one is for others, whereby one classifies oneself and is classified by others' (Bourdieu 2003: 56). On the other hand, they separate, as taste is first and foremost the distaste of the tastes of others: 'In matter of taste, more than anywhere else, all determination is negation; and tastes are perhaps first and foremost distastes, disgust provoked by horror and visceral intolerance ['sick-making'] of the tastes of others' (Bourdieu 2003: 56). Due to intensive campaigns valuing girl children and associating female foeticide with a backward mentality, condemning son preference openly and loudly has become a crucial mark of status in hospitals.

Both this ethnographical study and recent statistical data attest that son preference persists throughout society, despite at varying degrees. Yet, and as I have shown during the chapter by analysing the impact of awareness campaigns on girl discrimination, 'it is necessary to grasp the nature of change and not assume a straightforward continuity with tradition' (John et al. 2009: 18). In fact, public condemnation of son preference has ambivalent consequences in at least three respects. At the individual level, on the one hand, some nurses or auxiliaries blame women for expressing son preference but nevertheless, on the other hand, take more money from them when they have a boy. From a social point of view, the question of son preference has contributed to reinforcing stereotypes of social groups (Rajasthani urban and rural poor low-caste women) that are frequently singled out. And finally, at an institutional level, suspicions related to son preference practices have enhanced hospitals' mechanisms of surveillance and discipline that were already particularly prevalent within the field of obstetrics (for example, in relation to hygiene rules, breastfeeding choices, or the adoption of contraceptive measures), far exceeding official intentions of safe motherhood. By doing so, the question remains whether the significant rise of childbirth deliveries in Indian public hospitals over the last decade will be sustainable in the coming years.

Notes

1. Of the 1,036 ongoing cases related to the 1994 PC-PNDT Act, only 10% related to charges of communication of the sex of the foetus (Karat and George 2012).
2. In Rajasthan, the sex ratio went from 909 (2001) to 888 (2011).
3. I would like to thank the participants at the 'Transformation of Childbirth in South Asia: Ethical, Legal, and Social Implications' workshop held at the Department of Social Anthropology and Cultural Studies (ISEK), Zurich in October 2018, for their suggestions and discussion. I would also like to thank Shruti Chaudhry, Roger Jeffery, and Marie Schuler for their valuable and detailed comments on my work.
4. In order to guarantee anonymity, the name of the hospital and the names of the respondents have been changed.
5. https://www.nhp.gov.in/janani-suraksha-yojana-jsy-_pg

6. The low-performing states (UP, Uttaranchal, Bihar, Jharkhand, Madhya Pradesh, Chhattisgarh, Assam, Rajasthan, Orissa, and Jammu and Kashmir) get more funds from the central government to provide higher financial incentives to the women.

7. We can assume that some women caregivers might also have experienced such pressures during their own pregnancies.

8. As Pinto rightly outlined, while unregulated medical practice is often considered to be a sign of backwardness, boundaries between medicine and ersatz medicine are more blurred than it is thought, as the work of self-made doctors is 'interwoven with the structure and ethos of development' (Pinto 2004: 363).

9. See, for example, *DNA* (1 May 2015), *India Today* (1 May 2015), *Times New* (2 June 2016) or *Mumbai Mirror* (21 February 2018).

10. Percot (2005) clearly shows Indian nurses are first and foremost a 'speciality' of Kerala: more than a third of the schools that train nurses in India are located in Kerala, and the Malayalis make up the majority of the trainee nurses in the other Indian states (Percot 2005).

11. According to the Census of 2011, the literacy rate in Rajasthan is 67%. It is indeed below the national average (74%) and well below the literacy rate of Kerala (94%). Furthermore, Rajasthan has a large differential in literacy rates between men (81%) and women (53%).

12. Yet, it is worth noting that affluent and relatively educated states like Punjab or Haryana display a strong masculine child sex ratio.

13. This is particularly visible in Prime Minister Narendra Modi's speeches: 'Our mentality is still that of the 18th century' (2015); 'we cannot be counted as citizens of the 21st century' (2015).

14. The programme '*Lādlī Yojanā*' launched in Haryana is an exception: an amount of money is given to families who have at least two daughters, without taking their income into consideration.

References

Arokiasamy, Perianayagam. 2007. 'Sex Ratio at Birth and Excess Female Child Mortality in India: Trends, Differentials and Regional Patterns'. In *Watering the Neighbour's Garden: The Growing Demographic Female Deficit in Asia*, edited by Isabelle Attané and Christophe Z. Guilmoto, 49–72. Paris: Committee for International Cooperation in National Research in Demography.

Bhat, R.L., and Namita Sharma. 2006. 'Missing Girls: Evidence from Some North Indian States'. *Indian Journal of Gender Studies* 13 (3): 351–74.

Bhatnagar, Rashmi Dube, Renu Dube, and Reena Dube. 2005. *Female Infanticide in India: A Feminist Cultural History*. New York: SUNY Press.

Bourdieu, Pierre. 2003 (1984). *Distinction: A Social Critique of the Judgement of Taste.* Translated by Richard Nice. Cambridge, MA: Harvard University Press.

Croll, Elisabeth. 2000. *Endangered Daughters: Discrimination and Development in Asia*. London & New York: Routledge.

Das Gupta, Monica. 1987. 'Selective Discrimination Against Female Children in Rural Punjab, India'. *Population and Development Review* 13 (1): 77–100.

Dyson, Tim, and Mick Moore. 1983. 'On Kinship Structure, Female Autonomy, and Demographic Behavior in India'. *Population and Development Review* 9 (1): 35–60.

Foucault, Michel. 1963. *Naissance de la clinique: Une archéologie du regard médical.* Paris: Puf.

Foucault, Michel. 1995. *Discipline and Punish: The Birth of the Prison.* Translated by Alan Sheridan. New York: Vintage.

Foucault, Michel. 2004. *Sécurité, territoire, population: Cours au collège de France, 1977–1978.* Paris: Gallimard.

Gibson, Diana. 2004. 'The Gaps in the Gaze in South African hospitals'. *Social Science & Medicine* 59 (10): 2013–24.

Goffman, Erving. 1959. *The Presentation of Self in Everyday Life.* New York: Doubleday.

Government of India. 2016. 'National Family Health Survey, NFHS4, 2015–2016. State Fact Sheet: Rajasthan'. New Delhi: Ministry of Health and Family Welfare. Accessed 27 March 2020. http://rchiips.org/NFHS/pdf/NFHS4/RJ_FactSheet.pdf

Government of India. 2018. *Economic Survey 2017–2018.* New Delhi: Ministry of Finance.

Guilmoto, Christophe Z. 2008. 'L'inscription spatiale de la discrimination de genre en Inde: Effets des distances sociale et géographique'. *L'Espace géographique* 37 (1): 1–15.

Hudson, Valerie M., and Andrea den Boer. 2004. *Bare Branches: The Security Implications of Asia's Surplus Male Population.* Cambridge, MA & London: MIT Press.

Jeffery, Patricia. 2014. 'Supply-and-Demand Demographics: Dowry, Daughter Aversion and Marriage Markets in Contemporary North India'. *Contemporary South Asia* 22 (2): 171–88.

Jeffery, Patricia, and Roger Jeffery. 2010. 'Only When the Boat Has Started Sinking: A Maternal Death in Rural North India'. *Social Science & Medicine* 71 (10): 1711–18.

Jeffery, Roger, and Patricia Jeffery. 1983. 'Female Infanticide and Amniocentesis'. *Economic and Political Weekly* 18 (16/17): 654–6.

John, Mary E., Ravinder Kaur, Rajni Palriwala, and Saraswati Raju. 2009. 'Dispensing with Daughters: Technology, Society, Economy in North India'. *Economic and Political Weekly* 44 (15): 16–19.

Jullien, Clémence. 2017. '"Alors, à qui la faute?" Mort périnatale et accusations croisées dans une maternité au Rajasthan (Inde)'. *L'Homme* 22 (3–4):131–60.

Jullien, Clémence. 2019a. *Du bidonville à l'hôpital: Nouveaux enjeux de la maternité au Rajasthan.* Paris: Édition de la Maison des sciences de l'homme.

Jullien, Clémence. 2019b. '"Bien-être familial": une notion illusoire? L'envers de la rhétorique en milieu hospitalier indien'. *Collection Purushartha* 36: 57–79.

Karat, Brinda, and Sabu George. 2012. 'Don't Trash This Law, The Fault Lies in Non-implementation'. *The Hindu*, 4 February. Accessed 27 March 2020. https://www.thehindu.com/opinion/op-ed/dont-trash-this-law-the-fault-lies-in-nonimplementation/article2858004.ece

Lefebvre, Henri. 1991. *The Production of Space*. Translated by Donald Nicholson-Smith. Oxford: Blackwell.

Manier, Bénédicte. 2006. *Quand les Femmes auront disparu: L'élimination des filles en Inde et en Asie*. Paris: La Découverte.

Miller, Barbara D. 1987. 'Female Infanticide and Child Neglect in Rural North India'. In *Child Survival: Anthropological Perspective on the Treatment and Maltreatment of Children*, edited by Nancy Scheper-Hughes, 95–112. Dordrecht: Reidel.

Miller, Barbara D. 1997. *The Endangered Sex: Neglect of Female Children in Rural North India*. New Delhi: Oxford University Press.

Mills, C. Wright. 1940. 'Situated Actions and Vocabularies of Motive'. *American Sociological Review* 5 (6): 904–13.

Mitra, Aparna. 2014. 'Son Preference in India: Implications for Gender Development'. *Journal of Economic Issues* 48 (4): 1021–37.

Oldenburg, Philip. 1992. 'Sex Ratio, Son Preference and Violence in India: A Research Note'. *Economic and Political Weekly* 27 (49/50): 2657–62.

Patel, Archana B., Neetu Badhoniya, Manju Mamtani, and Hemant Kulkarni. 2013. 'Skewed Sex Ratios in India: "Physician, Heal Thyself"'. *Demography* 50 (3): 1129–34.

Patel, Tulsi, ed. 2007. *Sex-Selective Abortion in India: Gender, Society and New Reproductive Technologies*. New Delhi: Sage.

Percot, Marie. 2005. 'Les infirmières indiennes émigrées dans les pays du Golfe: de l'opportunité à la stratégie'. *Revue européenne des migrations internationales* 21 (1): 29–54.

Pinto, Sarah. 2004. 'Development Without Institutions: Ersatz Medicine and the Politics of Everyday Life in Rural North India'. *Cultural Anthropology* 19 (3): 337–64.

Rao, Mohan. 2004. *From Population Control to Reproductive Health: Malthusian Arithmetic*. New Delhi: Sage.

Robitaille, Marie-Claire, and Ishita Chatterjee. 2017. 'Mothers-in-Law and Son Preference in India'. *Economic and Political Weekly* 52 (6): 42–50.

Sudha, S. and S. Irudaya Rajan. 2003. 'Persistent Daughter Disadvantage: What Do Estimated Sex Ratios at Birth and Sex Ratios of Child Mortality Risk Reveal?' *Economic and Political Weekly* 38 (41): 4361–9.

Taylor, Laurie. 1972. 'The Significance and Interpretation of Replies to Motivational Questions: The Case of Sex Offenders'. *Sociology* 6 (1): 23–39.

Van der Geest, Sjaak, and Kaja Finkler. 2004. 'Hospital Ethnography: Introduction'. *Social Science & Medicine* 59 (10): 1995–2001.

Visaria, Leela. 2008. 'Improving the Child Sex Ratio: Role of Policy and Advocacy'. *Economic and Political Weekly* 43 (12/13): 34–7.

Vishwanath, L. S. 1983. 'Misadventures in Amniocentesis'. *Economic and Political Weekly* 18 (11): 406–7.

Vishwanath, L. S. 2004. 'Female Infanticide: The Colonial Experience'. *Economic and Political Weekly* 39 (22): 2313–18.

11

Politics of Childbirth in Nepal

The Case of the Maternal Mortality Ratio

Jeevan R. Sharma and Radha Adhikari

Introduction

Historically, childbirth has been a major cause of maternal mortality and
morbidity in Nepal. In the last two decades, women's chances of survival
during childbirth have greatly improved in the country. In international fora,
Nepal has been hailed as a global success in reducing maternal mortality because significant progress was made despite a decade-long civil war that se-
verely impacted the delivery of basic health services in rural areas (Devkota
and Teijlingen 2010; Engel et al. 2013). In 2010, Nepal won the Millennium
Development Goal (MDG) country award for its leadership, commitment,
progress, and achievement towards reducing maternal mortality. Data from
the Nepal Family Health Survey (1996) estimated Nepal's maternal mortality ratio (MMR) at 539 per 100,000 livebirths, which was highest among
the South-Asian countries at that time. Results from the Demographic and
Health Survey 2006 and 2016 suggested that this decreased significantly
to 281 in 2006 and 239 in 2016 (Hussein et al. 2011, Ministry of Health
et al. 2017).

According to Demographic and Health Survey data, more than half of
births (57%) took place in health facilities in 2016 compared to 19% in 2006
and only 8% in 1996. Skilled assistance during childbirth has increased from
9% in 1996 to 58% in 2016 (Ministry of Health et al. 2017). Over the last
two decades, there has been a major investment in building birthing centres
across the country and caesarean section facilities are available throughout
Nepal. In 2005, given that almost 80% of births took place at home, the
Nepali government approved, for home births, the use of the oral drug
misoprostol to tackle post-partum haemorrhage (PPH), considered to be one
of the leading causes of maternal deaths in Nepal as elsewhere in the world
(Sharma et al. 2018). Likewise, in 2002, abortion (or medical termination of

Jeevan R. Sharma and Radha Adhikari, *Politics of Childbirth in Nepal* In: *Childbirth in South Asia*.
Edited by: Clémence Jullien and Roger Jeffery, Oxford University Press. © Oxford University Press 2021.
DOI: 10.1093/oso/9780190130718.003.0011

pregnancy) was legalized to protect women's lives. Following this, termination of pregnancy is now legal, as long as it is not for sex selection, for any consenting Nepali woman, not dependent on age or marital status (Bhandari et al. 2011; Hussein et al. 2011). All these indicate that there has been a major shift in childbirth practices in Nepal.

Explanations for this notable achievement in MMR reduction have ranged from specific interventions in Nepal's health sector, such as its Safe Motherhood Programme built on result-based financing models, through a range of activities such as free antenatal and delivery services by skilled professionals and incentives to cover transport costs for mothers. Other technical interventions, such as community-based distribution of misoprostol after home births, were designed to reduce the risk of PPH of those women who could not come to health facilities for childbirth. A range of donor-funded projects have received significant technical and financial support from foreign agencies. However, it is important to note the contribution of non-health changes, such as the inflow of remittances, expansion of road networks and transportation, increased education of women and girls, and increase in girls' age of marriage, which are also believed to have brought improvements in overall health and well-being, including positive maternal and child health outcomes (Bhandari et al. 2011; Engel et al. 2013).

Based on the authors' long-term research and professional engagement on maternal health in Nepal,[1] this chapter begins with a brief social history of maternal and child health including childbirth services in Nepal, with a particular focus on the role and contribution of external donors. Donor-funded projects have fully shaped Nepal's maternal and child health priorities, policies, institutions, and programmes. The chapter, then, describes two donor-funded interventions that were designed and implemented around 2005 in an effort to address high maternal (and child) mortality by strengthening homebirth services and promoting institutional births in Nepal. First, we look at the US Agency for International Development (USAID) funded Nepal Family Health Program (NFHP) through which the oral drug misoprostol was piloted and later implemented through a national programme in Nepal. Second, we look at Aama Surakshya Karyakram (known as the Aama programme), which evolved through the Department for International Development (DfID) funded Nepal Safe Motherhood Programme (NSMP) and support for Nepal's Support for Safe Motherhood Programme (SSMP).

We analyse these two programmes and their different approaches to addressing high maternal mortality in Nepal. We also consider how these two interventions claim to have contributed to the rapid improvement in

MMR. Not only do these claims fail to acknowledge the wider sociocultural and political changes in Nepali society and their contributions to decline in MMR, but the data on MMR itself has also been highly contested. Nepal's *Population Monograph* (CBS 2014) suggested that MMR had not declined as much as is claimed by international actors and donor-funded projects.

We conclude this chapter by arguing that the push for institutional birth without adequate resources and capacity has not only led to a medicalization of childbirth but also that health services, including the provision of maternity services, have been systematically commercialized, leading to increased caesarean section rates in private health facilities in cities and towns.

A Social History of Maternal and Child Health Interventions in Nepal

While the country has a long history of Ayurvedic, homeopathic, and local shamanic practices, modern-day maternity and childbirth services are relatively new in Nepal. In 1928, the then Rana rulers sent four women (accompanied by their male guardians) to India for midwifery training.[2] Upon their return to Kathmandu in 1930, these midwives were posted in Kathmandu's Bir Hospital in the female ward (NAN 2002). Maternity and childbirth services at the time were offered entirely by local women, known as *Sudeni* or traditional birth attendants (TBAs) who did not have any formal training (Justice 1986; Maxwell with Sinha 2004; Pigg 1995).

Modern-day, Western-style maternity and childbirth services in Nepal emerged in the 1950s, triggered mainly by two key events: the first was the arrival of the Director of US mission Mr. Paul Rose with his pregnant wife in Nepal in 1951. Mr. and Mrs. Rose found no qualified midwife who could meet their expatriate standard and lifestyle to assist during the birth of their child in Nepal, so Mr. Rose requested an experienced Western-trained midwife to be sent from the British High Commission in Delhi, India (Maxwell with Sinha 2004; NAN 2002). A midwife called Ms. Junita Owen was sent to Kathmandu to assist the Roses during the birth of their baby. Ms. Owen felt that there was a pressing need to start training nurses and midwives in the country and recommended to His Majesty's Government of Nepal and to the World Health Organization (WHO) to set up a nursing and midwifery training programme. The government agreed to this request and, in 1954, the WHO sent two British nurses to Kathmandu to make all necessary preparations for training (Maxwell with Sinha 2004; NAN 2002). The second event was that in the 1950s, the then Princess Indra Rajya Laxmi Devi Shah died due to excessive bleeding, at the tender age of 24, when she already had given birth to six children. The present-day Maternity Hospital in Kathmandu was established in her memory in 1959 as the very first health facility offering maternity services in the country.

In Nepal, the fertility rate remained consistently high until the late-1960s—women were often having six or more children—and this began to come down only in the 1970s (Collumbien et al. 1997). The government's policy response to the high fertility rate in the country placed its initial focus on reducing the size of the family by offering family planning services. Nepal's Third Five-Year Economic Plan (1965–70) had family planning as a component (HMG 1962). A project was established in the maternal and child health section of the Ministry of Health and Population in 1968 with the support from USAID (Thapa 1989). In its early days, the focus of family planning was explicitly on population control to contribute to socio-economic development. The 1980s saw a more fundamental shift towards an increased emphasis on the norm of small family size and birth spacing for the health of the mother and her children (Thapa 1989).

Additionally, in the 1980s, the idea of Health for All (HfA) by 2000, through the core principle of primary healthcare was introduced. Nepal's first Long-Term Health Plan (LTHP) (1975–90) established maternal and child health services in six districts and began a movement towards an integrated primary healthcare system, which was later expanded to all 75 districts (Engel et al. 2013). Thereafter, maternal and child health services continued to remain a priority area in the national health system. In line with this, receiving support from USAID, the UN Fund for Population Activities (UNFPA) and the UN International Children's Emergency Fund (UNICEF), Nepal started a Female Community Health Volunteers (FCHV) programme in 1988, which was expanded to cover the whole of Nepal by 1995 (Glenton et al. 2010). Reports suggest that over 52,000 FCHV in Nepal not only provide health education on family planning and maternal and child health issues but also offer a number of other basic health services in their own localities (MoHP et al. 2014). These are unpaid volunteers who may nonetheless receive an allowance for taking part in training or participation in specific activities such as polio or Vitamin A tablet distribution.

The political transition in 1990 brought a further emphasis on the quality of health services including that of maternal and child health services (Bhandari et al. 2011; Engel et al. 2013). For this to be achieved, development donors increased their focus on maternal and child health. The sustained political interest on the part of the government was reflected in the National Health Policy (1991), the subsequent 5-year development plans, the Second LTHP (1997–2017), and many other policies, plans, and programmes.

In 1993, the Safe Motherhood policy and Plan of Action (1994–7) was developed. It set targets for the reduction of maternal mortality to 400 per 100,000 live births by 2000. The National Safe Motherhood policy formulated by the government in 1998 placed an emphasis on strengthening maternity services (including family planning), enhancing technical skills of healthcare providers at all levels, and strengthening referral services for the basic emergency obstetric care. Later, the Safe Motherhood Programme was integrated into the Reproductive Health Strategy (1998), with a central focus on avoiding the so-called three delays: in seeking, in reaching, and in receiving maternity and obstetric care (Bhandari et al. 2011; Engel et al. 2013).

The National Safe Motherhood and New-born Health Long Term Plan (2006–17) emphasized institutional birth and focused particularly on the development of functioning birthing centres with basic emergency obstetric care across the country. The National Policy on Skilled Birth Attendants (2006) defined who can be considered skilled birth attendants in Nepal, including competencies required for them (Engel et al. 2013).

What this account shows is that, in the past three decades, there has been a significant development in policies and interventions on maternal, child, and neonatal health services in Nepal, from almost no service available for ordinary women in the 1960s to numerous social and technical interventions being implemented in the country. One of our studies (Adhikari et al. 2018) found that development assistance in this sector is a messy assemblage of actors, institutional arrangements, and activities. It is a major challenge to get a comprehensive map of donor-funded interventions also because a large amount of aid is channelled outside the government system and runs through international and national non-governmental organizations (I/NGOs) and private consulting firms.[3]

As Nepal's long-standing development partner in the field of health and family planning, USAID has been a major player in the maternal and child health sector (Issacson et al. 2001). Given its high child mortality rate, USAID categorized Nepal among the Child Survival Priority Countries in 1990 (Issacson et al. 2001). It began to incorporate maternal and neonatal health into its assistance to Nepal in the mid to late 1990s (Issacson et al. 2001). A major $43 million 5-year project called the Child Survival/Family Health Services (CS/FHS) project was implemented between 1990 and 1998. This supported the government of Nepal's emphasis on basic needs, child survival, and reduction in population growth. It focused on services for and by women, extending services beyond the health posts and into communities, and extended the promotion of maternal and child health services. The project continued until 1998 (Issacson et al. 2001).

A notable USAID intervention in child health was the introduction of Vitamin A supplements through a programmatic intervention (Harper 2002). As a part of its effort to develop a replicable intervention that could save children's lives, USAID supported the Nepal Nutrition Intervention Project in Sarlahi district from 1988 to 1991. Implemented by Johns Hopkins University, the project looked at the impact of giving high-dose Vitamin A capsules to children between 6 and 72 months old. The success of this intervention led to the development of the National Vitamin A policy (Issacson et al. 2001). By November 1992, guidelines for implementation of the National Vitamin A Deficiency Control Program were adopted. Likewise, USAID supported a pilot programmatic intervention on Community Based Management of Acute Respiratory Infection in Jumla district, which was scaled up in 1994. It included using village health workers and FCHVs to diagnose and provide treatment (Issacson et al. 2001). USAID has funded several community-based interventions in addition to supporting health facilities in the first decade of 2000 through the NFHP phases I and II. These projects worked closely with the relevant family and child health departments to help formulate policy and guidelines (Justice et al. 2016).

Through NFHP, the government of Nepal's Family Health Division was also provided support for conducting regular Safe Motherhood Neonatal Sub-Committee meetings and various technical advisory group meetings (Justice et al. 2016). NFHP's support to enhance the knowledge and skills of health workers resulted in an increase in the number of functioning basic emergency and obstetric care sites and birthing centres, as well as improvement in the quality of care.

More recently, under the banner Health for Life Project (2012–17), USAID-funded interventions aimed to strengthen the Ministry of Health's capacity to plan, manage, and deliver high-quality family planning and maternal, neonatal, and child health services at the district and local levels. In addition to its support for the strengthening of health facilities at different levels of healthcare provision, USAID has had a strong focus on community-based interventions and its assistance has been consistently implemented through FCHVs (Justice et al. 2016). Overall, a key modality of USAID's assistance has been to generate evidence through its support for pilot programmatic interventions at the level of service delivery and to use the evidence generated to persuade policymakers to scale up those interventions (Justice et al. 2016; Sharma et al. 2018).

The UK's DfID is another key player in the field of Nepal's maternal and child health with its NSMP, which began in 1997 (Clarke et al. 2009). This resulted from a mission that recognized that the infrastructural and technical weaknesses in Nepal contributed to its high MMR. With a budget of UK£5.8 million, NSMP ran from 1997 to 2004 and was managed by London-based Options Private Limited (Barker et al. 2007). Its main objective was to reduce maternal deaths in Nepal by improving the quality of maternity services and encouraging more women to use health facilities for antenatal, childbirth, postnatal, and child health services (Bhandari et al. 2011). This was followed by the DfID-funded SSMP, which eventually led to the Aama programme.

Alongside USAID and DfID, UN agencies such as UNICEF, WHO, and UNFPA have been other major players in providing technical assistance in maternal and child health service provision in Nepal. I/NGOs and private sector organizations such as Save the Children, Care Nepal, Hellen Keller International, John Snow Inc., Research Triangle International, Plan, and JHPIEGO have worked with donors, local implementing partner NGOs, networks, and the government of Nepal to manage and provide managerial and technical assistance in improving maternal and child health services over this period in Nepal. All these actors and different interventions have played a key role in shaping the ideas and practices of childbirth in Nepal (Justice 1986; Justice et al. 2016; Sharma et al. 2018).

Two Case Studies

Below, we briefly describe and analyse two donor-funded interventions that aimed at reducing maternal death during childbirth in Nepal. Within the broad framework of reducing the maternal mortality rate in line with MDG targets, the discussion below shows that the two interventions adopted very different approaches to tackle the issues. These approaches are rooted in ideological struggles on women's agency and the politics of childbirth. As we discuss below, the distribution of misoprostol through FCHVs in Nepal was a community-based intervention aimed at addressing PPH in a resource-poor context like Nepal. The programme was based on the idea that it was possible that not all pregnant women would be able to reach health facilities and receive services offered by skilled birth attendants. It saw Nepal's FCHVs as a key cadre delivering life-saving misoprostol. The Aama programme, on the other hand, saw health institutions as the key site for childbirth, and was very much guided by a drive to bring women to health facilities to be assisted by skilled professionals. Despite differences in their approaches and ideological positions on where and who could (and should) provide life-saving services, both programmes aimed at reducing maternal mortality and were quick to claim that Nepal's success in reducing MMR resulted from their technical interventions.

Case #1: Introduction of Misoprostol through FCHVs in Nepal

Misoprostol, branded as *Matrisurakchya Chakki* in Nepali (literally translated as 'safety tablet for mothers'), was piloted and then introduced more widely in Nepal through the USAID-funded bilateral programme NFHP (Sharma et al. 2018).[4] For a resource-poor mountainous country with a high MMR caused mainly by PPH, oral misoprostol was introduced as a silver bullet to help meet the MDG target on MMR. The attraction of misoprostol was not just that it did not require a cold chain (needed for oxytocin, the existing medicine of choice for PPH), a key logistical challenge in Nepal, but also because it could be administered by FCHVs who lived in local communities (Sharma et al. 2018). In a patriarchal society, the involvement of female volunteers in the administration of misoprostol was also considered to be empowering and potentially revolutionary, although the voluntary dimension raises some questions about why it is that women contributing additional free labour should find this a form of empowerment (Glenton et al. 2010).

Initially, the government of Nepal was reluctant to start the misoprostol pilot. To address this, NFHP lobbied through several activities that included giving presentations to key stakeholders (Sharma et al. 2018). NFHP took a senior director responsible for family health to an international conference where the results of a study on community-based distribution of misoprostol in Indonesia were disseminated (Sharma et al. 2018). The managers of NFHP invited international experts to Nepal who presented the idea of using community-based distribution of misoprostol in the meeting of the National Safe Motherhood and Neonatal Sub-Committee in September 2004

(Sharma et al. 2018). There was widespread speculation that misoprostol use could undermine skilled birth attendance and institutional delivery. The use of misoprostol was a sensitive issue as Nepal did not have any legal provision for medical abortion when this discussion started in Nepal. This legal lacuna was important because misoprostol can be taken in the first and second trimesters of pregnancy to cause an abortion.

The lobbying led to the permission that the drug could be imported under recommendation by the Nepal Society of Obstetricians and Gynaecologists (NESOG) (Sharma et al. 2018). The pilot intervention was designed and implemented in Banke district in Nepal where NFHP had the necessary programmatic infrastructure and networks in place (Sharma et al. 2018).

The findings from the Banke pilot interventions were published in the *International Journal of Gynaecology & Obstetrics* in 2006 and 2010 (Rajbhandari et al. 2006, 2010). The study found that community-based distribution of misoprostol for PPH prevention can be successfully implemented under government health services in a low-resource, geographically challenging setting, resulting in much increased population-level protection against PPH (Rajbhandari et al. 2010). The government committed to a national-level programme for misoprostol and an action plan was announced. The findings of the study were further discussed in the National Safe Motherhood and Neonatal Sub-Committee meeting in September 2004, supported by the technical advisory group (TAG) (Sharma et al. 2018). The government of Nepal finally launched this as a national programme in 2009, and it is currently covering most communities in the country.

Case #2 Aama Surakshya Karyakram

The DfID-funded interventions NSMP and SSMP formed the background of the Aama programme, currently a national programme of the government of Nepal, which has two key components. Firstly, to offer free institutional childbirth services to women throughout Nepal, and secondly, to offer a cash incentive for women who travel to health facilities for childbirth services (Bhandari et al. 2011).

Initially, the NSMP, managed by London-based Options Private Limited, was piloted in three districts, and was later expanded to a further six districts. A key outcome of the project was that it highlighted for the officials at the Ministry of Health and Population and other key stakeholders the importance of skilled birth attendants and emergency obstetric care (Bhandari et al. 2011; Clarke et al. 2009). Although the direct outcome of NSMP was limited as it was only implemented in nine districts, it had a critical impact on the development of policies and programmes in the field of safe motherhood. Once NSMP came to an end, building on the same framework of NSMP, the DfID funded the SSMP, which worked closely with the government of Nepal from 2005 to 2010, with the aim of improving maternal and newborn health and survival, especially for the poor and excluded communities (Bhandari et al. 2011). The budget of this programme was UK£23 million and was again managed by Options Private Limited. SSMP supported the delivery of and access to quality maternal and newborn health services, including human resources, infrastructure investments, equipment and supplies, and comprehensive abortion care.

Under SSMP, the government started the Maternity Incentive Scheme (MIS) in 2005. This was implemented to help mitigate the high financial costs of childbirth (transport, loss of earnings, support and medical costs) so that poor women, many of them in remote rural areas, could reach health facilities (Bhandari et al. 2011). It was designed to ensure that there was no cost associated with child delivery in the institution (fees were waived), and that other costs associated with travel and purchasing of materials needed for childbirth would be compensated as incentives. A commentary authored by those associated with programme in the *International Journal of Obstetrics and Gynecology* stated:

> During the life of SSMP, CEOC expanded from 34 facilities in 26 districts in 2004/5 to 94 facilities in 33 districts in 2009/10 (including the private sector) and BEOC facilities from 18 in 2004/5 to 105 in 2009/10, almost all public sector. The met need for EOC grew by 2–3% per year, and by 2–9% for caesarean section. The number of health posts offering 24-hour delivery increased from almost zero to over 400 health posts and 137 subhealth posts. SSMP provided support to expand SBA training sites and invested in advanced training, advocating for the establishment of the Diploma in Gynaecology and Obstetrics course in 2010.[5]
>
> Bhandari et. al. 2011: 27

This intervention was directly based on the evidence generated through a study commissioned by NSMP (Clarke et al. 2009). This was probably the first time a policy to offer demand-side financing was introduced in Nepal. Later in 2007, the name was changed to SDIP (Safe Delivery Incentive

Programme). This time, provision was made to offer incentives also to health workers and health facilities offering childbirth services.

The experience of NSMP and SSMP was the genesis of the Aama programme in Nepal. The 'Aama Programme Implementation Guidelines', published by the Ministry of Health and Population in 2009, specifies the services to be funded, the tariffs for reimbursement, and the system for claiming and reporting on free maternity services (Family Health Division/ Department of Health Services 2009). For example, the payment to health staff per facility delivery was revised from NRs 200 to NRs 300. Similarly, for health facilities, the stated rates of NRs 1,000 per normal delivery, NRs 3,000 per complicated delivery and NRs 5,000 per caesarean section in the guidelines has been replaced, after consultation with providers, with: normal delivery at health facility with fewer than 25 beds, NRs 1,000; normal delivery at health facility with 25 and more beds, NRs 1,500; complicated delivery NRs 3,000; C-Section NRs 7,000. When Auxiliary Health Workers (AHWs) felt excluded and protested, it was agreed that they would also get a share of the incentive.

When the Aama programme started in 2009, the DfID funded 80% of its cost for the first 18 months. In addition to funding, the DfID provided technical assistance for implementation and monitoring. At present, there is no direct funding from donors to the Aama programme although technical support continues to be provided as a part of DfID's overall technical support to Nepal's Health Sector Plan.

Millennium Development Goal Targets And Ideological Struggle

With global development consensus on the MDGs and SDGs, MMR has become a major global health indicator (Storeng and Béhague 2017). While exact figures are not available—because maternal mortality is a relatively rare event and linking women's deaths to maternity-related causes (particularly where an abortion is involved) is difficult in the absence of death certification—global health institutions spend considerable resources to calculate and measure MMR. The growing significance of MMR and its use in programmatic interventions in global development is directly linked to new norms of 'evidence based development', 'value for money', and pressure to 'demonstrate or produce positive impact', and to do so in such a way that the results can be attributed to specific interventions (Adams 2016; Storeng and Béhague 2017).

Despite their decreasing share in the national budget, development donors command considerable policy leverage in resource-poor countries like Nepal. They are often at the forefront in attributing progress in MMR to the programmatic and technical interventions that they fund. USAID supported the NFHP, which, for example, has been credited with improving maternal and child health services in Nepal through interventions such as the promotion of family planning and distribution of misoprostol, among others. Likewise, the DfID-supported programmes such as NSMP and SSMP are cited as key contributors, by the programme implementers and donors, to increasing access to quality maternal health services, thereby impacting on MMR reduction.

In 2014, the government of Nepal published its *Population Monograph*, based on its decennial census of 2011. According to this report:

> The Nepal 2011 census reported a total of 9,654 deaths of women of repro-ductive age, of which 2,159 were deaths during pregnancy, childbirth and puerperium in the period 12 months prior to the census ... A total of 22.4% of deaths of women in Nepal are due to deaths during pregnancy, child-birth and puerperium. The highest proportion of maternal deaths (31.8%) is found in the age group 20–24 and declines with an increase in the age of women. Based on the observed maternal deaths and the observed female deaths, the MMR for Nepal was 663.
>
> CBS 2014: 153

The report confirmed Nepal's MMR at 480 (adjusted for mortality and fer-tility), considerably higher than the estimates of 190 that had been presented by a consortium of UN, WHO, UNICEF, and the World Bank (recall that data from the Demographic and Health Survey suggested that MMR was 281 in 2006 and 239 in 2016) (CBS 2014).[6] It is possible that the choice of dif-ferent independent variables in regression analysis resulted in the discrepan-cies from the figure produced by UN agencies (CBS 2014).

Nepal's census data on MMR should have caused alarm bells to ring for policymakers who had been hailing Nepal's success and for donor-funded programmes that had been attributing this decline in maternal mortality to their interventions. The data discrepancies raised uncomfortable questions about the existing narratives on the contribution of the interventions to the rapid reduction of MMR in Nepal (Sharma 2016). There has, however, so far been no official comment on this from government sources.

Although the data from *Population Monograph* suggests that the progress on MMR might not have been as impressive as claimed, there is very little debate on this discrepancy, beyond an implicit recognition that different metrics and computing methods produce different results. However, this explanation is uncritical, because data have powerful consequences on resource distribution, and more importantly in saving lives (Sharma 2016).

While MMR's popularity as an indicator can be linked to it being included as an MDG (Storeng and Béhague 2017), it should not be conflated with maternal health as a priority area in national health policy. Taking MMR as the target of interventions can disrupt more holistic approaches to maternal health. Programmes become shaped by what can be measured (Adams 2016), and not necessarily by what might bring the greatest and most sustainable improvements in women's health. Target-focused development results in so-called high impact interventions that have quick and obvious impacts, while less attention is given to those that contribute to strengthening efforts in the wider health system, broader gender inequalities, or structural issues. Further, while MMR helps give an aggregate longitudinal and global comparative picture, and helps in mobilizing global policy responses and resources, it is not necessarily the best way to understand maternal health and childbirth, which are rooted in gender politics (Morgan et al. 2017). For example, poor access to nutrition and healthcare, persistent high workload and, prevalence of anaemia make women more vulnerable to ill-health and specific maternal health complications (Furuta and Salway 2006, Brunson 2010).

In a country like Nepal, subnational data and data disaggregation by intersections of inequalities often give a very different picture than an aggregate picture offered by measurement of MMR. The 2011 Nepal Family Health Survey suggested that there was significant variation in reproductive health service uptake by women from different caste, educational, and economic backgrounds (Hussein et al. 2011; Pandey et al. 2013). This analysis showed that the unmet need for contraception among Muslims (39%), Dalits (35%), and Hill Janajati women (34%) was much higher than in other groups. Likewise, the Newars and Hill Bahun women have the highest percentages of delivery in a health facility and are supported by skilled birth attendants, while Tarai and Madhesi Dalits have the lowest levels for both services. Similarly, levels of undernourishment and anaemia are higher in women from all the Tarai-based castes and ethnic groups than in other categories. All this shows a different narrative based on persistent inequalities, rather than a simple overall success. Data disaggregation and acknowledging those who have been left out of 'Nepal's success' remain key challenges.

Conclusion

Childbirth in Nepal has been medicalized and institutionalized through a range of social, technical, and policy interventions. Linked to donor-funded programmes, and global policies and targets, particularly in the past two to three decades, the very idea and the practice of childbirth has gone through a profound transformation in Nepal. Within the broader humanitarian mission to save the lives of mothers and children, Nepal has become a site of experimentation of different social and technical interventions. The government of Nepal has warmly welcomed and received these interventions that have significantly shaped maternity and childbirth experiences in the country.

The accountability agenda has given preference to 'high impact' interventions where measurements get priority over structural determinants. Interventions are funded for their potential to demonstrate measurable results. Indicators such as MMR and their measurements have become key modalities for generating evidence, allocating resources and accounting for interventions. Consideration for tracking, monitoring, and generating evidence determine the feasibility and desirability of maternal and child health interventions. An emerging debate on how gender and intersecting inequalities of caste, ethnicity, class, region, and religion shape maternal health remains at the margins when 'high impact' interventions whose results can be measured are prioritized.

Despite a massive move to the institutionalization of childbirth, health facilities remain under-resourced and under-staffed to cope with the increased demand for services. While statistics show that home birth has declined, it has not completely disappeared. Legalization of abortion in 2002 and its widespread use through various private and non-profit outlets was another major shift that has possibly shaped the meaning of pregnancy and childbirth, which remains under-researched.

Another critical theme that remains under-researched is the systematic commercialization with increase in Caesarean section birth in private health facilities in cities and towns. Although comprehensive statistics are not available, media reports have indicated a steady rise in caesarean section births, particularly in private health facilities (such as private nursing homes and teaching hospitals). A report in the *Kathmandu Post* on 23 March 2019 quotes a focal person at the Family Welfare Division of the Ministry of Health and Population: 'In some private hospitals, 95 percent of the deliveries are caesarean'. A study in Patan Hospital found that the caesarean section rate increased from 23% in 2005 to 44% in 2014 (Lamichhane and Singh 2015). Professionals and activists working in the maternal and child health field have expressed great concern about this trend, and the potential harmful consequences for maternal and infant health, as well as suggesting that caesarean section birth has been seen as a commercial opportunity for private practitioners. Findings from some small-scale studies in Nepal also suggest the same (Dhakal Rai et al. 2018; Subedi 2012). Media reports suggest that some caesarean sections are apparently not medically required but chosen by relatively wealthy women to avoid labour pains (Poudel 2019). The caesarean section rate amongst poor rural women remains much lower than that of affluent urban women (Aryal 2012; Hussein et al. 2011; Lamichhane et al. 2011; Pandey et al. 2013).

Wider international literature also suggests that there is a global rise in caesarean section birth, particularly in affluent countries (Betrán et al. 2016; Boerma et al. 2018; WHO 2015). This potentially life-saving service has been overused in private sectors at the same time that it is not available in resource-poor contexts, indicating a huge disparity in maternal and child health service provision nationally as well as internationally (Betrán et al. 2016; Boerma et al. 2018). The alarming rate at which caesarean section is increasing in private healthcare facilities in Nepal appears to show the commercialization of childbirth in Nepal.

As indicated above, MMR statistics presented by various sources are not consistent. Estimates produced by UN agencies are based on a regression model, whereas Nepal Demographic and Health Survey data is based on the sisterhood method, and the data on MMR from the *Population Monograph* (CBS 2014) is based on the analysis of census data. It is not sufficient to attribute MMR figures to different data sources as these data have political implications when they are attributed to interventions and policies. The existence of three sets of data on MMR, all produced by or with the technical support of donors, raises a question on whether MMR is the right index to measure maternal health.

Many sociopolitical changes are happening in Nepal and its society has gone through profound transformations, including rising income levels, increasing school enrolments and education levels, expanding road networks and private sector healthcare providers, an increase in the average age for marriage, growing access to contraceptives, and changing gender dynamics. There has been a shift from a deeply hierarchical social order, where gender differences were supported by a combination of ritual, law, political economy, and state, to one where the call for women's rights is widespread (Adhikari and Sharma 2018). Yet, given ample evidence of how caste, class, ethnicity, religion, and political patronage shape gender relations in Nepali society, the benefits of social changes are not equally shared by all women and it is critical that anthropological and sociological inquiry focus on heterogeneity of childbirth experiences. Anthropological investigations are well suited to address this lacuna on the implications of these rapid changes alongside the changing landscape of global interventions and privatization of healthcare that are rapidly changing childbirth experiences and practices in Nepal.

Notes

1. The lead author has been researching the maternal and child health system in Nepal for over 15 years; the second author has practised as a professional nurse-midwife and has been researching maternal and child health for over three decades in Nepal.
2. The Rana dynasty ruled Nepal from 1846 to 1951 in a very autocratic fashion, providing limited education, health, or any other public services available for the general public (Whelpton 2005).
3. Between 1 May 2014 and 31 October 2016, both the authors were involved in a research project titled 'New Norms and Forms of Development: Brokerage in Maternal and Child Health Service Development and Delivery in Nepal and Malawi'. It was funded by a grant awarded by the Economic and Social Research Council and Department for International Development in the UK.
4. For further information on institutional arrangements of NFHP and the involvement of different organizations in it, see Sharma et al. (2018).
5. EOC is essential emergency obstetric care, either basic (B) or comprehensive (C). SBA stands for skilled birth attendant.
6. In the Nepal Census of 2011, information on death during pregnancy, childbirth, and puerperium (the 6 weeks following childbirth) was collected from all households in the country for the 12 months prior to the census (CBS 2014: 143)

References

Adams, Vincanne. 2016. *Metrics: What Counts in Global Health*: Durham NC and London: Duke University Press.

Adhikari, Radha, and Jeevan Raj Sharma. 2018. 'Stereotyping Women as Victims'. *Nepali Times*, 13 June. Accessed 30 September 2019. https://www.nepalitimes. com/uncategorized/stereotyping-women-as-victims/

Aryal, I. 2012. 'Sharp Rise in C-section: Let Women Deliver Babies Naturally'. *The Rising Nepal* 3 August.

Barker, Carol E., Cherry E. Bird, Ajit Pradhan, and Ganga Shakya. 2007. 'Support to the Safe Motherhood Programme in Nepal: An Integrated Approach'. *Reproductive Health Matters* 15 (30): 81–90.

Betrán, Ana Pilar, Jianfeng Ye, Anne-Beth Moller, Jun Zhang, A. Metin Gülmezoglu, and Maria Regina Torloni. 2016. 'The Increasing Trend in Caesarean Section Rates: Global, Regional and National Estimates: 1990–2014'. *PloS one* 11 (2). doi: 10.1371/journal.pone.0148343.

Bhandari, A., M. Gordon, and G. Shakya. 2011. 'Reducing Maternal Mortality in Nepal'. *BJOG: An International Journal of Obstetrics & Gynaecology* 118: 26–30.

Boerma, Ties, Carine Ronsmans, Dessalegn Y. Melesse, Aluisio J.D. Barros, Fernando C. Barros, Liang Juan, Ann-Beth Moller, Lale Say, Ahmad Reza Hosseinpoor, and Mu Yi. 2018. 'Global Epidemiology of Use of and Disparities in Caesarean Sections'. *The Lancet* 392 (10155): 1341–8.

Brunson, Jan. 2010. 'Confronting Maternal Mortality, Controlling Birth in Nepal: The Gendered Politics of Receiving Biomedical Care at Birth'. *Social Science & Medicine* 71 (10): 1719–27.

CBS (Central Bureau of Statistics/Nepal). 2014. *Population Monograph of Nepal*. vol. 1. Kathmandu, Nepal: Central Bureau of Statistics, Government of Nepal.

Clarke, Jeremy, Enrique Mendizabal, Henri Leturque, Veronica Walford, and Mark Pearson. 2009. *DFID Influencing in The Health Sector: A Preliminary Assessment of Cost Effectiveness*. DFID Working Paper 33. London: DFID.

Collumbien, Martine, Ian M. Timæus, and Laxmi Acharya. 1997. 'The Onset of Fertility Decline in Nepal: A Reinterpretation'. In *CPS Research Papers 97–2*. London: London School of Hygiene and Tropical Medicine.

Devkota, Bhimsen, and Edwin R. van Teijlingen. 2010. 'Understanding Effects of Armed Conflict on Health Outcomes: The Case of Nepal'. *Conflict and Health* 4 (1): 20. doi: 10.1186/1752-1505-4-20.

Dhakal Rai, S., Pramod Regmi, Edwin Van Teijlingen, Juliet Wood, Ganesh Dangal, and K. Dhakal. 2018. 'Rising Rate of Caesarean Section in Urban Nepal'. *Journal of Nepal Health Research Council* 16 (41): 479–80.

Engel, Jakob, Jonathan Glennie, Shiva Raj Adhikari, Sanju Wagle Bhattarai, Devi Prasad Prasai, and Fiona Samuels. 2013. 'Nepal's Story: Understanding Improvements in Maternal Health'. In *Research Reports and Studies*. London: Overseas Development Institute.

Family Health Division/Department of Health Services. 2009. *Safer Mother Programme Working Guideline-2065/2009*. Kathmandu: Ministry of Health & Population, Government of Nepal.

Furuta, Marie, and Sarah Salway. 2006. 'Women's Position within the Household as a Determinant of Maternal Health Care Use in Nepal'. *International Family Planning Perspectives* 32 (1): 17–27.

Glenton, Claire, Inger B. Scheel, Sabina Pradhan, Simon Lewin, Stephen Hodgins, and Vijaya Shrestha. 2010. 'The Female Community Health Volunteer Programme in Nepal: Decision Makers' Perceptions of Volunteerism, Payment and Other Incentives'. *Social Science & Medicine* 70 (12): 1920–7.

Harper, Ian. 2002. 'Capsular Promise as Public Health: A Critique of the Nepal National Vitamin A Programme'. *Studies in Nepali History and Society* 7 (1): 137–73.

His Majesty's Government. 1962. *Second Three-Year Plan (1962–65)*. Kathmandu: Government of Nepal.

Hussein, Julia, Jacqueline Bell, Maureen Dar Iang, Natasha Mesko, Jenny Amery, and Wendy Graham. 2011. 'An Appraisal of the Maternal Mortality Decline in Nepal'. *PloS one* 6 (5). doi: https://doi.org/10.1371/journal.pone.0019898

Isaacson, Joel M., C.A. Skerry, K. Moran, and K.M. Kalavan. 2001. *Half-a-Century of Development: The History of US Assistance to Nepal, 1951–2001*. Kathmandu, Nepal: United States Agency for International Development.

Justice, Judith. 1986. *Policies, Plans, and People: Culture and Health Development in Nepal*. Berkeley, CA: University of California Press.

Justice, Judith, S. Pokhrel, Jeevan Raj Sharma, M. Sharma, A. Shrestha, S.S. Thapa, G. Gautam, H. Shakya, and D. Shrestha. 2016. 'Twenty-Five Year Review of Assistance to Nepal's Health Sector'. In *Global Health Performance Cycle Improvement Project*. Washington DC: United States Agency for International Development.

Lamichhane, Basant, and A. Singh. 2015. 'Changing Trend of Instrumental Vaginal Deliveries at Patan Hospital'. *Nepal Journal of Obstetrics and Gynaecology* 10 (2): 33–5. doi: 10.3126/njog.v10i2.14333.

Lamichhane, Prabhat, Tabetha Harken, Mahesh Puri, Philip D. Darney, Maya Blum, Cynthia C. Harper, and Jillian T. Henderson. 2011. 'Sex-Selective Abortion in Nepal: A Qualitative Study of Health Workers' Perspectives'. *Women's Health Issues* 21 (3): S37–S41.

Maxwell, Mary, with Rebecca Sinha. 2004. *Nurses Were Needed at the Top of the World: The First Fifty Years of Professional Nursing in Nepal, 1951–2001*. Kathmandu: TU Institute of Medicine, Lalitpur Nursing Campus.

Ministry of Health, Nepal, New ERA, and ICF. 2017. *Nepal Demographic and Health Survey 2016*. Kathmandu, Nepal: Ministry of Health, Nepal.

Ministry of Health and Population (MoHP), Department of Health Services, Family Health Division. 2014. *Female Community Health Volunteer National Survey Report*. Kathmandu: Ministry of Health Nepal.

Morgan, Rosemary, Moses Tetui, Rornald Muhumuza Kananura, Elizabeth Ekirapa-Kiracho, and A.S. George. 2017. 'Gender Dynamics Affecting Maternal Health and Health Care Access and Use in Uganda'. *Health Policy and Planning* 32 (suppl_5): v13–v21.

NAN (Nursing Association of Nepal). 2002. *History of Nursing in Nepal 1890–2002*. Kathmandu: Lazimpat.

Pandey, Jhabindra Prasad, Megha Raj Dhakal, Sujan Karki, Pradeep Poudel, and Meeta Sainju Pradhan. 2013. *Maternal and Child Health in Nepal: The Effects of Caste, Ethnicity, and Regional Identity: Further Analysis of the 2011 Nepal Demographic* and Health Survey. *Kathmandu and Calverton*, Maryland, USA: Nepal Ministry of Health and Population, New ERA and ICF International.

Pigg, Stacy Leigh. 1995. 'Acronyms and Effacement: Traditional Medical Practitioners (TMP) in International Health Development'. *Social Science & Medicine* 41 (1): 47–68. doi: https://doi.org/10.1016/0277-9536(94)00311-G.

Poudel, A. 2019. 'Caesarean Section Rate is Alarmingly High in Nepal, but Officials Say They Can't Control It'. *Kathmandu Post*. March 23. Accessed 30 September 2019. https://kathmandupost.com/health/2019/03/23/test-20190323201101

Rajbhandari, Swaraj, Asha Pun, Stephen Hodgins, and Peeyoosh Kumar Rajendra. 2006. 'Prevention of Postpartum Haemorrhage at Homebirth with Use of Misoprostol in Banke District, Nepal'. *International Journal of Gynecology & Obstetrics* 94: S143–4.

Rajbhandari, Swaraj, Stephen Hodgins, Harshad Sanghvi, Robert McPherson, Yasho V. Pradhan, Abdullah H. Baqui, and Misoprostol Study Group. 2010. 'Expanding Uterotonic Protection Following Childbirth through Community-Based Distribution of Misoprostol: Operations Research Study in Nepal'. *International Journal of Gynecology & Obstetrics* 108 (3): 282–8.

Sharma, Jeevan R. 2016. 'Looking beyond Maternal Mortality Rates in Maternal Health Interventions: Lessons from Nepal'. *South Asia@ LSE*.

Sharma, Jeevan Raj, Rekha Khatri, and Ian Harper. 2018. 'Accountability and Generating Evidence for Global Health: Misoprostol in Nepal'. *IDS Bulletin* 49 (2): 49–64.

Storeng, Katerini T., and Dominique P. Béhague. 2017. '"Guilty Until Proven Innocent": The Contested Use of Maternal Mortality Indicators in Global Health'. *Critical Public Health* 27 (2): 163–76.

Subedi, Shanti 2012. 'Rising Rate of Caesarean Section—a Year Review'. *Journal of Nobel Medical College* 1 (2): 72–76.

Thapa, Shyam. 1989. 'A Decade of Nepal's Family Planning Program: Achievements and Prospects'. *Studies in Family Planning* 20 (1): 38–52.

Whelpton, John. 2005. *A History of Nepal*. Cambridge: Cambridge University Press.

SECTION 6
NEW TECHNOLOGIES

12

Discourses of Childlessness in Bangladesh

Power and Agency

Mirza Taslima Sultana

Jokhon take niya daktarer kache ber hoite parlam tokhon shomoi shesh
(When I could make him [my husband] agree to go to the doctor, then it was too late)

This excerpt is from my interview with Parul. She was expressing her frustration that she could not convince her husband to go to the doctor earlier. She thought that they needed to seek help from a doctor for two reasons: firstly, because her husband was not interested in having sexual intercourse with her; and secondly, because of their childlessness. According to her, biomedical treatment was needed to resolve both these problems. Nevertheless, in this excerpt 'age' emerges as a crucial issue for conception: when she said 'it was too late' she was referring to her age as the reason for the failure to seek treatments such as intra-uterine insemination (IUI) or in vitro fertilization (IVF).[1] It was also 'too late' as her husband had prioritized his extended family's interest, which was to marry off his sisters first. He was unwilling to have a baby earlier. The interview also sheds light on the discursive practices that render both sexuality and childlessness as medical problems in contemporary Bangladesh. While I was interviewing Parul, I was primarily concerned with how she was dealing with childlessness. However, she implied that her childlessness was the result of the absence of sexual relations with her husband. In this chapter, I explore the ideas and norms around medical treatment and alternative treatments that emerged in the accounts of my interviewees—the 11 middle-class Bengali women who sought treatment for their childlessness.[2] I conducted these interviews in Bangladesh (Dhaka and another big city)[3] in 2010 as a part of my PhD research. This investigation informs my analysis of the links between biomedical power and childlessness as they are emerging in Bangladesh.

Mirza Taslima Sultana, *Discourses of Childlessness in Bangladesh* In: *Childbirth in South Asia.* Edited by: Clémence Jullien and Roger Jeffery, Oxford University Press. © Oxford University Press 2021. DOI: 10.1093/oso/9780190130718.003.0012

Though the advent of IVF technology in Bangladesh is mostly celebrated, Farida Akhter, the director of Unnayan Bikalper Nitinirdharoni Gobeshona (UBINIG, the Policy Research for Development Alternatives) has contended that, through the turn to the procedures of IVF to solve the problem of childlessness, women's bodies have been undermined (Akhter 2010). UBINIG is an active organization associated with FINRRAGE (Feminist International Network of Resistance to Reproductive and Genetic Engineering), an international network of feminists. Members of FINRRAGE have characterized medicine as a patriarchal instrument and have argued that the female body has increasingly become the site of technological interventions in childbirth and other conditions associated with reproduction. FINRRAGE was the first collective agency organized at the international level to address the uses and abuses of 'new' reproductive technologies as they impact on women's bodies. They campaigned actively against 'population control programmes' in developing countries, including Bangladesh. Since 1950, there have been population control programmes in developing countries throughout the world, organized on the assumption that the world's population is increasing alarmingly, especially in poor countries. Excessive population was identified as contributing to the poverty of these countries. As a result, population control programmes have targets of population growth that have been met by processes of forced sterilization and other abusive initiatives. In her article, Akhter noted that the technologies and the doctors who 'direct' them are mainly given the credit for their successes. She has argued against the use of IVF in Bangladesh, invoking FINRRAGE's declaration of 1989:

> We protest the use of in vitro fertilization in countries that wish to increase or decrease births. It is a dangerous dehumanizing technology. It uses women as living test sites and producers of eggs and embryos as raw material to enable scientists to work towards further control over the production and quality control of human beings and international business to accumulate profit (Akhter 2010).[4]

In this declaration, scientists and doctors are framed as possessing sovereign power. In contrast, women who cannot have children 'naturally' are presented as being passive victims of this power. I acknowledge Farida Akhter's contributions in Bangladesh with regard to critically assessing reproductive technologies and contraception practices. Nevertheless, I cannot totally agree with her position on the procedures of IVF, which she argues are undermining women's bodies.

Throsby (2004) both acknowledges and challenges FINRRAGE's substantial criticisms of developments around assisted reproductive technology (ART). She argues that members of FINRRAGE failed to recognize that these technologies might not be bad for all women; rather, they might have different meanings for different women. In her research on IVF failure she showed how treatment failures have implications for women, producing a normalized form of childlessness that may be more socially acceptable and enabling some women to deal with childlessness. I find Throsby's approach more relevant than Farida Akhter's position.

Like Throsby (2004), other feminist scholars in the field of reproductive technologies, including Margaret Lock and Patricia Kaufert (Lock et al. 1998), Emily Martin (1991, 1992), and Charis Thompson (2005), do not consider women to be merely the victims of biomedicine or ART. For example, Lock and Kaufert consider that women are 'pragmatic' in relation to biomedicine, as in their constraints women always learn to choose the best use of what is available. In this chapter I show what meanings, within the prevailing meaning of childlessness, are being mediated by the women who sought help of the technology encountering the ART as well as IVF practitioner's construction of childlessness. It will be evident that these technologies are not the same for all women.

I describe the backdrop of this chapter in the first section. The second section addresses the accounts from my interviews that illustrate the different trajectories my interviewees pursued in dealing with childlessness. The third section focuses on the issue of the so-called perfect age for ART treatments and accounts of resistance. The fourth section explores my interviewees' stories of their experiences of IVF and of reports of malpractice among medical practitioners. This fourth section also includes my consideration of accounts of the side effects of biomedical treatments. In the fifth section I discuss the women's accounts of the restrictions that limit their technological options.

Background

Due to its population growth, Bangladesh has been the primary focus of various population control policies since its birth in 1971 (Mookherjee 2007a)[5] Social science and anthropological research has predominantly focused on the importance of motherhood for Bangladeshi women (Blanchet 1984; Kotalová 1993; Nahar 2007). However, this chapter will show that the middle-class Muslim women I interviewed did not always prioritize achieving motherhood over their career.

According to some Bangladesh medical journals (such as *Orion* and *Bangladesh*), infertility is defined as the inability to conceive a child after one year of 'regular' heterosexual intercourse (Haque 2010). There is, however, no agreement about this definition. According to one prominent gynaecologist (Chowdhury and Chowdhury 2009), infertility is a label that is applied after 1 or 2 years of regular intercourse without contraception. However, in parallel with modern medical discourses, childlessness is also recognized in various local perceptions. According to these, there is no specific time limit involved in recognizing the inability to conceive, nor is there a precise age limit.

There are also specific terms available in the Bengali language to designate the failure to conceive: women who cannot have children are referred to as *banja* or *bandha*, while men are referred to as *aatkura*. In general, these terms connote the stigmatized and derogatory status of the women and men who do not have children. Still, *banja* or *bandha* connote more stigmatization than aatkura. In Bangladeshi society, which is predominantly Muslim, having children is often regarded as being dependent not only on the state of the body, but also on divine wishes (Allah or God). So the meanings of banja or aatkura are not the same as the meaning of the biomedical term, infertility. Infertility designates a physiological condition. However, it is a common belief that the inability of the body to reproduce may be due to a curse or the unhappiness of Allah/God. Therefore, to overcome this problem, it is quite common to have recourse to both biomedical and various religious measures to ensure divine satisfaction and intervention.

In general, Bangladeshi society is portrayed as 'pronatalist' and reproduction is considered a primary goal for married people.[6] There is a widespread assumption that women's main role is to reproduce. Here women are highly valued as mothers. Indeed, there is a Bangladeshi proverb: '*Nari mayer jati*' ('woman belongs to the category of mother'), which implies that the term 'woman' is synonymous with the term 'mother'. Hence, achieving motherhood is deemed to be very important for most women. This chapter challenges this dominant view and investigates how some women consider motherhood in different ways for themselves.

In the context of the strong emphasis on motherhood in Bangladesh, the advent of IVF has been particularly significant. This technological development is related to the pattern of health provision in Bangladesh. Treatment for infertility is yet to be included in the public health sector in the country. Hence, those who seek infertility treatment must turn to private clinics and hospitals. Financially well-off couples went abroad to countries like India, Singapore, or Thailand to access IVF prior to 2001, when the first IVF triplets were born in Bangladesh, and many such couples continue to do so. More affluent couples go to the USA or European countries for their IVF cycles.

According to Akhter (1996) the public sector health service in Bangladesh is primarily focused on population control, based on a state programme established in 1965 (although there was short gap from 1971 to 1972 because of the liberation war). She traces how, since 1973, the government of Bangladesh has pursued population and family planning programmes with renewed vigour. Hence, fertility (rather than infertility) is regarded as the major problem of the country and excessive fertility is often identified as the main cause of poverty. This is portrayed as a circumstance that must be controlled to ensure national development. Therefore, the reproductive health services that the government of Bangladesh provides do not prioritize infertility.[7]

All big state medical college hospitals have provision for infertility treatment in their gynaecology sections, but IVF procedures are not provided in these hospitals. However, in 2020, an IVF center was established at the Dhaka medical college hospital. In Bangabandhu Sheikh Mujib Medical University (the only postgraduate medical college in Bangladesh) in Dhaka, there is a unit to deal with patients who present with infertility. Besides this, one other state institution, Mohammadpur Fertility Services and Training Centre (MFSTC) in Dhaka, also provides services for problems associated with infertility. However, neither of these have provision for IVF procedures.

The situation is different in the private sector. In 2001, the first births using ART occurred in Bangladesh when triplets were born at a private clinic in Dhaka. The event received huge media coverage (*Daily Janakantha*, 31 May and 1 June 2001; *Daily Jugantor*, 31 May 2001; *Daily Star*, 31 May 2001). Since then, several doctors have been practising ART in the capital city. By 2010, there were 20 private clinics or hospitals in Dhaka where IVF was available.

To understand health provision in Bangladesh it is necessary to take account of private sector initiatives. With limited resources, the public sector provides cheap and affordable health support to a large section of Bangladeshi society, but middle- and upper-class people in both rural and urban areas usually prefer not to use state services. There are two reasons for this: firstly, they generally do not find the medical care provided in those facilities to be of a sufficiently high standard. Secondly, many of them prefer to be treated in a segregated setting away from the working class and the poor. Health insurance is not institutionalized and few people who access private health facilities usually have any insurance. This relatively small section of the society, regardless of cost, is ready to spend on their health needs and it is this sector of Bangladeshi society who access and support ART initiatives in Bangladesh.

Daktar Dekhao ('Seek Advice from the Doctor'): Seeking Solutions

daktaarer kache jao, daktaarer kache jao (urgently seek help from a doctor)

This excerpt is again from the interview with Parul. She invoked this comment as advice from her mother-in-law, who had inquired '*bachha hoi na keno?*' ('why are you not conceiving?'). Parul added that her mother-in-law also said to Parul's elder sister, '*Bachha nite kao*' ('tell her to get pregnant'). Parul recalled disclosing to her mother-in-law that her husband was not interested in having sexual intercourse very often and that if he did, it did not last long. Besides her mother-in-law, one of her colleagues (meaning to wish her well) was also curious. She said: 'Why is it [conception] not happening, Parul? . . . We are eagerly waiting to hear something'. Here, we see that both her friend and her mother-in-law were concerned and anxious because, after a period of marriage, no children had been produced.

The statement also shows that these women considered not only childlessness but also problems with sexual relationships were biomedical issues. Parul's relatives' and her colleague's suggestions reflect the idea that biomedical treatment is the best solution for childlessness. They might have considered it best because in Bangladesh biomedicine is frequently portrayed as continually developing for human well-being. This emerged also in the interview with another participant, Nuri. She sought advice from her experienced neighbours about seeing a good doctor as she had been trying to conceive but without success.

Afrin Khan was also concerned about her failure to conceive a child after her second marriage and she decided to go to a doctor.[8] She had conceived twice in her first marriage, but had miscarriages; in her second marriage she had never conceived. She reported that, 'when it had been six months or one year, I felt bad as I still did not conceive, and then went to see a gynaecologist'. After a period of waiting to see if they could conceive, like Afrin Khan, the women I interviewed usually went to doctors for treatment.

Aakhi and Maya also continued seeing doctors, taking tests and medications and were continuously under the gaze of biomedicine. Likewise, Aleya took eight years to decide to have a baby. She said she prioritized finishing her PhD before starting to think about having a child. After her PhD she wanted to have a baby, but she found that she was unable to conceive and went to see a doctor.

My interviews revealed the strong hold of the idea that biomedicine is the best solution for childlessness. Moreover, at least in one case, biomedicine was also regarded as a means of resolving problems in the sexual relationship between a husband and wife. Among my eleven interviewees, nine went to see a doctor immediately after realizing they had problems in conceiving. The other two interviewees went to gynaecologists, but for different problems. These interviewees demonstrated that they placed great faith in biomedicine in dealing with their reproductive difficulties. These women themselves depended on biomedicine, in the hope that their reproductive capabilities could be optimized.

When Roksana sought treatment after only one year of her marriage, she said that the doctor was surprised and laughed at her as she was worried so early about not having a child. Throsby uses the idea of the 'rational' when she explained that an interviewee wanted to discursively situate herself in the realm of rationality, rather than identifying with uncontrolled desperation (Throsby 2004: 73). Borrowing from her idea of rationality, I see that although the knowledge around treating childlessness suggests that one should seek medical help as early as possible, a rational individual woman should select a 'perfect time' (neither 'too late' nor 'too early') for seeking biomedical help.

During my interviews I sensed that not only Roksana but all these women were keen to emphasize that they had never neglected their reproductive problems. Since they saw biomedicine as offering ways out of childlessness, seeking treatment early showed them to be 'responsible'. Some of them were frustrated as they took the issue of time seriously and wanted to be responsible, yet the results were not always positive.

For example, having sought treatment responsibly, within the 'proper time', Tandra found that she still could not conceive. Like all the other interviewees, Tandra had sought treatment from more than one doctor. This suggests that they were strategic in their relationships with doctors and in seeking medical advice. Their comments also showed that they weighed up the various suggestions made by these doctors before reaching a conclusion. Tandra's comments are indicative of her active role in seeking treatment: 'I didn't sit

[idle] ... I was running to doctors one after another and it is going on and on'. While this 'running' from one doctor to another makes Tandra subject to the decisions of the doctors, she was also strategizing about the various processes of her treatment. Even though the interviewed women tended to prefer biomedicine in seeking solutions for their childlessness, they did not only depend on it. While they underwent biomedical treatment, most concurrently sought other forms of help that were available in Bangladesh.

Alternatives to Biomedicine

Women sought different types of alternatives to biomedical solutions. These ranged from *kabiraji*, to *pir-fakir* and to deliver themselves to the mercy of Allah through their everyday prayer.[9] However, although most of my interviewees tended to inform me of the alternatives they had already explored, they did not seem to want to elaborate much on them. They may not have wanted to represent themselves as deviant or irrational. This is similar to Throsby's idea of rationality: her interviewees did not want to link themselves to disreputable therapies—in their case, these were identified with alternative medicine, which might make it appear that they were acting in uncontrolled desperation. Rather, the women she interviewed preferred to locate themselves in 'the realm of determined rationality' (Throsby 2004: 73).

From my interviews, I inferred that all these women who sought solutions for their childlessness were informed by some knowledge of biomedicine. In addition, it was not just the interviewed women, but also their relatives and friends who insisted that biomedical science was the best option. Here, the power of biomedicine was perceptible. It was demonstrated not only by women's own self-knowledge but also with how they were policed by relatives and friends to be responsible and rational. This power is traceable by exploring the challenges that emerged in the interviewed women's accounts. Specifically, while seeking treatment, the women themselves actively made comparisons between doctors and among the different advice they gave, using their judgement to appraise the information and guidance provided.

They also explored other options available in Bangladesh, although they mentioned such activities only briefly in the interviews. They presented their belief that Allah would solve their problems as responsible behaviour, and that there were no contradictions between seeking treatment from biomedicine and maintaining their religious beliefs. They believed that successful and unsuccessful outcomes of treatment also depended upon divine intervention. In the end they wanted to satisfy Allah and seek his support to have a child.

'Main Switch Tai Nosto' ('Your Main Switch Is Damaged'): Encountering Categorizations

aapnar main switch e noshto heye gese, aapni boyoshko ekjon fatty mohila, apnar abar bachha hobe ki kore! (Your main switch is damaged, you are a fat and aged woman, and how would you get pregnant!)

After her second marriage Aakhi had an operation to remove an ovarian cyst in India. Later on, at the age of 38, Aakhi went to see a famous doctor who made the comment quoted above. The comment labelled Aakhi with reference to three categories: a damaged 'main switch' (organ damage and ovaries and other reproductive organs that are the 'main switch' for women), fat, and aged. As the ovaries are crucial reproductive organs the doctor identified these as the 'main switch'. According to him these were 'damaged' because she had had an ovarian cyst removed from one of her ovaries. It seems that to this doctor, women's bodies are only for reproduction. He constituted Aakhi as an unfit reproductive female body, unfit to have a child. Aakhi indicated that, upon hearing this, she became very upset. She and her husband decided they would not see this doctor again.

In her second marriage Aakhi did conceive, but she had a miscarriage before realizing she was pregnant. She then went to different doctors, and they asked her to do all the available tests. One of the doctors suggested she was capable of conceiving at her age of 44, which she put forward as medical evidence coming from the doctor. The pathological tests and the doctor's explanation of the size of the follicle categorized her as fit for pregnancy. She reported that the doctor told her that 'if a follicle's size is 19 mm, it could be [transformed as] a baby', and she was told that her follicle's size was 23 mm. The doctor even had given her the hope that if she conceived in that month, she would have twins. Here the biomedical knowledge and tests influenced Aakhi to rethink her ability to have a child. Aakhi participated in the process of regulating her reproductive body. These processes and the doctor's opinion accentuated a desire for motherhood in Aakhi at an age when, usually, fertility decreased.

Aleya went to the same doctor Aakhi had gone to after her second marriage. Aleya reported that this doctor told her 'something', and as a result she had cried for 4 days. When I asked her what the doctor said, she could not remember it. She said:

> I might not want to remember this, so I forgot. I recall that I was crying for four days after listening to this comment. Another one came [a patient] after eight months of marriage. [So] the doctor commented on this, 'One comes after eight years of marriage [Aleya] and another comes after eight months' . . . [However] it was awkward that he dealt with two patients at a time, while he talked to one, another was waiting inside the room.[10] . . . I felt that as I was in a good job and held a good position, that might have influenced him to say such a comment. I usually do not forget, but I may have forgotten this because I wish to forget.

In this excerpt, Aleya was explaining her discomfort with the doctor. Aleya thought that as she was highly educated, seeking treatment from a doctor was an obvious step for her. However, when the doctor made a negative comment about her childlessness, Aleya was distressed. Nevertheless, she reported that she had 'forgotten' the details of the comment.

It was clear that the doctor did not like the 8-year gap between Aleya's marriage and her seeking treatment. Aleya also speculated that the doctor disapproved of the success she had had in her career and was thus, perhaps, implying that she had not prioritized motherhood. If so, this doctor might have been working within Bangladeshi society's prevailing idea that reproduction is women's prime function. Since Aleya was non-compliant, the doctor's discursive practices effectively disciplined her. Interestingly, Aleya had decided to try to have a child during the eighth year of her marriage, after finishing her PhD, suggesting that she was therefore already resisting such disciplining processes. However, she said:

> As I do not have this *hahakaar* (despair) for a baby, like many others around me, I was not like them. This is because I have a big world, without a child my world does not end. I never felt that if I do not have a baby I would die. Yet I was thinking, in the future if I have any regrets, when I would not have the time, as the time for having a baby is limited for women . . . I know it is a risk to have a baby after thirty-five. But I have passed thirty-five years to finish my PhD. I could do nothing, at that time . . . So I did not try for a baby at the *right hour*.

In this account Aleya resisted the idea that a woman's only purpose in life was reproduction. However, at the same time, she was reasserting that trying for a baby is legitimate at a late age because it might allay any future regrets. This means that she agreed on the importance of reproduction, but that she did not prioritize it above all else. Moreover, if she did not conceive at the ideal age, she knew what the medical account of the consequences were. While Aleya was resisting the idea that a woman's prime task is reproduction and that there is a fixed age limit for reproduction, she still desired a baby. That did not stop her prioritizing the completion of her PhD. Aleya's case shows that the women I interviewed did not necessarily follow medical advice about the ideal age for having a baby, because they make decisions according to their own circumstances. Nevertheless, Aleya did conceive with IUI.

I have been focusing on two interviewees, both of whom had experiences of different ARTs. However, they did not undergo IVF. Aakhi could not pursue IVF as she was beyond the age limit for such treatment in Bangladesh, although she did indicate that one of her doctors had encouraged her to seek technological help. Aleya was ready to have IVF but she conceived with the prior procedure of IUI that had been suggested by the doctor. Both women had experienced unsettling behaviour from a doctor related to their age. These doctors talked as if reproduction was the prime function for women. Aakhi had been undergoing medical treatment during her first marriage for a long time because she had prioritized reproduction. Also, in the second marriage, due to the gap for having child and treating an ovarian cyst, she went to a doctor who considered her effort at too 'late' an age. Aleya also believed a woman's primary role is reproduction, even though completing her PhD was her priority. These narratives show the forms of body discipline and the impact of the norm that women should prioritize reproduction: they were complying with this to some extent although neither of these women was totally submissive to these ideas. Hence, they also developed strategies to defy them and establish other priorities in their lives.

Roksana, Tandra, Fatema, and Ruby went through the processes of IVF cycles. Roksana was told that the pathological tests showed that because of her previous suffering from tuberculosis, her fallopian tubes were blocked, and IVF could be the only solution for her. However, the other three were suggested IVFs after undergoing treatment for some years without any result. They were told that for an 'unexplained reason' they could not conceive naturally.

All the women I interviewed, whether they had undergone IVF or not, were disciplined as well as convinced that one of women's key roles is to reproduce. With all the different tests they underwent they were under continuous surveillance. They confirmed, in their accounts, biomedical explanations of their childlessness, and thus they were influenced by the specific version of the knowledge of biomedicine that they were offered by their doctor(s). It is also evident that they all depended on biomedical treatment to identify and solve their problems. Only one of the interviewees had a child with IUI. Among the interviewed women, eight were considered too old to pursue IVF. Both of those who did not get the chance to undergo IVF because of their age and those who had undergone IVF without success still considered that this technology was helpful to the women who wanted to have baby but could not conceive. I will discuss in the following section what some of these women told me about their terrible encounters with ART practitioners while they were searching for ways to conceive.

'Shob Prescription Puraye Fellam' ('I Burnt All the Prescriptions'): Frustration with, and Resistance to, Biomedical Treatments

Aakhi: I had changed my doctor . . . I had been seeing this doctor continuously for seven years . . . She gave me medicine and asked me to go to see her at the thirteenth day of my period for an internal ultrasound image. Then she gave me an injection with the explanation that my follicles needed to be matured . . . By doing this, taking the hormonal injections repeatedly, my body was swelling up. After each three-month gap in each month, I was given these hormonal injections . . . I had been taking the medicine for the entire month, but conception was not occurring. By this I was frustrated. One day I burnt all the prescriptions and said that 'I won't go to see this doctor anymore'.

Aakhi describes an instance that occurred during her first marriage. When I met her, I found her to be overweight. She told me that before this treatment she was known as a pretty woman. During the process of ART treatment, she had undergone 7 years of a bodily regimen involving various medicines, such as injections, as well as regular ultrasound images of her body. Aakhi herself depended on biomedicine, which she thought would solve the problem of her childlessness. This said, she was very critical of the treatment, as she thought she had lost her feminine appeal because of it. Since the treatment was unsuccessful, burning the prescriptions was clearly an act of despondency and frustration. During all this, she had conceived with bio-medical aid, but she lost the child after the birth, claiming negligence on the part of the gynaecologist.

Nuri also shared with me an account of bad experiences during her treatment. She said that she had consulted a doctor who was well known for the treatment of infertility. After one year of treatment the practitioner told her that he wanted to check her internal system, and that this would require a laparoscopy. She was informed that they would make a small hole around her navel for the investigation, which proved inconclusive. The doctor said he could not find the source of her problems and he consulted her husband about operating on her stomach (conducting a laparotomy). Despite Nuri being unconscious, her husband gave consent to the procedure. This was an operation that she later found out was inappropriate.

Nuri consulted doctors in Madras, India, and Dubai, UAE, where both doctors expressed the opinion that the 'laparotomy' was the incorrect procedure. The doctor in Dubai also informed her that, because of the operation, her reproductive organs were not in a 'normal' place. This explanation made her believe that her reproductive organs were no longer 'perfect' and, as a result, that her possibilities of conception were hindered. She subsequently underwent three courses of IUI, and two IVF, all without success.

Nuri also relayed a story of a terrible experience in one of the IVF procedures she underwent. During the first IVF cycle, she suffered from an overdose of egg stimulating injections.[11] She spent three lakh Bangladeshi Taka (nearly £3,000) for this cycle. Nuri felt frustrated by the expense, and the high levels of intervention she had experienced. She also indicated that her doctor had suggested that she have another cycle soon. She expressed her dissatisfaction with this proposal as she evaluated that her body would not permit this. She did have another cycle of IVF, but in a different clinic. There she said she had to spend three and half lakh Taka (around £3,500).[12] She was happier about that experience, as the clinic did not pressurize her to undergo an IVF cycle, although the cycle was unsuccessful.

Ruby also told me about her experience of a wrong (bhul) treatment.[13] She recalled:

I was so desperate, so I did not think [about an after effect]. One white-skinned doctor came, she just wanted to test her instruments, she got [me as] a live specimen. To treat endometriosis she did a laparotomy. She opened the stomach! . . . She did the operation and told me that 'there was a cyst in you'. She removed the cyst . . . This lady was actually testing hormonal drugs.

This excerpt shows how mistrust circulates around the doctors and clinics, although generally they believe in biomedicine but at the practice level this doubt prevails. As the doctor was a foreigner, this might have further increased mistrust of the clinic. Moreover, there is a general awareness that the state does not oversee the activities of private clinics and, therefore, that they may violate ethical standards. Ruby was thus speculating that the 'foreign doctor' might have used her body as a vehicle for testing drugs.

In all the above cases, these women not only evaluated the clinics but also medical practice as a whole. They describe the medical provision they experienced in Bangladesh as not always reliable and sometimes problematic. Also, as Ruby's comments suggest, while the presence of a foreign doctor might have connoted better treatment, her derogatory reference to the doctor as 'white-skinned' highlights suspicions about the presence of a foreigner. Ruby was not a passive recipient of medical surveillance. While undergoing biomedical procedures, she was continually evaluating the services of the doctors and clinics in Bangladesh as substandard. Later in 1988, she had one failed IVF cycle in Manchester, after which she did not want any further treatments.

In both Nuri's and Ruby's cases biomedical practices had brought them suffering, resulting in damage to their bodies that made conception less likely. Yet this did not stop them from seeking further treatment: they repeatedly enrolled for medical treatment and continued believing that biomedicine is a progressive force. Aakhi, Aleya, Nuri, and Ruby reported negative experiences either with doctors or clinics. They were clearly active in the processes of these treatments. They made judgements of the clinics, staff, and the doctors. In the following subsection I will continue this discussion considering my interviewees' accounts of their experiences of IVF failure.

Failure in IVF: Hope and Pain

Nuri underwent three IUI and two IVF procedures. When I asked about her feeling about the treatments, she replied:

Each time the feeling was not same. After the first unsuccessful result, I thought maybe it will work next time. Maybe the hope was there but when it fails for the second time and the third time then I felt really bad, I was psychologically shattered . . . after the unsuccessful last cycle . . . they told me you can have another cycle but, because of your age, the possibility is very thin. I was then mentally and physically exhausted; I did not want to go through this again.

The production of hope for the potential success of IVF is apparent in this excerpt. In the first IVF cycle her hope for a positive outcome was strong. Yet she was less enthusiastic in subsequent cycles. In addition, she reflected upon the economic burden that she and her husband undertook. With savings and some economic support from family members they could arrange a certain number of cycles (she meant both IUIs and IVFs), even one abroad. After these failures, the burden was, of course, more than financial and Nuri comments about the psychological trauma she felt. While there had been possibilities of a negative result, the desire to undergo the regulatory process for a biological, 'natural' child outweighed these concerns.

Ruby also said that after the first cycle of IVF in Manchester, in 1988, she did not want to try again, despite the doctor's suggestion. She said: 'I did not go back next time. I was shattered. Rather I told my husband that if you want to take another wife, [you] go for it. I do not want to go through this'. Ruby had IVF treatment when it was not available in Bangladesh. She told me at the beginning of this statement that she had consented to her eggs being used in research. She described this fact, laughing embarrassedly, and said that it was a matter of 'desperateness'. Here again, Ruby may be constructing 'desperateness' as the action of a person who is not 'normal' or 'rational', and pointing out that consenting to her eggs being used in research was neither normal nor rational according to the norms of Bangladeshi society.

Throsby's analysis suggested that, because of the unproven nature of alternative therapies, one of her interviewees in the UK rejected them as an option. Throsby contends that this interviewee seemed anxious to avoid identification with the category of 'irrational' and 'uncontrolled desperation' (Throsby 2004: 73). In Ruby's case the issue was not about turning to unproven alternative therapies but consenting to her eggs being used in scientific research. Although science is not considered an unproven realm, consenting to her body parts being used in scientific experiments seems to have contradicted her beliefs and practices. Therefore, she described her 'consent' as an act of desperation, a position that may be associated with 'irrationality'.

Roksana had undergone two cycles of IVF. She reported that she and her husband had taken a bank loan for the first IVF cycle. After the unsuccessful cycle she was upset. She described her experiences when she decided to stop the treatment: 'I would not go through this procedure again, [because] there is no guarantee [of a positive outcome], it is an uncertain procedure, isn't it? And when it fails the mental and physical burden is too tough to bear'. She mentioned both mental and physical suffering. Roksana was regulated by injections, various tests, and measurements. In fact, the bank loan had contributed to instability in her marriage, as did the unsuccessful IVF treatment. Interestingly, Roksana knew the procedure did not promise conception, but that it still created a sense of expectation, or hope for a positive result. She underwent another cycle that also proved to be unsuccessful. Fascinatingly, Roksana discussed her last miscarriage laughingly. Failure to have a child might be painful but she described it, nevertheless, in a relaxed way. However, she was critical of the practitioners. She suggested that they were not adequately concerned about IVF failures as they did not monitor or analyse the success of the procedures.

After having undergone three cycles of IVF, Tandra reflected that, 'it [the procedure] is painful and our body degenerates as we get older, how can I bear the side effects of IVF?' Fatema similarly said: 'I could not accept mentally that I would have the treatment again. At the beginning, there was an expectation'. While both Tandra and Fatema were concerned about bodily discomfort, we can see here that stopping IVF served as a way of restoring their lives to 'normal'. Moreover, money was an important issue for them. They did not want to continue being 'abnormal', childless, and yet enduring endless bodily discomforts and the high cost of recurrent treatments.

Most of the women I interviewed provided one or two examples of unpleasantness they had had while seeking or having treatment. Moreover, they also told me about the side effects of the different treatments they experienced. The way they have evaluated the performances of the doctors, clinics, and nurses, as well as their experiences of using different medications, demonstrate that they were active and were strategic. While they were often critical about some of the treatments they received, they did not, as whole, reject biomedical practices entirely. Rather, they expressed a desire for changes in biomedical practice that would eliminate suffering from the malpractices of doctors in future.

'Donor Dhormiobhabe Acceptable Na' ('A Donor Is Not Religiously Acceptable'): Boundaries In Technological Options

Nuri: *Na onno donor theke neoar prosnoi ashe na jehetu eta acceptable na* (no, accepting from a donor [relating to sperm, egg, surrogacy] is out of question as it is not acceptable [religiously])

The comment quoted above was Nuri's reply to my question about donor sperm and eggs, and surrogacy. When I inquired further about the religious issues she mentioned, she explained: 'No, you just try to imagine the marital relationship. How shall we explain [to some woman about] bearing the sperm of another man [not her husband]? Though sexual intercourse has not occurred . . . sperm of an unknown man needs to be carried. The religious bar is there but I feel it is also unethical'. She drew my attention to the general conventions about marital relationships in Bangladesh. She seemed to imply that taking a donor's sperm was like committing 'infidelity'. Although, as she states, intercourse is not involved, the relationship with the donor and the child would raise issues for her, and socially the child would be considered illegitimate. Similarly, she mentioned that surrogacy was problematic for her.

At the end of our conversation she declared that 'life is too short to make these kinds of decisions'. She might, therefore, have also been concerned about her afterlife. According to Islam, every person will be resurrected after death and will be judged based on how they conducted their lives. Therefore, she decided that she would not opt for donor's eggs or sperm or surrogacy. Nuri's account was like Roksana's. She said she would prefer to adopt a child. Roksana was affirming the discourse that children should be born within heterosexual marriage and gestated in the wife's body. Likewise, Fatema said she was offered options of donation and surrogacy in the UK, which she refused as she considered them prohibited by Islam.

In her work, Inhorn (2003) refers to a fatwa issued at Al-Azhar University, an important Islamic religious institution in Egypt. Her interviewees denied any third-party donation (sperm or egg donation and surrogacy) following the fatwa directed at the university, even though IVF and intracytoplasmic sperm injection (within IVF treatment) were not generally regarded as illicit. As Inhorn explained, the official body of Al-Azhar University represents a dominant strand within the Sunni sect of Islam (Inhorn 2003: 106, 107). Islam et al. (2013), analysing Islamic bioethics, argue that Islam prohibits all third-party involvement in IVF procedures, so in Bangladesh, they should not be practised.

Nuri, Fatema, Tandra, Roksana, and Ruby all went through IVF cycles. However, all of them said that they did not want to take the options of egg or sperm donation, or surrogacy. These women are subjected through the axis of knowledge, which includes social norms and religion. Although Tandra and Nuri said that they were never offered the option of donor eggs and sperm, or surrogacy, Roksana assumed that these options were actually being used by the clinic. She commented:

> Of course, the uses of these [options] are frequent . . . secretly they [clinics/ doctors] are employing these options. Because when I did IVF for the first time, the lab assistant of the clinic called me and said: 'the condition of your eggs is very good, you do not need so many [eggs], if you donate a few eggs, many cannot produce one egg even, and in that case you need to spend only fifty percent of the fee to have another cycle. Both you and other people will benefit'. Now why did she tell me this? . . . These are procedures which are at odds with our religious precepts, which is not possible for me because where my egg will go, who would be (receiving) it . . . The whole social relationships will be broken down; which is actually happening secretly.

Roksana was clearly convinced that egg donation is occurring in the clinic she visited. She speculated about the availability of other options as well. She confirmed her belief in the importance of the relationship of the married father and mother who produce children. Beyond this she was not comfortable, and she assumed that by taking up options of egg and sperm donation, the proper forms of familial relationship could be eroded. In this respect, women like Roksana were adhering to the socio-religious discourse that children should be born only within heterosexual marriages. Hence, they considered that sperm and egg donations, as well as surrogacy, were in direct conflict with this.

Roksana's concern is primarily religious. I could not find any Bangladeshi laws that clearly acknowledged her concern. In exercise of the power conferred under section 5 (22) of the Bangladesh Medical and Dental Council Act 2010, the Bangladesh Medical and Dental Research Council, a regulatory body under the Ministry of Health and Family Welfare (MOHFW), sets out the professional conduct and ethics to be followed by registered medical practitioners. At article 2.3.4.3, there is a code of conduct regarding prenatal diagnosis and intervention, scientifically assisted reproduction, and related technology that says:

1. Doctors who perform any human reproductive technology procedure or conduct research on human embryos or other harvested fertilized ovum should ensure that it complies with relevant National law and regulations, if there is any.

2. Informed consent for artificial insemination should be taken only after disclosure of risks, benefits and likely success rate of the method proposed and potential alternative methods to the patients/ clients. Any individual or couple contemplating artificial insemination by husband should be counselled about the full range of infectious and genetic diseases for which the donor or recipient can be screened for including communicable disease agents and diseases.[14]

However, there is no national law or regulation yet regarding human reproductive technology procedures. In the second rule, whether there is any third-party involvement in the procedure is vague or unclear. Though here only 'and' is mentioned regarding artificial insemination, this possibility is applicable to both the individual or the couple. Hence, this procedure might be possible to use for the individual who is out of wedlock.

Conclusion

In Bangladeshi media, IVF procedures are portrayed as an important development in biomedical practices and as offering potential solutions to the problem of childlessness (*Daily Jugantor*, 31 May 2001; *Daily Star*, 31 May 2001). I have noted that biomedical solutions, particularly IVF, spurred hope and inspiration among the women I interviewed. Here, I have presented the discourses that emerged in these women's accounts of how they negotiated a path through their reproductive difficulties. Following Foucault's idea of biopower, I have indicated how these women were categorized and standardized in terms of having 'fit' or 'unfit' reproductive bodies.[15] I identified four different discourses that emerged in my interviews: biomedical science is progressive and benevolent; reproduction is subject to Allah's wishes; reproduction is women's prime function; and finally, children should be born within the framework of a heterosexual marriage.

While the exercise of biopower is implicit in the power of technological assistance when dealing with childlessness, these technological practices do not operate from a single centre, nor are the women I interviewed passive in engaging with treatments. Rather, I see the women I interviewed as actively negotiating their relationship to their difficulties in reproduction and to ART, particularly IVF.

Moreover, it has emerged that biomedicine and religion are two institutions that are sometimes in tension concerning reproduction in

Bangladesh. I argue that hopes for technological solutions for childlessness did figure prominently in the accounts of the women I interviewed. However, I have also shown that biomedical discourses are often incompatible with established religious discourses. The women I interviewed operated within the existing discourses, but on occasion did challenge them.

This discussion has showed how the interviewed women actively negotiated the options available in, around, and outside of IVF procedures. They evaluated, criticized, and even challenged some biomedical practices and some forms of assisted reproductive technologies. Nonetheless, the interviewed women's experiences of suffering from malpractices by the ART (including IVF) practitioners suggest that both guidelines and a regulatory body are necessary in Bangladesh to supervise ART practices. I have also shown that not all the technological options were acceptable for reasons of religious belief in Bangladesh. Therefore, the women I interviewed often tried IVF with the hope that, if Allah wished it, the technology would be successful.

Notes

1. For IUI, doctors place prepared sperm into a woman's womb (uterus) at the time of ovulation, often combined with fertility drugs to increase the chances of conception. For IVF, eggs are removed from a woman's ovaries and mixed with sperm (fertilized) in a laboratory culture dish (in vitro).

2. I selected 11 women who could not conceive 'naturally' and who are from affluent and solvent backgrounds, so they can afford IVF procedures. These women are established, and some are well known in Bangladesh. To keep them anonymous, I removed all the information that could disclose their identities.

3. For the sake of anonymity of the interviewees, the name of the city is omitted.

4. http://www.ubinig.org/index.php/home/showAerticle/26/english, accessed 6 March 2020.

5. Various scholars have also highlighted how Bangladesh has been a laboratory for population control (Murphy 2012) and vaccine trials (Das and Dasgupta 2000).

6. Marcia Inhorn also identifies 'non-western societies' as being 'pronatalist' (Inhorn 2003: 7, 8).

7. In policy documents, such as the National Health Policy 2011, 4th Health, Population and Nutrition Sector Programme 2017–22, and the 7th Five-Year Plan 2016–20, fertility reduction is the main concern. In addition to reducing maternal

mortality, ensuring safe childbirth is the next priority. None of these policy documents considered childlessness as a problem worthy of attention.

8. Afrin Khan's first marriage was ended by her as she could not get along with her mother-in-law, who tried to control her movements and her involvements with the outer world. Being an MA from a public university, Afrin Khan could not agree with this. She had a good relationship with her husband. However, he did not have a stable job, and also when difficulties arose with her mother-in-law, he used to keep quiet. Therefore, she got a divorce.

9. Kabiraji are religious healers who usually attribute healing power to food and drink by uttering verses of the Qur'an; pir-fakir are healers who combined the knowledge of Ayurveda and Unani in treating patients.

10. In Bangladesh, it is common that during busy hours in a doctor's private practice more than one patient might be attended to at the same time. Occasionally, besides a consultant doctor, a junior doctor is present to assist.

11. Nuri explained to me that generally certain amounts of injections are given to the patients to stimulate egg production, but the dose she had been given had exceeded the usual limit.

12. In 2012, at the time of my research, 1 Taka = $0.0122 or £0.0079.

13. Ruby mentioned this wrong treatment at a time when there was no infrastructure to lodge a complaint against the medical practitioners and clinics. However, in 2018, under the *Shastha Batayon*, citizens can make complaints against any public or private health service by calling 16263: http://www.dghs.gov.bd/images/docs/Health%20Bulletin/Health%20Bulletin%202018%20Pre%20print%20version.pdf, accessed 10 May 2019.

14. http://bmdc.org.bd/wp-content/uploads/2017/10/EthicsBookMakeupfinal.pdf, accessed 12 May 2019.

15. Biopower, according to Foucault, denotes the 'numerous and diverse techniques for achieving subjugation and control of population' (Foucault 1978: 140). This concept means the constructive machinery of power over life through the regulation of birth, health, sex, and mortality. Biopower is not associated with violent imposition; rather, it revolves around rendering bodies malleable. Foucault's proposition is that, since the eighteenth century, many techniques have been developed to make the body docile so that it can be 'subjected, used, transformed and improved' (Foucault 1991: 136).

References

Akhter, Farida. 1996. *Depopulating Bangladesh: Essays on the Politics of Fertility.* Dhaka: Narigrantha Prabartana.

Akhter, Farida. 2010. 'Commercialisation of Women's Infertility'. Accessed 10 March 2021. http://www.ubinig.org/index.php/home/showAerticle/26/english

Bangladesh Medical and Dental Council. 'Code of Professional Conduct Etiquette and Ethics'. Accessed 12 May 2019. http://bmdc.org.bd/wp-content/uploads/2017/10/EthicsBookMakeupfinal.pdf

Blanchet, Thérèse. 1984. *Meanings and Rituals of Birth in Rural Bangladesh: Women, Pollution and Marginality*. Dhaka: University Press.

Chowdhury, T. A., and T. J. Chowdhury. 2009. 'An Overview of Infertility'. *Orion Medical Journal* 32 (1): 610–11.

Das, Veena, and Abhijit Dasgupta. 2000. 'Scientific and Political Representations: Cholera Vaccine in India'. *Economic and Political Weekly* 19 (26): 633–44.

Foucault, Michel. 1978. *The History of Sexuality*. vol. 1. London: Penguin Books.

Foucault, Michel. 1991. *Discipline and Punish*. London: Penguin Books.

Government of People's Republic of Bangladesh. Ministry of Health and Family Planning. 'Health Population and Nutrition Sector Development Program (HPNSDP)'. 2011–16. Accessed 22 December 2012. http://www.mohfw.gov.bd/index.php?option=com_content&view=article&id=166&Itemid=150&lang=en

Government of People's Republic of Bangladesh. Directorate General of Health Service, Ministry of Health and Family Planning. 2010. 'National Guidelines on Medical Biotechnology'. Accessed 16 June 2013. http://www.dghs.gov.bd/en/index.php/medical-biotechnology/114-medical-biotechnology-resource-book

Government of People's Republic of Bangladesh, Ministry of Health and Family Welfare. 2018. 'Health Bulletin'. Accessed 10 May 2019. http://www.dghs.gov.bd/images/docs/Health%20Bulletin/Health%20Bulletin%202018%20Pre%20print%20version.pdf

Haque, Shahara. 2010. 'Role of Hysterosalpingography for Evaluation of Infertility'. *Bangladesh Medical Journal* 39 (1): 16–23.

Inhorn, Marcia. 2003. *Local Babies Global Science: Gender, Religion and In-Vitro Fertilization in Egypt*. New York & London: Routledge.

Islam, Shamim, Rusli Bin Nordin, and Hanapi Bin Mohammed. 2013. 'Ethical Considerations on In Vitro Fertilisation Technology in Bangladesh'. *Bangladesh Journal of Medical Science* 12 (2): 121–8. doi: 10.3329/bjms.v12i2.14938.

Kotalová, Jitka. 1993. *Belonging to Others: Cultural Construction of Womanhood in a Village in Bangladesh*. Stockholm: Uppsala University.

Lock, Margaret, Patricia Alice Kaufert, and Alan Harwood. 1998. *Pragmatic Women and Body Politics*. Cambridge: Cambridge University Press.

Martin, Emily. 1991. 'The Egg and the Sperm: How Science Has Constructed a Romance Based on Stereotypical Male–Female Roles'. *Signs: Journal of Women in Culture and Society* 16 (3): 485–501. doi: http://www.jstor.org/stable/3174586.

Martin, Emily. 1992. *The Woman in the Body: A Cultural Analysis Of Reproduction*. Boston: Beacon Press.

Mookherjee, Nayanika. 2007. 'Available Motherhood: Legal Technologies, "State of Exception" and the Dekinning of "War-Babies" in Bangladesh'. *Childhood* 14 (3): 339–54. doi: 10.1177/0907568207079213.

Murphy, M. 2012. *Seizing the Means of Reproduction: Entanglements of Feminism, Health, and Technoscience*. Durham, NC: Duke University Press.

Nahar, Papreen. 2007. 'Childless in Bangladesh: Suffering and Resilience among Rural and Urban Women'. PhD, Medical Anthropology, University of Amsterdam.

Thompson, Charis. 2005. *Making Parents: The Ontological Choreography of Reproductive Technologies*. Cambridge, MA & London: MIT Press.

Throsby, Karen. 2004. *When IVF Fails: Feminism, Infertility and the Negotiation of Normality*. Basingstoke: Palgrave Macmillan.

13

Digitalizing Community Health

Mobile Phones to Improve Maternal Health in Rural India

Marine Al Dahdah and Alok Kumar

Introduction

In 2015, Samia, 7 months pregnant, is working in the fields close to her house in Samastipur district, Bihar. Her mobile phone rings, she picks up and listens to Dr Anita, who encourages her to go to the hospital for her final antenatal visit. Samia has never given birth at the hospital, but, encouraged by the community health worker of her village, she is paying one rupee to receive this message. Dr Anita is a voice recorded on a platform developed in the United States. She is the central character of the Motech Programme implemented by the Bill and Melinda Gates Foundation in partnership with the government of India. Samia's story is not a fiction. We met many women in rural Bihar who, like Samia, did not have electricity, running water, or toilets in their homes, but had a mobile phone, and thereby became the targets for new policies, using mobile technology as a central instrument. With the widespread use of mobile phones in the Global South, digital tools are attracting growing interest from international aid actors as well as local governments—positioning digital technology as an essential driver of economic growth and an obvious solution to many social problems. Initiated by multiple actors from the digital industry, these policies revive old questions about technological development, relations between the market sector and states, and the role of knowledge and techniques in inequalities between North and South. Often undertaken in the name of the fight against corruption or to improve failing public services, these initiatives reconfigure the state, the perimeter, and access to health services—in this case, to maternal and reproductive health.

Since 2010, mobile operators, pharmaceutical companies, philanthropic foundations, and NGOs have been massively investing in 'mHealth' projects

Marine Al Dahdah and Alok Kumar, *Digitalizing Community Health* In: *Childbirth in South Asia*.
Edited by: Clémence Jullien and Roger Jeffery, Oxford University Press. © Oxford University Press 2021.
DOI: 10.1093/oso/9780190130718.003.0013

involving the use of mobile technologies to improve women's health. Several international initiatives have suggested using mobile phones to intervene in maternal health issues (Philbrick 2013). The field of maternal health has been a priority target for mHealth programmes and is therefore particularly relevant to explore the development of mHealth and its associated transformations. Nevertheless, so far these interventions have been little researched. The available articles on the subject consist in literature reviews of existing mHealth projects (Noordam et al. 2011; Tamrat and Kachnowski 2012), or reports on the use of mobile phones by a group of midwives in Northern Indonesia (Chib 2010) and in Thai border areas (Kaewkungwal et al. 2010). Our research mobilizes a wide literature combining Science, Technology, and Society studies (STS) and Information and Communication Sciences to reveal inequalities at work in these new socio-technical artefacts. It focuses on assemblages of people, techniques, and institutions that are shaped by dynamics of power in an increasingly digitally mediated world. It is based on empirical data collected between 2014 and 2018 in Ghana and India, and it focuses particularly on the case of Mobile Technology for Community Health (Motech).[1]

Motech was launched in Ghana in 2010. Its goal is to improve maternal and child health in rural areas in developing countries by supporting women during pregnancy and up to the first birthday of the newborn. The project combines health information modules, SMS alerts, and vocal messages for women and community health workers. The aim of Motech is to become a 'global' platform used worldwide to support and improve the quality and accessibility of health information and care. From 2012, the Motech project was exported to Bihar on the basis of the Ghanaian experience. In previous articles, we have discussed the promise of easier access to health information thanks to mobile phones that emerged with Motech's implementation. Far from the original assumption of a cheap, ubiquitous, and universal tool, we have shown, firstly, that the accessibility of mobile phones and of Motech for women in rural Bihar was not obvious, and, secondly, that mobile phones as gendered technologies were enhancing rather than reducing gender inequalities (Al Dahdah and Kumar 2018). We also unpacked the participation of states, funders, and implementers in such technological partnerships, to highlight the philanthropic as well as commercial interests that fuel mHealth projects like Motech, by focusing on the role of private foundations and technology providers involved in it (Al Dahdah 2019). This article focuses specifically on the Bihari deployment of Motech, and allows us to study in detail the significant involvement of community health workers in such a digital programme.

Motech officials regularly remind their interlocutors that the aim of the programme is to save the lives of women and children and that 'information' is at the heart of this humanitarian endeavour. Thus, in this chapter we analyse two different information strategies and mobile applications developed by the Motech programme to 'save lives' in Bihar, and their specific forms and content. These two strategies both involved community health workers as intermediaries to subscribe women to the messaging system and one even required them to deliver the mobile-based messages to women; both needed these workers to use mobile phones on a daily basis. The main difference between the two strategies is the extent to which the community health workers are active agents in disseminating information. For Motech, the mobile phone is central to the patient–carer relationship as the community health worker uses the mobile to interact with the patient. This vision of the health worker assisted by the mobile is twofold; on one hand, it would make the community health worker efficient and omniscient; on the other hand, it calls into question the knowledge of health workers and their autonomy by introducing an automated system of communication. Is the community health worker enhanced or replaced by mobile applications? Can their role as intermediaries between the patient and the machine be challenged? In order to answer these questions we will focus specifically on the particular role attributed to community health workers in the deployment of these mobile applications. Indeed, three mobile applications were tested in Bihar through the Motech project, but we propose to analyse the two that were dedicated to health information, involving both patients and health workers: Mobile Kunji and Kilkari.[2] Kilkari is the application we described at the beginning of the chapter; a fully automated system that sends vocal health messages once a week to registered numbers of women for 1 rupee per message. Mobile Kunji is a set of illustrated cards given to community health workers that contain short codes that community health workers dial on their mobile phone in order to make pregnant women listen to the same vocal health messages. These vocal messages have information on care during pregnancy, childbirth, and childcare practices. Both applications are perfect illustrations of two very different paths that mHealth devices can take, and they have been evaluated very differently. Whereas Mobile Kunji will never be extended outside Bihar, Kilkari has been chosen to be nationally implemented in India. In the conclusion, we reflect on the consequences of such decisions for community health.

Weak Community Health Infrastructures to Support Digital Programmes

The International Conference on Primary Health Care, organized by WHO and UNICEF in 1978 in Alma-Ata, highlighted the crucial role of community health workers (CHWs) in linking individuals and healthcare systems in developing countries (WHO and UNICEF 1978). Since then, more and more health projects in developing countries have been trying to place community participation at the heart of improving the health situation of rural populations (Chorev 2012). The refinement of this concept and the various attempts of planners to incorporate it into new or existing maternal health programmes have resulted in an abundant literature (Fournier and Potvin 1995; Rifkin 1990; Rosato et al. 2008). These community health systems, whose missions are to empower patients and change their health behaviour, play a key role in the implementation of mHealth interventions like Motech. Community health workers were targeted by Motech to become agents to promote devices, collect information, and relay messages through mobile phones. Indeed, Motech relies exclusively on the community level, a system that already faces many difficulties in its functioning. It is essential to understand the peculiarities of this level at the periphery of the health system that manages, on a daily basis, important expectations and challenges. Thus, the introduction of new devices such as Motech in this context necessarily involves transformations, for, as Nelly Oudshoorn rightly points out, technologies transform problems more than they solve them (Oudshoorn 2011).

In India, two different ministries deliver community health programmes (Kosec et al. 2015). On one side, since 1975 the Ministry of Women and Child Development has been handling a community service for women and children called the Integrated Child Development Services (ICDS). On the other side, in 2005 the Ministry of Health and Family Welfare invested the community level with a new programme called the National Rural Health Mission (NRHM), involving trained accredited social health activists (ASHAs—(an acronym that also means 'hope' in Hindi). The ICDS programme provides services for the development of mothers and children, and one of its main tasks is to improve the health of pregnant and lactating mothers and children under 6 years by providing vaccinations, health check-ups, nutritional and health advice, and referrals to primary health centres (PHCs). This national programme relies on village-based structures, the Anganwadi Centre (AWC) and their employees the Anganwadi workers (AWW), and it provides one AWC for a community of 400 to 800 inhabitants. Since 2005, AWWs have been present in almost all Indian villages. The AWC provides some basic village health services but—contrary to PHCs or sub-centres—it is not a place of clinical practice. There are neither doctors nor nurses, and the AWWs who manage them are not employees of the health system. The main mission of the centre is to welcome children from 3 to 6 years of age for informal education and one meal per day, as well as food distribution to a limited number of families and the most vulnerable pregnant women of the community. Children are regularly weighed and vaccinated. The AWW are always women from the surrounding area. They must have a minimum level of education to apply (10th standard, secondary school, equivalent to the middle of high school). In Bihar, they have a fixed 'honorarium' of 3,750 rupees ($58.5) per month; they can also receive wage supplements, called 'incentives', based on their involvement in some activities like Vitamin A supplementation and polio immunization. They are present in the morning at the centre and must ensure home visits in the afternoon. In 2014, an AWC covered an average of 68 malnourished children, with large differences between states: from 24 children per centre in Himachal Pradesh to 198 per centre in Bihar; a sad national record that shows both the inadequacy of overloaded community structures and the severity of child under-nutrition in Bihar.

The second pillar of community health in India is the NRHM, through which the Ministry of Health wishes to expand its presence in village-level settings. To improve maternal and child health, the purpose of the NRHM is to deploy an ASHA in each village (or for a community of about 1,000 people). The ASHA is the health system entry point; she must coordinate with the AWW at the village level to conduct community outreach activities together. The ASHA also works in coordination with nurses at the sub-centre or PHC. Although since 2011 every village in India should have an ASHA, in Bihar, many ASHA positions remain vacant (Bajpai and Dholakia 2011; Gill 2009). These auxiliaries are local health actors, appointed by the Gram Panchayat (village government) and trained to mobilize the community on health issues and to encourage the use of public health infrastructures. They do not have any workplace but are expected to go once a month to the PHC on which they depend, and to regularly visit the nearest AWC. The ASHAs must be residents of the village and have as a minimum level of education 8th Standard, middle school, equivalent to the end of secondary school. But in Bihar, the most illiterate state of India, very few women have reached this minimum level of education and ASHAs were still appointed. Indeed, 20 to 30% of ASHAs in the studied blocks did not reach this minimum level of schooling. Considered as volunteers, they have no fixed salary in Bihar and are financially compensated based on their activities through 'incentives'. For example, by bringing children to the AWC for vaccination they earn roughly 150 rupees ($2.3), and they receive 600 rupees ($9.3) if they bring a woman to the PHC for delivery.

The activities of the AWW and ASHA overlap on maternal health issues, but the head of the AWC is more educated and well off and has more influence in the community than a more recently named ASHA whose legitimacy has not yet been established. The AWW also has access to the material resources of the centre and rations are under her responsibility, which also gives her more power than the ASHA. AWWs and ASHAs, however, have no means of transportation to make their visits and are expected to travel several kilometres a day to meet a few beneficiaries. The few weekly home visits done by AWWs are irregular because they must primarily take care of the AWC and activities there, such as immunization days. For their part, the ASHA is expected to visit an average of 30 homes per month, each visit lasting at least 30 minutes. In the Motech Programmes, both AWWs and ASHAs receive phone credits as incentives to become promoters and intermediaries of Motech in a very competitive as well as dysfunctional system.

The Indian health system has regularly been blamed for the low level of central and regional government involvement in public health spending, chronic dysfunctions in the structures and supply chains of health goods, and the very large geographical inequalities of health and in accessing healthcare reinforced by caste, class, religion, or gender. Numerous studies show that the quality and accessibility of health services have deteriorated overall in the country (Das 2015; Deaton and Drèze 2009; Drèze and Sen 2013; Pinto 2008). Some even estimate that the Indian government has simply abandoned any policy to make the health system accessible (Hodges and Rao 2016). Even if PHCs and AWCs exist, the allocated resources are squandered, centres are understaffed and understocked, and their accessibility is poor (Drèze and Sen 2002). This situation is not new: researchers who have been working on maternal health in northern India for more than 30 years, have denounced the many dysfunctions in women's care (Jeffery et al. 1984, 1987; Jobert 1985) and the gap between the promises of national programmes undermined by the almost impossible access to quality maternal health services (Jeffery and Jeffery 2010).

These general observations apply to Bihar, in a very exacerbated manner. The government of Bihar has been introducing new policies aimed at strengthening the health sector and several health indicators rose substantially between 2005 and 2015. For example, the percentage of women delivering at a health facility increased from 22 to 67% between 2005 and 2006, and 2015 and 2016 (National Family Health Survey 2005–6, 2015–16). Nevertheless, important gaps persist in the health practices of households and in service provisions, and the health outcomes of Bihar's population still need considerable improvement. Bihar's situation is particularly dramatic because records of poverty and corruption go hand in hand with a multitude of health services run by competing private organizations that come to assist a 'sick' system and propose alternative paths for healthcare and health products.

In Bihar, as in the rest of India, block (sub-district) administration is chronically understaffed. One third of the block manager positions are vacant across the country but more than half in Bihar (Centre for Policy Research 2015). In the blocks surveyed, half of the positions of block community manager, in charge of supervising community health, were not filled and, therefore, had to be assumed by the manager of the PHC, the block health manager (BHM). This dual responsibility entails an important overload of work for this administrative officer who devotes little time to the community health workers and favours the supervision of the PHC instead. In addition, the sums allocated to finance community health very often never reach the block level. Even if the funds do arrive, the complexity of the compensation system causes multiple delays of payments and also allocation errors, as explained by this manager: 'If funds for incentive is allocated and are available to me, I would pay the incentives right away. If the fund is not available then I face problem. Also, it is difficult to make incentives for 229 frontline workers working in 6–7 programs receiving incentive from all these programmes' (H, Block 02, Patna, 15/9). Because of this, and despite their work, a quarter of the ASHAs in our studied blocks had not received any financial compensation called 'incentives' for the past 10 months: 'We do not even have a regular salary. We survive on incentives and even for that we keep running in the field. When we do not get even this, it becomes very difficult' (HWFGD01, Patna, 15/10).

The situation is no better on the side of the AWWs and the ICDS programme, which is crossed by considerable territorial inequalities and major dysfunctions, thoroughly analysed by Akhil Gupta (2012). This situation has worsened since 2015, because in 2015–16 the national budget of the ICDS, which covered 90% of AWW and AWC expenses in Bihar was cut in two by the central government, which asked the states to take care of these expenses (9,918 crore less or 1.5 billion dollars to be filled by the states from then on) (Yadav 2015). In Bihar, this decision resulted in irregular payments for rents and wages for the AWWs, and a lack of food to prepare children's meals, leading to the shutdown of several AWCs, as explained by this AWW: 'We have not been receiving payments for last two rounds' (HWFGD01, Patna, 15/10). Community health workers report that health system failures are the main source of tension with people in the community. The pressure AWWs and ASHAs may face from women in the village are often linked to the difficulties these women encounter in obtaining information, health products, benefits, or access to basic health services. Thus, the community health workers are held responsible when women do not receive financial compensation promised by the government or when the community centre is out of stock of drugs or equipment. Infrastructures, amenities, and staff are insufficient to meet the health needs of rural populations.

In Bihar, health facilities are dysfunctional and public money and goods do not always reach the district, the block level, and even less the villages. In this way, the community health level is the weakest and least supported level of the health system. Presented as the transmission belt of the health system, community health workers face difficult working conditions: irregular incomes, overloaded hierarchical superiors, and tense relations with villagers due to lack of resources and inequalities in accessing them. They receive all the complaints and reproaches that are in fact addressed to an unequal and failing health system, and at the same time they are the ones bearing new innovative programmes—such as those based on mHealth—on the top of this.

Mobile Technologies for Community Health Work in Bihar

For the ASHAs and AWWs we met in India, the acquisition and use of mobile phones was related to their position: they have invested in a mobile for their community work. In India, community health workers almost exclusively use mobile phones for calling and have very basic phones. The use of SMS is not common, and smartphones are not there yet. Still, they are unanimous that the mobile plays a fundamental role in their daily lives: the mobile simplifies their life and work. Thanks to the mobile, community health workers easily contact beneficiaries, their officers, ambulances, or PHC, and no longer need to travel all the time. This is a significant gain of time in areas where road infrastructure is very poor and where most villages are accessed along unpaved dirt roads.

The mobile is a strategic object for most of these workers, one that could help them in their professional activity, even if their employer does not supply it. Until 2017, these workers had to assume the full financial burden of this tool. That way, most AWW had their own mobile phone, but not all ASHAs have access to a mobile. Indeed, for workers without a fixed salary, mobile usage was too much of an expense to assume. Moreover, the spending levels depended on professional obligations, as this ASHA explains:

> Our employer does not pay the mobile phone bills, it's bought personally by us. According to their roles, each category of frontline worker recharges their mobile with different amounts. ASHA facilitator spends at least 500 INR (7,8$) a month since she makes calls to all ASHA under her. AWW spend 200–250 INR (3,5$) since they make calls to their supervisors. ASHA spend 100–150 INR (1,9$) in a month at an average.
>
> HWFGD01, Patna 15/09

According to their level of responsibility, staff have different mobile expenses. Those in charge of the coordination of other workers spend more than those who do not have to provide this coordination. None of them gets any financial support to meet those expenses. In 2017, things changed for ASHAs when the Department of Health in Bihar provided them SIM cards from BSNL (an Indian mobile network operator) to call only their immediate supervisors and the other ASHAs for free, with also 50 free minutes available to call outside this closed user group per month, but no phone is provided, only the SIM card. The mobile is anyway a professional investment, an expense regarded as necessary by many workers. And Motech reinforces the role of the mobile, making it essential to the functioning of the maternal health programme. Our study allowed us to better understand the special status of mobile phones and mHealth applications for community health workers and how their use changes the practice of community health. Here we consider community health workers as intermediaries of mHealth, sometimes augmented and sometimes overshadowed by mobile technology.

Enhancing the Community Health Worker: Mobile Kunji

mHealth promoters present the possession or use of mobile phones as a benefit for the caregiver. According to them, health workers are more competent or credible with mobile phones, hence the multiplication of mobile devices to help them to 'better' do their job and to support them in the care relationship (Agarwal et al. 2016). In India, Motech positioned the mobile as a central working tool in a professional environment where resources are lacking. The community health workers on which the Motech project is relying are the least qualified workers, the least equipped and the least considered of the health system. They have very few professional tools. When asked about their work 'tools', some evoke a bowl and spoon provided by a programme on nutrition, sometimes a preparation kit for childbirth, and often 'Mobile Kunji', one of the mobile phone devices developed by Motech, as reported by this ASHA: 'Care India has provided us with a bowl and spoon to demonstrate complementary feeding. We got soap, blade and other clean items to be demonstrated for birth preparedness. We have Mobile Kunji to show cards and make them listen to the messages through mobiles' (HWFGD01, Patna, 15/09).

Mobile Kunji, this set of picture cards linked to voice messages accessible via the frontline workers' mobile phones, is the most developed working tool that ASHAs ever handled in their daily work. It was also the first mobile-enabled communication strategy put in place by the Motech programme in Bihar to improve maternal health.

mHealth promotes and strengthens interdependence of health workers and mobile phones. Indeed, the various applications of Motech depend more or less heavily on community health workers to function. In the case of Mobile Kunji, this strong interdependence is particularly evident, as during home visits community health workers show the deck of cards to beneficiaries and it is through their mobile phones that vocal messages are transmitted. So community health workers constitute the single entry point to access Mobile Kunji messages. According to its promoters, Mobile Kunji fills the knowledge deficits of community health workers and increases their performance. Like a bionic leg, Mobile Kunji would enhance their working capacities (Claverie 2010; Le Dévédec and Guis 2013). In India, stakeholders of Motech explain that health workers are not trained or educated enough and that Mobile Kunji allows them to enhance their knowledge and improve their 'soft skills':

We felt that while there is a strong reliance on the health workers to be the health providers at the village level, in terms of imparting, training, or technical information to them, they lag behind in this area . . . Mobile Kunji is a tool for the frontline workers, to address their knowledge gap and to improve their communication with the beneficiaries.

S, Private Foundation, Delhi, 15/02

Mobile Kunji's mission is to strengthen the skills of workers, to make them more efficient in their interactions, and also to transmit intact messages to the beneficiaries. According to Motech administrators in India, Mobile Kunji guarantees fair information, ensures that the right message is delivered in time, something that the health worker alone could not guarantee: 'Earlier whatever the frontline workers said was coming from her. It was not warranted that what they say is technical or right and appropriate. Now, with these two programs, there is certain technical credibility in these, (H, Block 02, Patna, 15/09); 'Before, the time taken to explain things was more. Also, the discussion was not structured. The FLW [frontline worker] would say few things that were not required or not applicable. Mobile Kunji talks only about few things and focuses on things that are essential. So, it is very focused' (CLC, BBC, Block 01, Patna, 15/09).

Recorded messages are preferred by the programme designers, on the grounds that they guarantee access to the same comprehensive health information for all, when it could be truncated or incomplete from one patient to another, depending on community workers' abilities. Moreover, they argue, the message will be more effective than the simple interaction between CHWs and beneficiaries because 'Doctor Anita', the speaker of the recorded messages, seems a more credible interlocutor than community health workers: 'Listening from doctor makes the messages more credible. Since ASHA is also from the community and may not be considered as an outsider so sometimes she may not be taken seriously with the information given by her. If the same thing is told by a person who is from outside, they feel that it is important or special' (B, Block 02, Patna, 15/09).

For others, the messages of Dr Anita and those transmitted by community health workers are similar and this redundancy effect mixed with the medical authority embodied by Dr Anita would strengthen the effectiveness of health messages doubly conveyed: 'What the FLW said is also said by Dr Anita, so people have more credibility around it, the FLW feels much more confident and respected, because she is being seen by the community as a person who talks the same language as the doctor over there' (N, BBC, Patna, 15/09).

This enhanced worker, a symbol of efficiency, will that way convince people to adopt healthy behaviour and thereby improve maternal and child health in the community, as explained by this Motech administrator in Patna: 'How to communicate with the beneficiaries, how to negotiate those behaviours with beneficiaries was something that was not there. So they were not equipped for that. That was one of the major barriers to people actually erupting those behaviours' (N, BBC, Patna, 15/09).

Mobile Kunji thus promises an improvement in the interactions between community health workers and individuals, and more effective health messages. But does this promise of an enhanced worker really materialize? At the end of 2013, according to the mid-term study by Ananya programme, 39% of women recalled being exposed to Mobile Kunji in the last 6 months and 45% of workers reported using Mobile Kunji during home visits (Borkum et al. 2014). If the women we met in Bihar stated that ASHA and AWW are their central referees for health issues in their village and that they gave them help and support during their pregnancy, some spontaneously quoted Mobile Kunji as a reliable source of health information: 'We access information related to health from ASHA and AWW through mobile, audio messages at Anganwadi centre [Mobile Kunji]' (BFGD01, Patna, 15/09).

Women explained that ASHAs visit them more often and stay longer since they have been using Mobile Kunji: 'ASHA comes more now since Mobile Kunji has come. ASHA has started visiting us more often than earlier' (BFGD01, Patna, 15/09). Some women were thus sensitive to this device, because it makes interaction with community health workers more frequent and longer. Is this due to the mobile phone or due to Dr Anita?

In fact, Mobile Kunji supports the knowledge and skills of community health workers, above all, because women hardly understand Dr Anita's messages. Indeed, many of these women have had very little schooling and don't understand the level of Hindi spoken by Dr Anita, so frontline workers serve as intermediaries and translators of the messages, as this beneficiary explains: 'The information on mobile and on cards is the same. ASHA explains more than what she makes us listen in her mobile. ASHA explains in a better way' (BFGD13, Samastipur, 15/10).

For some women, Mobile Kunji is seen as a way to strengthen and increase interaction with community health workers, an excuse to talk about health topics that the worker would perhaps not have mentioned spontaneously. However, the mobile is not the central tool. Indeed, the illustrated cards and the feedback from community workers are regularly cited by women as more useful than voice messages: 'Photos on the Mobile Kunji cards are interesting and we look at them attentively and it is more understandable than messages from the phone' (BFGD02, Patna, 15/09).

Moreover, some frontline workers use only the Mobile Kunji card set and have virtually no use of audio messages; they use the cards to talk about a specific topic and to organize the discussion. Others believe that Dr Anita's message alone provides very little interaction and that the message makes sense only once the cards have been discussed before, as explained by this

ASHA: 'Though it is easier for us to make them listen to the calls, it is more effective to show the card first and then make them listen to the call. This way they understand it more' (HWFGD01, Patna, 15/09).

Thus, Mobile Kunji proposes a tripartite technical assemblage between the community health worker, the illustrated cards, and Dr Anita's messages and offers a rather positive representation of mHealth devices, where non-human and human complement each other. The other Motech application we are analysing in this chapter—Kilkari—offers a very different picture where the non-human takes over from the human. Our research shows how this mobile automated system can sometimes be used to replace the community health workers and thus reduce the interactions between patients and the health system.

Replacing the Community Health Worker: Kilkari

Launched in Bihar one year after Mobile Kunji, the second communication strategy experimented by Motech—Kilkari—addresses vocal messages directly to women. Each week, voice messages are sent to Motech clients for 1 rupee per message. These messages depend on the progress of the pregnancy or the age of the newborn. The 64 Kilkari messages start at 6 months of pregnancy and continue up to 1 year of the child. In India, a client can be registered at any time with Kilkari and can also unsubscribe themselves after each message. The messages are in Hindi, the official language of India and Bihar, and not in the local dialects of Bihar (such as Bhojpuri or Magahi). They are referenced by theme and linked to one of the nine key behaviours on which Motech must intervene: 1) preparation for birth; 2) prenatal follow-up; 3) birth care; 4) postnatal monitoring; 5) exclusive breastfeeding; 6) immunization; 7) family planning; 8) hand washing; and 9) complementary feeding practices. Families are subscribed to Kilkari by ASHAs and AWWs, and they receive talk time on their own mobile phones whenever they subscribe women to this paid service.

During our fieldwork, we discovered that unlike Kunji, Kilkari was used as a replacement for community health workers and thus reduced the caregiver–patient interactions. One employee of the implementing partner of Motech in Bihar explained that during training for Kilkari, community health workers were encouraged to tell women that they would conduct home visits only in an emergency and that the rest of the time Kilkari messages would be sufficient to obtain the information they need on their pregnancy: 'We ask FLW to tell the beneficiaries that they go for home visits only when needed. So, the FLWs tell them that they would get time appropriate message in Dr Anita's voice weekly with Kilkari' (CLC, BBC, Patna, 15/09).

A project manager explained that this was not the original goal but the similarity between Kilkari and Mobile Kunji led health workers to substitute Kilkari for home visits to save time:

> They are confusing Kunji and Kilkari because those services are very similar, it's the same messages coming again through Kilkari. So the confusion that came along the way, is if I subscribed a beneficiary to Kilkari I don't need to go to their house to talk the same message to them with Kunji, so it's a substitute. Instead of actually complementing each other, they became substitutes
>
> N, BBC, Patna, 15/09

In any case, the path proposed by Kilkari is that of the substitution of home visits. The beneficiary is directly put in contact with the machine and the health worker is no longer an intermediary required for the functioning of the device.

In January 2016, the central government announced the national extension of Kilkari in India, but not of Mobile Kunji.[3] A new version of Kilkari provides free and automatic enrolment of pregnant women listed in the national maternal health database (MCTS). In this version of Kilkari, selected for the national extension, community health workers no longer have any role to play. This total disappearance of community health workers in the process is considered by the administrators of Motech to be problematic:

> The scenario for the national rollout is to be free and automatically set up for pregnant women. There won't be anyone to explain the relevance of the service, how to use it, what are the benefits, nothing. The incentives for health workers will not be maintained for national roll out. Nobody will explain the service in the national scheme. You'll get a message saying you've been subscribed to this service and you don't know what to expect from it
>
> A, BBC, Delhi, 15/08.

Some managers explain the low success of Kilkari in Bihar by its cost but also by the fact that women could get the same information through the community health workers: 'After 2–3 calls, when she [the beneficiary] realizes that the information given from Kilkari is same as what ASHA tells her and she is also getting charged one rupee a week for this, she may continue with it for less than a month and then deactivate it. Mobile Kunji has no such problems' (Health Department, Block level, Patna, 15/09).

The implementers of Motech in Delhi also recognize that women are not interested by Kilkari because of the rigidity of a completely automated device with no possible interaction or feedback: 'We found out that people are not so interested in Kilkari because in Kilkari you cannot talk back, ask questions, it's just one way' (A, BBC, Delhi, 15/03).

The doubts that appeared related to the relevance and effectiveness of a fully automated device contradict the initial proposal of Motech to transmit perfect information, free of the alterations induced by human transmission. These doubts also underlie the evidence that Dr Anita's messages are not listened to or appreciated until they have been proposed or shared by the community health workers.

Conclusion

Mobile Kunji and Kilkari illustrate two very different paths that mHealth devices can take: one that supports a communication system that enhances interpersonal exchange around health information, and the other dedicated to a fully automated information system. A reduction of mHealth to automated information systems presents the risk of creating technologies that fail to support care or improve it because they neglect the importance of the emotional and social dimension of care provided remotely. This is the fundamental difference between Kunji and Kilkari.

The linear model, without intermediary, chosen for Kilkari eclipses the human part of community work; it favours automation and depersonalization of the transmission of health information. Studying similar digital health projects, Ruth Malone recalls the importance of face-to-face and physical presence in care practices. Care is a human practice for which interpersonal relationship is essential (Malone 2003). In her analysis of telemedicine devices, Nelly Oudshoorn confirms the importance of direct contact between carers and patients. She explains that only communication technologies with a virtual co-presence (a phone conversation or a video conference between the patient and the caregiver) can maintain this indispensable relationship. Two-way oral communication is fundamental in order to create a digital proximity (Oudshoorn 2011).

As described very well by Annemarie Mol, care is not a finished product, it is the result of negotiations and discussions, a continuous process of adaptation:

Care is a process: it does not have clear boundaries. It is open-ended. This is not a matter of size; it does not mean that a care process is larger, more encompassing, than the devices and activities that are a part of it. Instead, it is a matter of time. For care is not a (small or large) product that changes hands, but a matter of various hands working together (over time) towards a result. Care is not a transaction in which something is exchanged (a product against a price); but an interaction in which the action goes back and forth (in an ongoing process)

Mol 2008, 31

In her study on the management of diabetes in Holland, Mol examines the 'logic of care', that is, the elements and values that guide care. Mol states that the 'logic of care' relies on adaptability and collective perseverance of both patients and caregivers; for her the essence of care is in interactions (Mol 2008, 2). She concludes her research on the management of diabetes with the idea that 'good care' does not depend on individual choices but on elements that support in the long run this collective process of care, this perseverance and adaptability.

The deployment of mHealth at the community health level can take many forms and paths. We have discussed in this chapter two different paths, which are not under the same logic. The role of community health workers to support the understanding of Motech messages is necessary to the care process, but it has been denied by the recent developments of Motech and the preference for Kilkari over Mobile Kunji. Some mHealth promoters remain silent on this work of accompaniment and 'translation' that community health workers do, and favour a total delegation of responsibilities to the patient and the technical device. They claim that the messages are immediately understandable, acceptable, and cause a connection and action from their listeners. The recent decisions taken to ensure the future of Motech support these views and confirm the fully automated approach of the programme. The model proposed by Mobile Kunji allows co-construction of care: a joint effort between community health workers, patients, and mHealth device. The fully automated path without intermediaries offered by Kilkari offers no interactions and can even pull patients away from public health infrastructures. This second path highlights the insensitivity, limits, and shortcomings of automation applied to care. Unfortunately, it is this path that was chosen for future developments of mhealth in India.

Notes

1. One hundred individual interviews were conducted with professionals involved in mHealth in those two countries, including: ministries, public health agencies, United Nations agencies, NGOs, digital agencies, mobile operators, and private foundations. Among these interviews, 40 stakeholders were directly engaged in the implementation of Motech. A qualitative survey dedicated to Motech was also conducted in two districts of Ghana in 2014 and two districts of Bihar in 2015 and 2018. Thirty-five Motech project administrators, 20 health managers, 50 community health workers, and 200 women enrolled in the programme were interviewed in focus groups or face-to-face interviews conducted in English or in local languages (Fanté and Hindi).
2. The third application called 'Mobile Academy' was a recorded course of less than 2 hours to train community health workers on maternal health issues.
3. According to our interviews, Mobile Kunji was not extended because of cost issues: the required training of health workers and the printed set of cards were too costly to be sustainable for central government.

References

Agarwal, Smisha, Leona Rosenblum, Tamara Goldschmidt, Michelle Carras, Neha Goal, and Alain B. Labrique. 2016. *Mobile Technology in Support of Frontline Health Workers*. Baltimore, MD: Johns Hopkins University Global mHealth Initiative.

Al Dahdah, Marine. 2019. 'Between Philanthropy and Big Business: The Rise of mHealth in the Global Health Market'. *Development and Change* (online). doi: 10.1111/dech.12497.

Al Dahdah, Marine, and Alok Kumar. 2018. 'Mobile Phones for Maternal Health in Rural Bihar'. *Economic & Political Weekly* 53 (11): 50–7.

Bajpai, Nirupam, and Ravindra H. Dholakia. 2011. *Improving the Performance of Accredited Social Health Activists in India*. Accessed 27 August 2015. http://academiccommons.columbia.edu/catalog/ac:152281.

Borkum, Evan, et al. 2014. 'Midline Findings from the Evaluation of the Ananya Program in Bihar. Draft Report Submitted to the Bill & Melinda Gates Foundation. Princeton, NJ'. *Mathematica Policy Research*.

Centre for Policy Research. 2015. 'NHM GOI, 2015–2016'. *Budget Briefs* 7 (4):1–12. Accessed 3 November 2016. http://accountabilityindia.in/sites/default/files/nhm_2015.pdf

Chib, Arul. 2010. 'The Aceh Besar Midwives with Mobile Phones Project: Design and Evaluation Perspectives Using the Information and Communication Technologies for Healthcare Development Model'. *Journal of Computer-Mediated Communication* 15 (3): 500–25.

Chorev, Nitsan. 2012. *The World Health Organization Between North and South*. Ithaca & London: Cornell University Press.

Claverie, Bernard. 2010. *L'homme augmenté: Néotechnologies pour un dépassement du corps et de la pensée*. Paris: L'Harmattan.

Das, Veena. 2015. *Affliction: Health, Disease, Poverty*. New York: Fordham University Press.

Deaton, Angus, and Jean Drèze. 2009. 'Food and Nutrition in India: Facts and Interpretations'. *Economic and Political Weekly* 44 (7): 42–65.

Drèze, Jean, and Amartya Sen. 2002. *India: Development and Participation*. Oxford & New York: Oxford University Press.

Drèze, Jean, and Amartya Sen. 2013. *An Uncertain Glory: India and Its Contradictions*. Princeton, NJ: Princeton University Press.

Fournier, Pierre, and Louise Potvin. 1995. 'Participation communautaire et programmes de santé: Les fondements du dogme'. *Sciences sociales et santé* 13 (2): 39–59.

Gill, Kaveri. 2009. *A Primary Evaluation of Service Delivery under the National Rural Health Mission (NRHM): Findings from a Study in Andhra Pradesh, Uttar Pradesh, Bihar and Rajasthan*. New Delhi: Planning Commission of India, Government of India.

Gupta, Akhil. 2012. *Red Tape: Bureaucracy, Structural Violence, and Poverty in India*. A John Hope Franklin Center book. Durham: Duke University Press.

Hodges, Sarah, and Mohan Rao, eds. 2016. *Public Health and Private Wealth: Stem Cells, Surrogates, and Other Strategic Bodies*. Delhi: Oxford University Press.

Jeffery, Patricia, and Roger Jeffery. 2010. 'Only When the Boat Has Started Sinking: A Maternal Death in Rural North India'. *Social Science & Medicine* 71 (10): 1711–18.

Jeffery, Patricia, Roger Jeffery, and Andrew Lyon. 1987. 'Contaminating States: Midwifery, Childbearing and the State in Rural North India'. In *Women, State and Ideology*, edited by Haleh Afshar, 152–69. London: Macmillan.

Jeffery, Roger, Patricia Jeffery, and Andrew Lyon. 1984. 'Only Cord-Cutters? Midwifery and Childbirth in Rural North India'. *Social Action* 34 (3): 229–50.

Jobert, Bruno. 1985. 'Populism and Health Policy: The Case of Community Health Volunteers in India'. *Social Science & Medicine* 20 (1): 1–25.

Kaewkungwal, Jaranit, Pratap Singhasivanon, Amnat Khamsiriwatchara, Surasak Sawang, Pongthep Meankaew, and Apisit Wechsart. 2010. 'Application of Smart Phone in "Better Border Healthcare Program": a Module for Mother and Child Care'. *BMC Medical Informatics and Decision Making* 10 (1): 69. doi: 10.1186/1472-6947-10-69.

Kosec, Katrina, Rasmi Avula, Brian Holtemeyer, Parul Tyagi, Stephanie Hausladen, and Purnima Menon. 2015. 'Predictors of Essential Health and Nutrition Service Delivery in Bihar, India: Results from Household and Frontline Worker Surveys'. *Global Health: Science and Practice* 3 (2): 255–73.

Le Dévédec, Nicolas, and Fany Guis. 2013. 'L'humain augmenté, un enjeu social'. *SociologieS*. Accessed 8 August 2016. http://journals.openedition.org/sociologies/4409

Malone, Ruth E. 2003. 'Distal Nursing'. *Social Science & Medicine* 56 (11): 2317–26.
Mol, Annemarie. 2008. *The Logic of Care: Health and the Problem of Patient Choice.* London & New York: Routledge.
Noordam, A. Camielle, Barbara M. Kuepper, Jelle Stekelenburg, and Anneli Milen. 2011. 'Improvement of Maternal Health Services through the Use of Mobile Phones'. *Tropical Medicine & International Health* 16 (5): 622–6. doi: 10.1111/j.1365-3156.2011.02747.x.
Oudshoorn, Nelly. 2011. *Telecare Technologies and the Transformation of Healthcare.* Basingstoke & New York: Palgrave Macmillan.
Philbrick, William C. 2013. *mHealth and MNCH: State of the Evidence: Trends, Gaps, Stakeholder Needs, and Opportunities for Future Research on the Use of Mobile Technology to Improve Maternal, Newborn, and Child Health.* Washington, DC: UN Foundation.
Pinto, Sarah. 2008. *Where There Is No Midwife: Birth and Loss in Rural India.* New York & Oxford: Berghahn Books.
Rifkin, Susan B. 1990. *Community Participation in Maternal and Child Health: An Analysis Based on Case Study Materials.* Geneva: World Health Organization.
Rosato, Mikey, Glenn Laverack, Lisa Howard Grabman, Prasanta Tripathy, Nirmala Nair, Charles Mwansambo, Kishwar Azad, Joanna Morrison, Zulfiqar Bhutta, and Henry Perry. 2008. 'Community Participation: Lessons for Maternal, Newborn, and Child Health'. *The Lancet* 372 (9642): 962–71.
Tamrat, Tigest, and Stan Kachnowski. 2012. 'Special Delivery: An Analysis of mHealth in Maternal and Newborn Health Programs and Their Outcomes around the World'. *Maternal and Child Health Journal* 16 (5): 1092–1101. doi: 10.1007/s10995-011-0836-3.
WHO and UNICEF. 1978. *Primary Health Care: Report of the International Conference on Primary Health Care, Alma-Ata, USSR, 6–12 September 1978.* Geneva: World Health Organization.
Yadav, Anumeha. 2015. '"Children Are Worst Affected": Budget Cuts Are Taking a Toll on a Crucial Nutrition Scheme'. *Scroll.in.* Accessed 26 November 2015. http://scroll.in/article/767475/children-are-worst-affected-budget-cuts-are-taking-a-toll-on-a-crucial-nutrition-scheme

Glossary

ALLOPATHY	In South Asia, the use of the terms 'allopathy' or 'Western medicine' or sometimes 'medicine' persists in lieu of 'biomedicine'
ANTENATAL CARE	Set of measures and tests undertaken to ensure a healthy pregnancy for a mother and her baby
AYUSH	In India, a term encompassing all recognized non-allopathic systems of medicine: Ayurveda, Yoga, Unani, Siddha and Homoeopathy
DAI	A woman who has learned midwifery through apprenticeship (typically with female relatives) and who earns an income from assisting at births
ECLAMPSIA	A disorder of pregnancy that is characterised by high blood pressure and convulsions
EPISIOTOMY	A vertical cutting of the perineum during the last phase of childbirth to quickly enlarge the opening for the baby to pass through
IATROGENIC	Caused by medical treatment
MATERNAL MORTALITY RATIO	Deaths of women due to complications from pregnancy or childbirth per 100,000 live births in a given year
MHEALTH (OR MOBILE HEALTH)	Practice of public health supported by mobile devices
MILLENNIUM DEVELOPMENT GOALS	Eight development goals, set by the United Nations in 2000, that countries should have achieved by 2015
MISCARRIAGE	Cessation of a pregnancy before delivery of the baby's head at less than 22 weeks of gestation
NEONATAL MORTALITY RATE	Death of a liveborn infant within 28 completed days of birth, per 1,000 live or still births
POST-PARTUM CARE	Set of measures and tests undertaken during the first 6 weeks following childbirth to ensure a mother and her baby are safe and healthy

STILLBIRTH	Death prior to the complete expulsion or extraction from its mother of foetus, after 20 weeks gestation
SUSTAINABLE DEVELOPMENT GOALS	Seventeen development goals, set by the United Nations in 2015, that countries should achieve by 2030
UTEROTONICS	Agents used primarily during labour to intensify uterine muscle contractions

About the Authors

Radha Adhikari is a Lecturer in the School of Health and Life Sciences, University of the West of Scotland. She works on international migration of healthcare professionals, maternal and child health, gender and global health inequality. She has published extensively on international nurse migration from Nepal and global health workforce challenges. She is the author of *Migrant Health Professionals and the Global Labour Market: The Dreams and Traps of Nepali Nurses* (2019).

Marine Al Dahdah holds a PhD in Sociology from Paris University. She is a CNRS research fellow at CEMS (Centre for Studies on Social Movements). In recent years, she has worked on the use of mobile phones and digital technology to improve health in South Asia and Sub-Saharan Africa. She is the author of several articles dedicated to mobile health and digital health in the Global South.

Sunita Bhadauria worked in an administrative capacity for 15 years and developed an interest in translation. She has been working as a freelance translator (Hindi–English) for the past 19 years. She enjoys her work as a freelancer as it gives her freedom to work with different people, on different issues, and on her own terms. Most of her work has been in the development sector. She believes that sometimes one needs a little support or helping hand to make life better and she was lucky to have some such friends in her life. Today she wants to be that support for someone else to help them make life better. She also believes nothing is impossible—you only need to dream, believe in yourself, and work hard to achieve it.

Deepra Dandekar (PhD) works as a researcher at the Leibniz-Zentrum Moderner Orient, Berlin on a project about Hindu-Muslim interactions in the vernacular history writing of Maharashtra. Her doctoral dissertation and first book on the politics of reproductive health in rural Maharashtra was published by Zubaan Books (2017), followed by research on religious minorities and conversion in Maharashtra that includes her latest publications in 2019 and 2021, entitled *The Subhedar's Son: A Narrative of Brahmin-Christian Conversion from Nineteenth Century Maharashtra*, Oxford University Press, and *Baba Padmanji: Vernacular Christianity in Colonial India*, Routledge.

Pascale Hancart Petitet, PhD, is a medical anthropologist, senior researcher at the International Unit TransVIHMI (Institut de Recherche pour le Développement, INSERM, Université de Montpellier). Her research in India and Cambodia explored the historical constructions, the production and the circulation of ideologies, norms and practices in the field of human reproduction and reproductive health. Since 2013, her research in Laos stands at the intersection of reproduction politics, national and transnational migrations and infectious vulnerabilities. She has developed a strong interest in the co-construction of transdisciplinary research. She is the author of 50 articles and book chapters, and experiments with innovative approaches to scientific mediation (radio programmes, films, and theatre).

Roger Jeffery was Professor of Sociology of South Asia, University of Edinburgh, from 1997 to 2020. He carried out sociological research in Pakistan, Delhi, and Uttar Pradesh (UP), and lived for extended periods of time in villages and a small-town 160 kms north-east of Delhi. He has published *The Politics of Health in India* (1988) and is a co-author of *Labour Pains and Labour Power: Women and Childbearing in India* (1989). Currently, he is a Professorial Fellow with a collaborative research project on nitrogen-based pollution in South Asia. He is also pursuing his interests in the 'footprint' of India in Scotland: how did India influence the city of Edinburgh? His recent publications include 'Health policy and federalism in India', in *Territory, Politics, Governance.*

Clémence Jullien has been a CNRS research fellow in anthropology in Paris since 2021. She completed her PhD in Anthropology at the University Paris Nanterre in 2016 and carried out post-doctoral research at the University of Zurich, in Switzerland between 2017 and 2021. Both her research and her teaching have focused on reproductive healthcare in India, analysing particularly the articulations between health policies, narratives of development, gender relationship, and the medicalization of childbirth. Based on 15 months of ethnographic fieldwork in Rajasthan, her work resulted in several publications, including a book *Du bidonville à l'hôpital: Nouveaux enjeux de la maternité au Rajasthan*. She is currently working on the so-called crisis of masculinity and marriage in northern India, with a special emphasis on rural Punjab.

Jocelyn Killmer, PhD, is a lecturer in Anthropology and Asian Studies at San Diego State University. She is a cultural anthropologist with a research focus on gender, space, and healthcare in North India. Her most recent research compares urban and rural healthcare in doctors' narratives. She is currently working on projects to promote equity in university teaching.

Alok Kumar has worked on maternal and child nutrition and health in Indian states (extensively in Bihar). His research interests include a sociological approach to health systems and digitalization of health. He has been trained in Health Administration from the Institute of Health Management Research (IIHMR), New Delhi

Isabelle L. Lange is a medical anthropologist working on maternal health, hospital environments, quality of care and global health policy adaptation at the London School of Hygiene and Tropical Medicine (LSHTM) in the Department of Global Health and Development and in the Department of Infectious Disease Epidemiology. Her further research interests surround questions of identity and health seeking, and the logics of humanitarian aid organizations.

Neha Madhiwalla is a senior researcher at ARMMAN, Mumbai. She has previously served as the Co-ordinator for the Centre for Studies in Ethics and Rights, Mumbai. She was also a member of the editorial board of the *Indian Journal of Medical Ethics*. Her specific research interest areas are medical education and human resources in health. She has been involved in several initiatives to mainstream gender, social sciences, and humanities in medical education.

Mirza Taslima Sultana is a professor of Anthropology, Jahangirnagar University, Dhaka, Bangladesh. Her main research interest is gender relations in Bangladeshi female domestic workers to the Gulf Countries, and women's experiences of sexual harassment and violence. She also likes to enquire into the higher education system. She also works with national and international organizations in search of the sustainable policies that mitigate the situation of marginal communities. Along with academic publications, she has been regularly publishing articles in dailies and periodicals and taking part in electronic media discussions on gender as well as on contemporary issues in Bangladesh. She has been involved in a small group that is named 'Public Nribijayan [Anthropology]' and is publishing a book series in Bengali. As an activist she always stands for social justice and raises her voice against inequality in society.

Loveday Penn-Kekana is a medical anthropologist who works in the field of health systems and maternal/newborn health. She worked most of her adult life in South Africa, as a researcher and as a government advisor. For the last 10 years she has been based at the London School of Hygiene and Tropical Medicine, working on projects in India, Tanzania, and Brazil. For the last few years, she has seen too much superficial 'qualitative' work as part of mixed methods teams.

Samiksha Sehrawat has researched the historic link between health and governance in South Asia, with particular attention to women's health. Her publications include *Colonial Medical Care in North India: Gender, State and Society, c. 1840–1920* (OUP 2013). Her research interests include the history of colonial healthcare in India and its legacy for contemporary medical care, medical professionalization, the history of human development, and colonial expertise. She has received funding from the British Academy and was awarded a Leverhulme Fellowship for her research on the historical transplantation of hospitals and biomedicine in the Global South. Her research has also explored the impact of gender, race, and ethnicity in shaping the experiences of medical professionals and patients historically. She has published on environmental history, urban history, First World War, gender history, Indian princely states, and the press. She is a Senior Lecturer in History at Newcastle University.

Jeevan R. Sharma is Senior Lecturer in South Asia and International Development at the University of Edinburgh. He is the author of *Crossing the Border to India: Youth, Migration and Masculinities in Nepal*, Temple University Press, 2018/Bloomsbury 2019, and *Political Economy of Social Change and Development in Nepal*, Bloomsbury, 2021. His research interests include changing norms and forms of international development, global health, human rights, and humanitarian response. He has carried out field research in western Nepal, including following Nepali migrants to India, and among low-income migrants in Indian cities.

Sunita Singh is a doctoral student of Demography with the Institute for Population and Social Research (IPSR), Mahidol University. Before her affiliation with IPSR, she worked with the London School of Hygiene and Tropical Medicine as a consultant researcher. Sunita has over 16 years of work experience, including surveys, project planning, and management. She has been involved in many qualitative and quantitative research studies on health, specifically with a focus on mental health, gender, and reproductive health. Her areas of expertise are health systems, reproductive health, women's rights, community accountability, maternal mental health, and qualitative and quantitative research.

Fouzieyha Towghi is a medical anthropologist in the School of Archaeology and Anthropology, Australian National University. Her scholarship focuses on the politics of reproduction, medicine, science, and technologies and their implication on women's corporeal and social bodies in South Asia. Building on her postdoctoral research on the localization of the HPV-vaccine in India, her current research explores the global circulation of molecular biology and the diagnostic and therapeutic norms of reproductive cancers and their impact on public health policy and

women's health. Drawing from over 10 years of public health work and doctoral re-
search in Pakistan, she is currently completing her ethnography, *Midwifery 'In the
Time of the Lady': Contesting Modern Imaginaries of Childbirth, Midwives and the
Tribal in Rural Balochistan*. In 2015, her article 'Normalizing Off-Label Experiments
and the Pharmaceuticalization of Homebirths in Pakistan', was awarded the Rudolph
Virchow Professional Award, by the American Anthropological Association.

Helen Vallianatos is a Professor of Anthropology and Associate Dean, Office of the
Dean of Students at the University of Alberta. Her research and teaching, on the
topics of food, gender, body, and health, involves collaborating with communities
and working in interdisciplinary teams. Much of her work is focused on experiences
of migration and settlement, with past and ongoing research on immigrant women's
experiences in Canada, applying intersectionality theory and analyses to understand
how racialized, gendered, and classed identities are (re)created, and how family and
household dynamics change as sociocultural identities shift. She has also worked on
applying anthropological lenses to understand post-secondary student experiences,
including assessing students' perceptions of health, mental health, and wellness, and
incorporating this information into improving student mental health services.

Index